Animal Communication Theory

Information and Influence

The explanation of animal communication by means of concepts such as information, meaning and reference is one of the central foundational issues in animal behaviour studies. This book explores these issues, revolving around questions such as:

- What is the nature of information?
- What theoretical roles does information play in animal communication studies?
- Is it justified to employ these concepts in order to explain animal communication?
- What is the relation between animal signals and human language?

The book approaches the topic from a variety of disciplinary perspectives, including ethology, animal cognition, theoretical biology, evolutionary biology, philosophy of biology and philosophy of mind. A comprehensive introduction familiarises non-specialists with the field and leads on to chapters ranging from philosophical and theoretical analyses to case studies involving primates, birds and insects. The resulting survey of new and established concepts and methodologies will guide future empirical and theoretical research.

ULRICH E. STEGMANN is a Lecturer in Philosophy at the University of Aberdeen, UK. After training initially as a biologist, he subsequently switched to philosophy and now specialises in Philosophy of Biology. He was awarded a British Academy Postdoctoral Research Fellowship and has previously worked at King's College London and at the Universities of Cambridge and Bristol.

Animal Communication Theory

Information and Influence

Edited by

ULRICH E. STEGMANN

University of Aberdeen, UK

CAMBRIDGE
UNIVERSITY PRESS

CAMBRIDGE
UNIVERSITY PRESS

University Printing House, Cambridge CB2 8BS, United Kingdom

One Liberty Plaza, 20th Floor, New York, NY 10006, USA

477 Williamstown Road, Port Melbourne, VIC 3207, Australia

314-321, 3rd Floor, Plot 3, Splendor Forum, Jasola District Centre, New Delhi - 110025, India

79 Anson Road, #06-04/06, Singapore 079906

Cambridge University Press is part of the University of Cambridge.

It furthers the University's mission by disseminating knowledge in the pursuit of education, learning and research at the highest international levels of excellence.

www.cambridge.org
Information on this title: www.cambridge.org/9781108464727

First published 2013
First paperback edition 2018

A catalogue record for this publication is available from the British Library

Library of Congress Cataloging in Publication data
Animal communication theory : information and influence / edited by Ulrich Stegmann, University of Aberdeen.
pages cm
ISBN 978-1-107-01310-0
1. Animal communication. I. Stegmann, Ulrich, E. 1968–
QL776.A537 2013
591.59–dc23

2012036000

ISBN 978-1-107-01310-0 Hardback
ISBN 978-1-108-46472-7 Paperback

Contents

Preface

> Central to the notion of communication is the reception of information through a stimulus that an organism perceives from the external environment.
>
> Peter Marler (1967, p. 769)

> [W]e prefer to avoid the very idea of information, whether true information or false ... [T]he traditional views of the functions of communication – transmission of information as to species, sex, breeding condition, etc. – are pitifully inadequate to account for the musical elaboration of bird song ... Oratory is unnecessary if the purpose is simply to convey information.
>
> Richard Dawkins and John Krebs (1978, pp. 304 and 308)

This book is about a familiar view in animal behaviour studies: the idea that animal communication is a matter of conveying information. On this view, interacting animals are construed as senders, who emit signals that carry information, and receivers, who pick up the information in order to guide their behaviour. Communication systems as diverse as the waggle dance of honeybees, the alarm calls of vervet monkeys and the light pulses of fireflies are all regarded as sharing the same basic means of regulating behaviour. That is, animals respond to signals in certain ways because the signals carry useful information: worker bees fly to a particular location because the dance informed them about the whereabouts of a valuable resource, vervet monkeys hide in a bush because the alarm call signalled an approaching eagle and so on. This is the view that Peter Marler's remark encapsulates so well. But it has not gone unchallenged. Some 30 years ago, Richard Dawkins and John Krebs suggested banishing the information concept from the study of animal communication. Since then there have been occasional calls for replacing, or at least supplementing, information with concepts such as manipulation and influence.

One motivation was the thought that information is, at bottom, merely an empty metaphor, and a harmful one at that. More recently, when the preparations for this volume were already under way, this lingering tension came to the fore and attracted wider attention.

The criticisms of the information view raise some fundamental questions about the study and nature of animal communication. How are concepts such as 'information' and 'meaning' employed? Which theoretical roles are they meant to play? Do they live up to these roles? Do they adequately conceptualise animal communication and, if so, to what extent and why? And ultimately: what do information, reference and meaning consist in? Do these phenomena feature in interactions between animals? Similar questions can be asked of the purported alternatives: manipulation, persuasion and influence.

The goal of this volume is to address these issues head-on and, more broadly, to improve our understanding of the conceptual and methodological foundations of animal behaviour studies. The volume aims to achieve this goal in several ways. First, it brings together key proponents and opponents of the informational approach, offering an opportunity to engage directly with the arguments, for example by means of peer commentaries to individual chapters. Second, it broadens the way in which the topic is addressed by considering advances in related fields, such as the neuroscience of signal processing, signal evolution, the relation between animal signals and human language, and statistical decision theory. Third, it adds a philosophical point of view. Inviting philosophers to the table may strike many practitioners as a risky move. The concern may be that it blows out of proportion moderate, and as some believe insignificant, disagreements, engulfing the topic in unproductive sophistry. However, I believe that philosophy has specific and valuable resources to offer. Theories of information, for instance, can help articulate what information is, or plausibly could be, and what role it might play in animal communication.

A few remarks about the structure of this book. The Introduction is intended for readers who are new to the topic. It surveys informational and non-informational approaches to animal communication and sketches some philosophical concepts and distinctions. The 18 chapters are divided into five parts.

Part I explores the key notion of information. Horn and McGregor use the perspective of communication networks to operationalise information. Scarantino defends a probabilistic theory of information and applies it to animal communication. Kight, McNamara, Stephens and Dall recommend the use of statistical decision theory in order to understand signalling. Wiley defends both qualitative and quantitative notions of information. Millikan advances a solution to the reference problem for probabilistic theories of information.

Part II subjects the information concept to criticism and advocates alternative approaches. Rendall and Owren bolster and extend their previous criticisms with doubts about current views of human language and communication. Sarkar challenges the utility of both qualitative and quantitative notions of information in explaining animal signalling. Morton and Coss, and the late Professor Owings, argue that information is an empty metaphor, best replaced with a 'management' approach. Ryan focuses on sexual communication to argue that informational explanations are impoverished.

Part III addresses the topic from the point of view of specific case studies, which range from insects and birds to meerkats and monkeys. Horisk and Cocroft consider vibrational communication in treehoppers and conclude that information transfer is optional. Botero and de Kort argue that manipulation cannot adequately explain song consistency in birds. Fischer explores the attractions and limits of understanding primate vocal communication in terms of information. Allen uses work on meerkats to defend the informational approach. Christison-Lagay and Cohen review how primates process the vocalisations of conspecifics at the neural level and stress the activation of multiple brain areas.

Part IV provides an evolutionary perspective on animal signalling. Lachmann ties quantitative information measures to fitness consequences. Godfrey-Smith explores the properties of sender–receiver systems at equilibrium and concludes that information and influence are complementary.

Part V explores the relation between animal signals and human language. Adams and Beighley regard animal communication as a matter of information transfer and reserve meaning for human languages. With a view on evolutionary linguistics, Scott-Phillips and Kirby propose an inferential model of communication that revolves around influence as its basic component.

The idea for this volume was hatched in 2008. It was part of a grant application to the British Academy for a project on informational and non-informational approaches to animal communication (SG-51996). I gratefully acknowledge the Academy's support. It allowed me, among other things, to visit Carel ten Cate, Lars Chittka, Rufus Johnstone and Nick Davies, and to hold conversations with Eugene Morton, Donald Owings, Michael Owren, Drew Rendall and Klaus Zuberbühler. Their patience and openness greatly helped me to better understand animal communication and prepare this book, for which I am very thankful. I would also like to thank the authors of this volume for their willingness to participate in a joint project, about which some have strong views, and to expose their chapters to public peer commentary. The external reviewers provided invaluable and constructive feedback on the individual chapters. For this I am indebted to Dorit Bar-On, Michael D. Beecher, Carl T. Bergstrom,

Guiseppe Boncoraglio, Jack W. Bradbury, Gordon M. Burghardt, Matthew Campbell, Rosa Cao, Erica A. Cartmill, Sarah Collins, Torben Dabelsteen, Hilmi Demir, Stephen M. Downes, Simon Fitzpatrick, Patrick Forber, Todd Freeberg, T. Ulmar Grafe, Justin Garson, Steven Hamblin, Anne Leonard, Ola Olsson, Jessica Pfeifer, Carolyn Price, Rafael L. Rodríguez, Gregg Recanzone, William A. Searcy, Nicholas Shea, Andrew D. M. Smith, Mitchell Steinschneider, Robert M. Seyfarth, Brandon C. Wheeler and three reviewers who preferred to remain anonymous. Special thanks are owed to the ever-encouraging Jack Bradbury, who provided extensive comments on a range of issues, especially statistical decision theory, and gave valuable advice in preparing this volume. I am also very grateful to Robert Seyfarth for sharing, despite some reservations, his immensely constructive suggestions. Any remaining shortcomings are, of course, my responsibility. I thank my colleague Nathaniel Jezzi for stylistic suggestions, as well as Martin Griffiths and Lynette Talbot from Cambridge University Press for their guidance through this project, and Lindsay Nightingale for her superb copy-editing.

Dawkins, R. & Krebs, J. R. (1978). Animal signals: information or manipulation. In J. R. Krebs & N. B. Davies, eds., *Behavioural Ecology: An Evolutionary Approach*, 1st edn. Oxford: Blackwell, pp. 282–309.

Marler, P. (1967). Animal communication signals. *Science*, **157**, 769–774.

Contributors

Professor Fred Adams
Department of Linguistics and Cognitive Science
University of Delaware
Newark, DE 19716
USA

Professor Colin Allen
Department of History and Philosophy of Science
Indiana University
1011 East Third Street
Goodbody Hall 130
Bloomington, IN 47405
USA

Steven M. Beighley
Department of Psychology
University of Delaware
Newark, DE 19716
USA

Dr Carlos A. Botero
Initiative in Biocomplexity and Global Change Center
North Carolina State University
Raleigh, NC 27695
USA

Kate L. Christison-Lagay
Department of Otorhinolaryngology: Head and Neck Surgery
University of Pennsylvania School of Medicine
3400 Spruce – 5 Ravdin
Philadelphia, PA 19104
USA

Professor Reginald B. Cocroft
Division of Biological Sciences
University of Missouri
105 Tucker Hall
Columbia, MO 65211
USA

Professor Yale E. Cohen
Department of Otorhinolaryngology: Head and Neck Surgery
University of Pennsylvania School of Medicine
3400 Spruce – 5 Ravdin
Philadelphia, PA 19104
USA

Professor Richard G. Coss
Department of Psychology
University of California
Young Hall, CA 95616
USA

Dr Sasha R. X. Dall
Centre for Ecology and Conservation
Biosciences, College of Life and Environmental Sciences
University of Exeter
Cornwall Campus, Tremough
Penryn
Cornwall TR10 9EZ
UK

Professor Julia Fischer
Cognitive Ethology Laboratory
German Primate Center
Kellnerweg 4
37077 Göttingen
Germany

Professor Peter Godfrey-Smith
Philosophy Program, The Graduate Center, CUNY
365 Fifth Avenue
New York, NY 10016
USA

Professor Claire Horisk
Department of Philosophy
University of Missouri
437 Strickland Hall
Columbia, MO 65211-4160
USA

Dr Andrew G. Horn
Department of Biology, Life Science Centre
Dalhousie University
Halifax, Nova Scotia
B3H 4J1
Canada

Dr Caitlin R. Kight
Centre for Ecology and Conservation
School of Biosciences, College of Life and Environmental Sciences
University of Exeter
Cornwall Campus, Tremough
Penryn
Cornwall TR10 9EZ
UK

Professor Simon Kirby
School of Psychology, Philosophy and Language Sciences
University of Edinburgh
3 Charles Street
Edinburgh, EH8 9AD
UK

Dr Selvino R. de Kort
Division of Biology and Conservation Ecology
School of Science and the Environment
Manchester Metropolitan University
Chester Street
Manchester, M1 5GD
UK

Dr Michael Lachmann
Department of Evolutionary Genetics
Max Planck Institute for Evolutionary Anthropology

Deutscher Platz 6
04103 Leipzig
Germany

Dr Peter K. McGregor
Reader in Applied Zoology
Cornwall College Newquay
Centre for Applied Zoology
Wildflower Lane
Trenance Gardens
Newquay TR7 2LZ
UK

Professor John M. McNamara
School of Mathematics
University of Bristol
University Walk
Bristol BS8 1TW
UK

Professor Ruth Garrett Millikan
University of Connecticut
Philosophy Department
Storrs, CT 06269-2054
USA

Professor Eugene S. Morton
Hemlock Hill Field Station, Cambridge Springs, Pennsylvania
and Department of Biology, York University, Toronto
4700 Keele Street
Toronto, ON, M3J 1P3
Canada

Dr Michael J. Owren
Department of Psychology
Emory University
Atlanta, GA 30322
USA

Professor Drew Rendall
Behaviour and Evolution Research Group
Lab of Comparative Communication and Cognition

Department of Psychology
University of Lethbridge
Lethbridge, Alberta T1K 3M4
Canada

Professor Michael J. Ryan
Section of Integrative Biology
University of Texas
Austin, TX 78712
USA

Professor Sahotra Sarkar
Department of Philosophy
and Section of Integrative Biology
University of Texas
Waggener Hall 316
Austin, TX 78712 -1180
USA

Professor Andrea Scarantino
Department of Philosophy and Neuroscience Institute
Georgia State University
PO Box 4089
Atlanta, GA 30302-4089
USA

Dr Thomas C. Scott-Phillips
Department of Anthropology
Durham University
Dawson Building
South Road
Durham, DH1 3LE
UK

Professor David W. Stephens
Ecology, Evolution, and Behavior
University of Minnesota
1987 Upper Buford Circle
St Paul, MN 55108
USA

Professor R. Haven Wiley
Department of Biology
University of North Carolina
Chapel Hill, NC 27599-3280
USA

Introduction: A primer on information and influence in animal communication

ULRICH E. STEGMANN

What is surprising is that, despite this intensive study, the whole subject [of animal communication] is extremely confused, largely because of the definitions of the various terms that have been used. While this was already true when the first edition of this book was written, the confusions have now reached monumental proportions, with leading theorists even disagreeing as to what should properly be called 'a signal' or 'communication'.

Marian Dawkins (1995, p. 72)

[T]here is widespread and often unrecognized confusion about the kinds of signal that exist, the mechanism responsible for their evolution, and the terms to be used to describe them ... So it may be that a disagreement about terminology in a particular case is not about theories, or the words used to describe them, but about what the world is like.

John Maynard Smith and David Harper (2003, p. 2)

Introduction

A midsummer evening in a temperate forest: male fireflies emit pulses of light from specialised organs as they fly about in search of females. Females respond by emitting their own light pulses, which prompt males to approach them. A dialogue of light pulses ensues until the males have located the females (Lewis & Cratsley, 2008). Mate recognition in fireflies illustrates some basic features of animal communication: a *sender* sends a physical *signal*, which is perceived by a *receiver* who responds to it. In fireflies the initial sender is the male, whose signal is the light pulse, and the receiver is the responding female.[1]

[1] The roles of sender and receiver reverse when the female emits her own light pulse.

Animal Communication Theory: Information and Influence, ed. Ulrich Stegmann. Published by Cambridge University Press.

Signals are physical events, behaviours or structures to which receivers respond. Yet they are more than that, according to the standard view in ethology (e.g. Hauser, 1996; Bradbury & Vehrencamp, 2011a). As the colloquial meaning of 'signal' suggests, animal signals are events that convey *information* to receivers, where information is the *content* of a signal, or what the signal is about. For instance, the light pulses of fireflies reveal information about location, motivational state and species identity; the light pulses of a male convey, "Here I am in time and space, a sexually mature male of species X that is ready to mate. Over." (Lloyd, 1966, p. 69).

However, such explicit specifications of information contents are rare (e.g. Owren & Rendall, 1997), not least because identifying specific contents is difficult (Cheney & Seyfarth, 1990; Hauser, 1996). Normally contents are circumscribed in vaguer terms, such as 'information about food', or they are invoked indirectly by classifying signals as, for instance, predator or alarm calls. Yet the underlying assumption is always that signals carry information in the sense of having some more or less specific content. Unsurprisingly then, information has found its way into formal definitions of signals and communication: *communication* is often defined as the process of conveying information from senders to receivers by means of signals, and *signals* as the behaviours or structures that senders evolved in order to convey information (Table 1).

Table 1 *Examples of informational and non-informational definitions of animal signals and communication. Note that both Wilson (1975) and Maynard Smith and Harper (2003) excluded information only for the purposes of defining signals and communication; they did not reject the idea that both phenomena involve information.*

	Informational	Non-informational
Signal	"[Signals are] behavioral, physiological, or morphological characteristics fashioned or maintained by natural selection because they convey information to other organisms." (Otte, 1974, p. 385)	"We define a 'signal' as any act or structure that alters the behaviour of other organisms, which evolved because of that effect, and which is effective because the receiver's response has also evolved." (Maynard Smith & Harper, 2003, p. 3)
Communication	"I consider communication to be any sharing of information between entities – in *social* communication, between individual animals." (Smith, 1997, p. 11)	"Biological communication is the action on the part of one organism (or cell) that alters the probability pattern of behavior in another organism (or cell) in a fashion adaptive to either one or both the participants." (Wilson, 1975, p. 176)

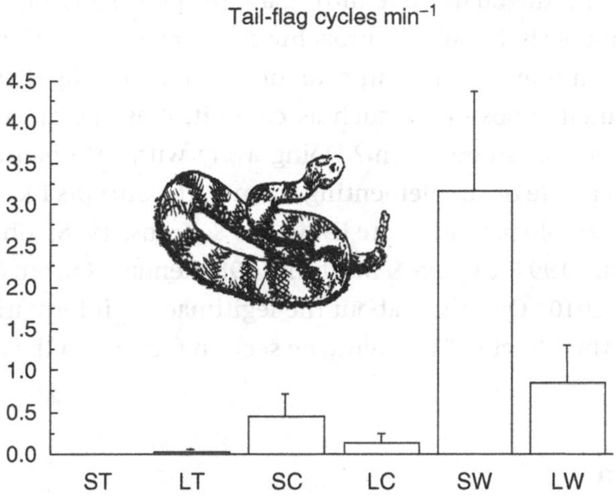

Figure 1 Mean rate (+SE) of tail flagging by squirrels during the first 2 minutes following playback of soft and loud tones (ST and LT, respectively) and of rattling sounds of small (S) and large (L) as well as cold (C) and warm (W) rattlesnakes. Squirrels flagged their tails significantly more in response to rattles than to tones, and more to rattles from warm snakes than to rattles from cold snakes. Warm snakes produce rattles that are both louder and have a higher click rate than those produced by cold snakes, which are less dangerous to squirrels. Graph reproduced with permission from Swaisgood *et al.* (1999); rattlesnake reproduced with permission from Richard Coss.

As structures that *evolved* to convey information, signals are typically contrasted with *cues*, which are behaviours or structures that convey information without having evolved for this purpose (e.g. Otte, 1974; McGregor, 1993; Hasson, 1994; but see Hauser, 1996). Rattling by rattlesnakes has probably evolved to ward off predators by conveying the information that the snake is venomous, i.e. rattling is a signal. But rattling can be a cue as well (Swaisgood, Rowe & Owings, 1999). The click rate and dominant frequency of the rattling sound of Pacific rattlesnakes correlate with a snake's body temperature and size, respectively (Rowe & Owings, 1990). California ground squirrels use these sound properties to adjust their degree of vigilance. Squirrels become more vigilant in response to rattling sounds from warmer snakes (Figure 1; Swaisgood *et al.*, 1999), which are more agile and therefore more dangerous. For the squirrels, click rate and dominant frequency thus carry information about snake temperature and size, and they are cues because they did not evolve in order to convey such information.

Although information is a central and entrenched concept in animal communication studies, it seems possible to describe communication without it. The first paragraph of this introduction sketched firefly communication simply in terms of what some individuals do (emitting a light pulse) and how others respond (emitting another light pulse/approaching). We can even *define* signals and communication without appeal to information (Table 1). Why then introduce apparently intangible postulates such as content, message, meaning or information? Why not do without them? Doing away with information concepts, minimising their role or supplementing them with concepts like manipulation is what some ethologists advocate (Dawkins & Krebs, 1978; Johnstone, 1997; Owren & Rendall, 1997; Owings & Morton, 1998; Rendall, Owren & Ryan, 2009; Carazo & Font, 2010). Questions about the legitimacy of information will be addressed later in this chapter. The following section focuses on the concept of information itself.

Information

Colloquial information

Signals are taken to convey information in the sense that they are about something, or have content (e.g. Halliday, 1983; Dawkins, 1995). But what does it mean to say that signals *have* content? This question is rarely addressed explicitly. Yet judging by how terms such as 'information' are employed in practice, it appears that much work in animal communication is based on three distinct but closely related answers (I will refer to these as 'content 1' etc. later in this introduction).

(1) Predictions and knowledge

Many authors use 'information' interchangeably with what receivers come to know (e.g. Krebs & Dawkins, 1984; Seyfarth & Cheney, 2003; Bradbury & Vehrencamp, 2011a), what they infer (e.g. Krebs & Dawkins, 1984; Slocombe & Zuberbühler, 2005) or what they predict when perceiving a signal (e.g. Smith, 1997; Seyfarth *et al.*, 2010). In other words, a signal's information content is often equated with what receivers predict, infer or learn from it. And this practice suggests a first answer to what having content consists in: signals have content (or, equivalently, carry information) when they enable receivers to predict something from their occurrence.

Predicting is frequently understood in a qualitative sense (e.g. Krebs & Dawkins, 1984; Smith, 1986; Seyfarth *et al.*, 2010). There is, however, a quantitative framework for modelling predictions: statistical decision theory (Bradbury & Vehrencamp, 2011a; see also Ch. 3). The basic idea in applying statistical decision theory is that animals constantly face decisions about how to act and that they use information (knowledge) to choose among alternative courses of action. Animals come equipped with some degree of background knowledge about the probability of certain events, which derives from earlier experiences and/or from heritable biases due to past selection. In order to achieve optimal decisions, animals continually update their prior information by attending to appropriate current events.

Consider contests among red deer stags over access to females. Frequent components of stag contests are roaring matches, which are usually won by the more frequently roaring male (Clutton-Brock & Albon, 1979). Faced with a roaring harem-holder, a challenger must decide whether to retreat or keep roaring. Stags base their decisions on an estimate of their opponent's fighting ability. Fighting ability comes in degrees, but let us assume for illustrative purposes that rivals categorise one another as being either weak (*W*) or strong (*S*). If prior knowledge suggests to a male that its rival is as likely to be weak as he is strong [$P(W) = P(S) = 0.5$], then such knowledge is of little help in deciding whether or not to retreat. However, fighting ability correlates with roaring: weak males roar less frequently than strong males (Clutton-Brock & Albon, 1979; Reby *et al.*, 2005). Males can use knowledge of this correlation to predict the fighting ability of opponents (Box 1).

Box 1 A simple application of statistical decision theory

According to statistical decision theory, predicting or inferring something from the occurrence of a signal amounts to calculating a *conditional* probability. A conditional probability is the probability of an event or state on the condition that some other event or state has occurred. Inferring something from a signal involves calculating the conditional probability of an event on the condition that the animal has observed that the signal has occurred. So, when a stag infers the fighting ability of a rival (the state) from his roar (the signal), he effectively 'calculates' the conditional probability that his rival has a certain fighting ability on the condition that he roars with a certain frequency.

Suppose that stags are either weak (*W*) or strong (*S*) and they either roar frequently (*F*) or infrequently (*I*). If a stag perceives his rival roar frequently, then the stag calculates two conditional probabilities: the probability that (1) the rival is weak on the condition that he roars frequently and the probability that (2) the rival is strong on the condition that (again) he roars frequently. To simplify matters, we will only consider how the stag calculates probability (1), which is written $P(W|F)$, where '|' means 'given' (not to be confused with '/', the symbol for division). One way to calculate $P(W|F)$ is to use Bayes' theorem:

$$P(W|F) = \frac{P(W) \times P(F|W)}{P(W) \times P(F|W) + P(S) \times P(F|S)}$$

In order to calculate $P(W|F)$, the stag needs some background knowledge. First, he needs to know how probable it is to encounter rivals that are weak and rivals that are strong. These are the 'prior probabilities', $P(W)$ and $P(S)$. They are independent of having heard a rival's roar.

Second, the stag needs to know how strongly roaring correlates with fighting ability. Such correlations are estimated as the conditional probabilities that a certain type of signal will be produced by the sender (or perceived by the receiver) given a certain state of the world. With two types of signal and two states there are four conditional probabilities:

	State or event in the world	
Signal	Strong male (S)	Weak male (W)
Frequent roaring (F)	$P(F\|S)$	$P(F\|W)$
Infrequent roaring (I)	$P(I\|S)$	$P(I\|W)$

This table is a coding matrix. It specifies the degree to which a state or event in the world affects the probability that a signal will be produced (or perceived). For instance, it specifies how the fact that a male is weak affects the probability that he roars frequently, $P(F|W)$ (this is the converse of the probability the stag needs to calculate, $P(W|F)$).

The stag can now 'update' his prior probability that the rival is weak. This process can be modelled with Bayes' theorem. Suppose the stag's prior probability that the rival is weak is $P(W) = 0.5$. So, without having heard the rival's roar, the rival is equally likely to be weak or strong [$P(S) = 0.5$]. Suppose also that the stag knows about the following correlations between roaring and fighting ability: strong males roar frequently 80% of the time and infrequently 20% of the time [$P(F|S) = 0.8$, $P(I|S) = 0.2$], whereas weak males roar infrequently 95% of the time and frequently 5% of the time [$P(I|W) = 0.95$, $P(F|W) = 0.05$]. Inserting these values into Bayes' theorem yields:

$$P(W|F) = \frac{0.5 \times 0.05}{0.5 \times 0.05 + 0.5 \times 0.8} = 0.06$$

The result shows that the stag has learned something from the rival's frequent roaring. Hearing the rival roar frequently reduces the stag's estimate of the probability that his rival is weak from an initial 50% to a mere 6%. In other words, the stag can now be fairly confident that the rival is not weak. He can adjust his behaviour accordingly.

Two points are worth emphasising. First, when a receiver has used a signal to update its estimate of the probability of certain events, it has just made the first step. In order to use what it has learned to guide its behavioural response, the receiver also needs to take into account the fitness costs of making correct as opposed to incorrect choices of action (Bradbury & Vehrencamp, 2011b). Second, updating critically depends on what the receiver knows about the correlations between signals and world states (the coding). From the point of view of statistical decision theory, the signal by itself, without the coding, carries no information (J. Bradbury, personal communication). As mentioned in the main text, a signal's carrying information can be understood as enabling receivers to infer something from it. Since without coding receivers cannot infer anything from a signal, the signal itself carries no information.

Statistical decision theory is not only a quantitative tool for modelling how and what receivers predict from signals. Ecologists studying foraging behaviour, too, understand the idea that *cues* carry information/content as a matter of allowing predictions, and they employ statistical decision theory to model this process (e.g. Valone, 1989; Giraldeau, 1997; Danchin *et al.*, 2004; Stephens, 2007; Wagner & Danchin, 2010). Indeed, a rich and partly controversial taxonomy of types of information has been developed along these lines (e.g. Danchin *et al.*, 2004; Wagner & Danchin, 2010). One of the proposals is to distinguish between *private* and *public* information. European starlings probe the ground for insects and so acquire knowledge about patch quality, which is then used in foraging decisions, for instance when to leave the current patch for another (private information: knowledge of *x* gathered from direct contact with *x*). Instead of probing for insects themselves, individuals may also gain this information by observing their flockmates' probing success (Templeton & Giraldeau, 1996). The latter is public information: knowledge of *x* gathered from a cue of *x*.

It is tempting to believe that predictions, inferences and knowledge imply cognitive or psychological processing on the receiver's part, perhaps even conscious awareness. Indeed, key steps of decision-making have neural correlates (reviewed in Lee, 2010, and Bradbury & Vehrencamp, 2011c). But cognitive capabilities are implied in neither foraging ecology nor animal communication. Quantitative and informal work in these areas remains explicitly neutral on the mechanistic aspects of deriving predictions (Danchin *et al.*, 2004; Stephens, 2007; McNamara & Dall, 2010; Bradbury & Vehrencamp, 2011a). In some species, inferences from signals may just consist in simple learned associations or evolved dispositions (Krebs & Dawkins, 1984; Smith, 1997). Likewise, predictions from cues may consist in non-cognitive processes (Danchin *et al.*, 2004; McNamara & Dall, 2010).

(2) Mental representations

A more demanding view about the nature of signal content emerged in work on 'referential' signals. Referential signals allow receivers to infer features of the external environment instead of, or in addition to, features of the sender (variously labelled "semantic", "referential", "symbolic"; reviewed in Hauser, 1996). The alarm calls of vervet monkeys are a well-known example (Seyfarth, Cheney & Marler, 1980). Vervets emit three acoustically different types of calls in response to three different types of predators: leopards, eagles and snakes (Figure 2). Listeners respond to the calls in a way appropriate for the type of predator. For example, calls emitted in response to approaching eagles prompt vervets to seek cover in bushes, whereas calls emitted in response to snakes elicit upright posture and scanning of the ground. These calls appear to function like labels for things in the world, in this case types of predators, much like some words in human languages (Hauser, 1996; Cheney & Seyfarth, 2007).

Animal signals are called "functionally referential" when they function like labels (e.g. Marler, Evans & Hauser, 1992; Macedonia & Evans, 1993; Fischer *et al.*, 1995; Evans & Evans, 1999; Manser, Bell & Fletcher, 2001). This leaves open whether the signals are like words in the additional sense of eliciting mental representations of the referent in the minds of receivers, i.e. internal representations which mediate receiver responses. Such "representational" (Hauser, 1996; Evans & Evans, 2007) or "conceptual" signals (Zuberbühler *et al.*, 1999) are taken to be close to human words on the basis of assuming that human words refer to things indirectly, via something in the mind of receivers, an abstraction or concept (e.g. Cheney & Seyfarth, 1990; Hauser, 1998) or a mental representation (Evans, 1997; see also Box 2). According to the most demanding view of informational communication, referential signals have content only in the case that receivers infer or predict something from it by means of internal representations, or even mental "images" (Maynard Smith & Harper, 2003; Seyfarth & Cheney, 2003; cf. Fedurek & Slocombe, 2011; Wheeler *et al.*, 2011). Accordingly, the term 'information' is sometimes used to denote whatever a receiver's mental representations encode (Maynard Smith & Harper, 2003; Seyfarth & Cheney, 2003).

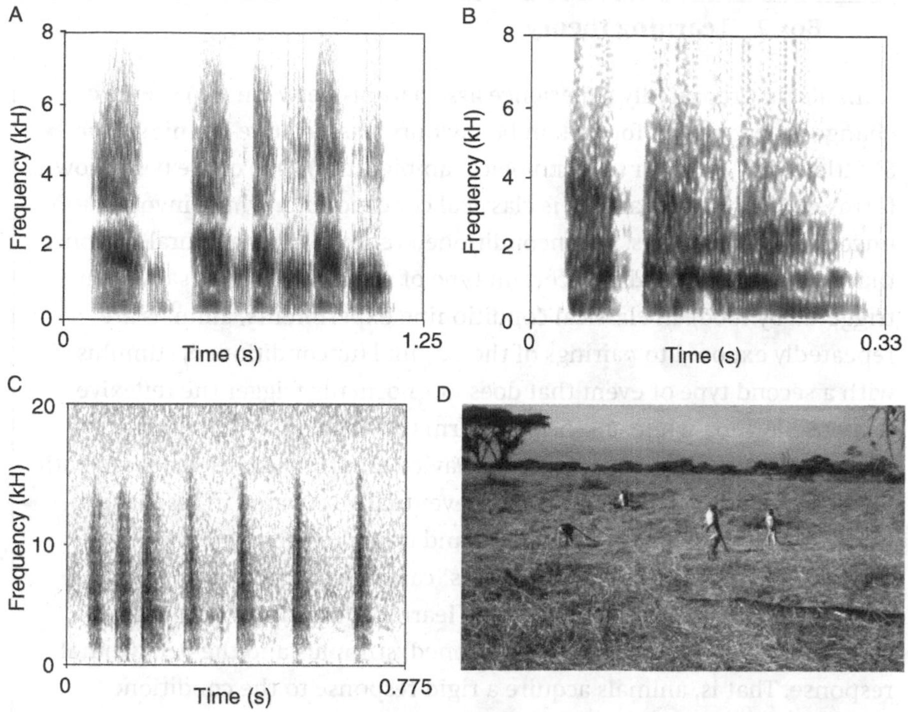

Figure 2 Vervet monkeys (*Chlorocebus aethiops*) give acoustically distinct alarm calls in response to leopards (A), eagles (B) and snakes (C). The acoustic features of alarm calls also differ from the predators' own vocalisations (e.g. vervet eagle alarm calls do not sound like eagle shrieks). When encountering one of these predators directly, vervets react in a manner specific and adaptive to the kind of predator involved, e.g. standing upright and scanning the ground when perceiving a python (D: python approaching from the lower right-hand side of the photo). Playback experiments in the wild showed that simply hearing an alarm call given in response to one type of predator, without perceiving the predator itself, triggers the appropriate behavioural response. Variations in acoustic features that may be associated with a sender's fear (e.g. call amplitude, or loudness) have no significant effect on the type of response. For these reasons, vervet alarm calls are considered to be "referential" or "semantic", i.e. "signs [that] refer to objects in the external world" (Seyfarth *et al.*, 1980, p. 1070). The study by Seyfarth *et al.* (1980) generated much interest in the presence of referential signalling in other species (reviewed in Seyfarth *et al.*, 2010; Fedurek & Slocombe, 2011; see Radick, 2007 for a history of playback experiments). A–C: Sonograms provided by Robert Seyfarth. D: Photo by Richard Wrangham.

(3) Correlation

What enable animals to make predictions from signals are correlations between signals and other states or events. In some contexts, correlations are deemed sufficient for signals to have content. The state or event with which the

Box 2 Learning theory

Animals that repeatedly experience associations between two events can change their capacity for certain behaviours ("associative learning"; see Shettleworth, 2001, for terminological ambiguities). One of the best-known forms of associative learning is classical conditioning, which involves unconditioned reflexes. An unconditioned reflex is a behavioural response that is always triggered by a certain type of stimulus (such as salivation triggered by food). In classical conditioning experiments, animals are repeatedly exposed to pairings of the original (unconditioned) stimulus with a second type of event that does not normally trigger the reflexive response. After a while, animals perform the behaviour simply after perceiving the new event on its own. Pavlov famously exposed dogs to both food and a ringing bell, and the dogs eventually salivated in response to hearing the bell. What psychological and neural mechanisms are responsible for this change in the dogs' capacity to react?

According to associative theories of learning, training 'stamps in' the association between the new (conditioned) stimulus and the behavioural response. That is, animals acquire a rigid response to the conditioned stimulus by establishing an excitatory or inhibitory connection between them (S–R theories). Representational or cognitive theories of learning propose instead that training creates a connection between the conditioned stimulus and an 'expectation' of the unconditioned stimulus (S–S theories). The bell triggers a neural representation of food (or a representation of the relation between the two), and the animal reacts on the basis of this representation (reviewed in Lieberman, 2003; Shettleworth, 2010). The classic debate between associative and representational theories of learning is the background for the contrast some ethologists draw between rigid (or automatic) and representation-mediated responses (see 'Colloquial information').

Current research favours cognitive theories (Shettleworth, 2010). But it is acknowledged that there is evidence on both sides (Lieberman, 2003) and that the nature of the posited neural representations remains elusive (Gallistel, 2008). One of the strongest lines of evidence in favour of cognitive learning theories is thought to come from alarm calls in Diana monkeys (Shettleworth, 2001). Diana monkeys react in the same way to acoustically distinct vocalisations, e.g. to the shrieks of an eagle and to the eagle alarm calls of their conspecifics (see figure). This suggests that despite their differences, the two types of vocalisations evoke the same kind of mental

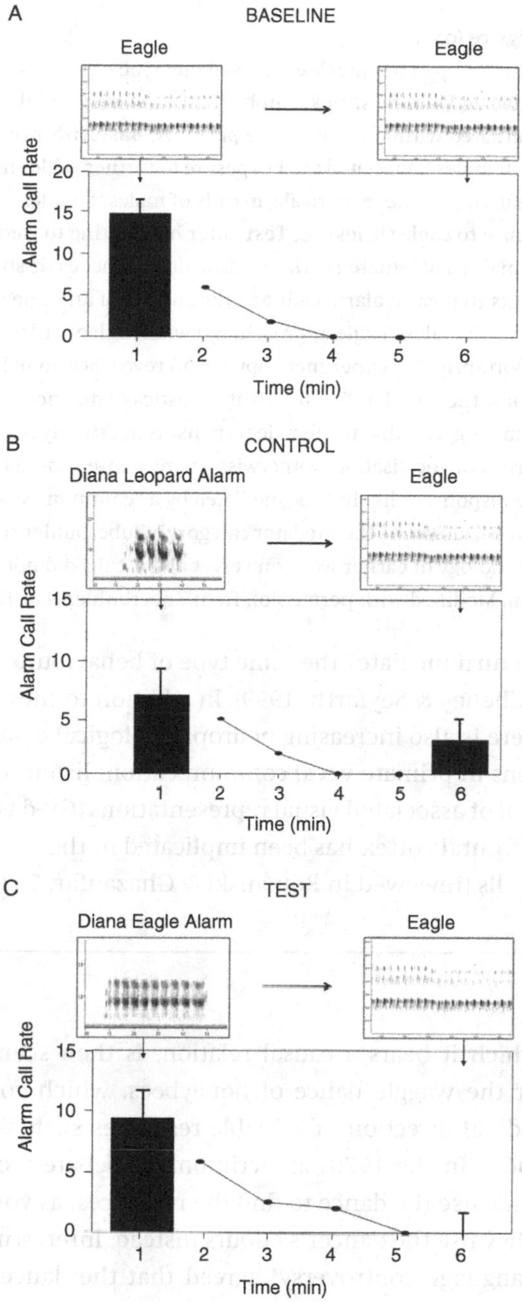

Figure Evidence for mental representations of signal referents by receivers (Zuberbühler *et al.*, 1999). Diana monkeys produce different alarm calls in response to their predators (eagles and leopards). Females also call in response to the alarm calls of their male conspecifics. In this set of prime–probe experiments

Caption for Box 2 Figure (cont.)
conducted in the wild, a group of females were played one type of vocalisation (prime) for 5 mins, followed by eagle shrieks (probe). After a strong initial response, females habituated within 5 mins to the prime. A, **Baseline**: primed with eagle shrieks, the females habituated after exposure to further eagle shrieks. B, **Control**: after habituating to the leopard alarm calls of males, females dishabituated in response to eagle shrieks. C, **Test**: after habituating to eagle alarm calls, females remained habituated to the acoustically distinct eagle shrieks. The experiment suggests that eagle alarm calls and the shrieks of an eagle carry the same information for females ('eagle approaching') whereas leopard alarm calls do not. More importantly, the experiment appears to reveal *how* females process the vocalisations: the fact that females treat acoustically distinct vocalisations as the same suggests that the female response is not simply triggered by the acoustic properties of vocalisations (otherwise the response should be different). Instead, the response is likely to be mediated by a "common associate, possibly a mental representation, of the predator category" (Zuberbühler *et al.*, 1999, p. 41). The methodology of earlier work on vervet alarm calls did not allow this further conclusion. Modified with permission from Zuberbühler *et al.* (2009).

representation, which in turn mediates the same type of behavioural response (Zuberbühler, Cheney & Seyfarth, 1999). In addition to these behavioural findings, there is also increasing neurophysiological evidence for mental representations in primate vocal communication: listening to calls activates the retrieval of associated visual representations (Gil-da-Costa *et al.*, 2004), and the pre-frontal cortex has been implicated in the semantic processing of calls (reviewed in Romanski & Ghazanfar, 2010; see also Ch. 14).

signal correlates, or to which it bears a causal relation, is then seen as the signal's content. Consider the waggle dance of honeybees, which correlates with the distance and cardinal direction of valuable resources such as flower stands (e.g. von Frisch, 1967). In the 1970s an acrimonious debate arose over whether bee recruits actually use the dance to find the resources, as von Frisch had claimed, or whether they use the dancer's odours instead. Interestingly, all participants of the 'bee language controversy' agreed that the dance carries spatial information; the contentious issue was only whether the recruits *use* its information (Dyer, 2002; Munz, 2005). Correlations obtain even if they are not exploited by receivers. This suggests that all sides of the debate implicitly agreed that the dance carries spatial information simply in virtue of its correlations with certain external factors.

Smith's (1965) distinction between the "message" and "meaning" of signals is relevant here. The distinction is influential but also fairly unclear and controversial (e.g. Philips & Austad, 1996; Bradbury & Vehrencamp, 2011b). Perhaps Smith's "message" is best understood as what signals correlate with (content 3), and "meaning" as what receivers infer from signals (content 1).

Mathematical information

As has often been noted, information is sometimes employed in a quantitative sense, in addition to its colloquial meaning (e.g. Marler, 1961; Smith, 1965; Krebs & Dawkins, 1984; Markl, 1985). Quantitative information features in studies which apply Claude Shannon's (1948) mathematical theory of communication to animal signals. Such studies measure what we know today as the Shannon entropy of a signal, as well as its conditional entropy and its transinformation – all quantities of the mathematical theory of communication. One of the earliest studies of this kind explored the visual displays of hermit crabs. Hermit crabs perform several kinds of displays when other crabs intrude into their personal space (Hazlett & Bossert, 1965; Laidre, 2009). They may, for instance, raise their chelipeds up and outwards, or raise one of their walking legs, or perform some other type of display (Figure 3).

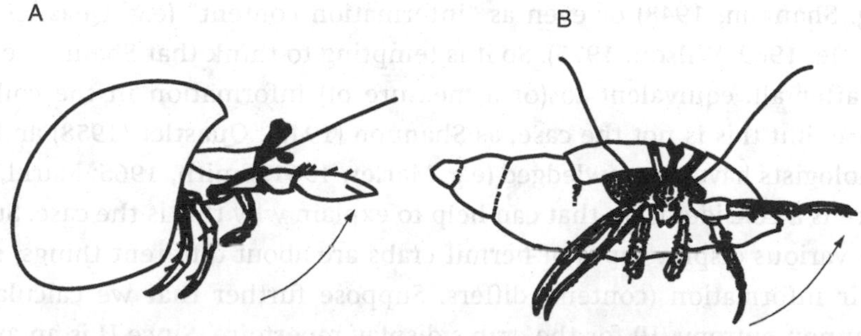

Figure 3 Hermit crabs can deter intruders by raising their limbs up and outwards. (A) Raising of the cheliped (clawbearing leg) in *Anisopagurus pygmaeus*. (B) Raising of a walking leg in *Clibanarius cubensis*. These visual displays were regarded as examples of threat signals, conveying the sender's intent for future agonistic opposition (e.g. Hazlett & Bossert, 1965). The view that threat signals convey information about sender intentions was undermined subsequently by findings of poor correlations between signalling and future aggression, as well as theoretical analyses suggesting that signals of intent are particularly susceptible to invasion by cheaters. More recent studies, however, support the viability of intention signalling in hermit crabs. The lack of correlations is likely to have been due to ignoring confounding variables, especially receiver responses: when intruders retreat, senders do not back up their displays with attack (Laidre, 2009). Reprinted with permission from Hazlett and Bossert (1965).

Hazlett and Bossert (1965) arranged encounters between pairs of crabs and counted how often crabs performed the various display types. They observed 6138 performances in total, of which 1121 were "major cheliped extensions". The cheliped rise therefore had a relative frequency of 1121/6138 = 0.18. And since relative frequencies can serve as estimates of probabilities, the probability of a crab raising its cheliped was $P(d_1) = 0.18$ (where d_1 stands for cheliped rise). The probabilities of the other displays (such as raising a walking leg) were calculated in the same way. Hazlett and Bossert (1965) then calculated the Shannon entropy of the entire signal repertoire by, first, multiplying the probability of a given display type with the logarithm of its probability, e.g. multiplying $P(d_1)$ by $\log_2 P(d_1)$, $P(d_2)$ by $\log_2 P(d_2)$, and so on for all display types. For each type they thus obtained a product. They then summed the products to yield the Shannon entropy,

$$H = -\sum_i P(d_i) \times \log_2 P(d_i)$$

where d_i denotes a kind of display (taking the logarithm to the base of 2 ensures that the unit is a 'bit'). Another important quantity is transinformation, which measures statistical dependencies between two sets of events (e.g. signals and responses).

Shannon entropy is sometimes referred to as a "measure of information" (e.g. Shannon, 1948) or even as "information content" (e.g. Quastler, 1958; Dingle, 1969; Wilson, 1975). So it is tempting to think that Shannon entropy is, after all, equivalent to (or a measure of) information in the colloquial sense. But this is not the case, as Shannon (1948), Quastler (1958) and many ethologists have acknowledged (e.g. Marler, 1961; Smith, 1965; Markl, 1985). Here is a consideration that can help to explain why this is the case. Suppose the various display types of hermit crabs are about different things, so that their information (content) differs. Suppose further that we calculate the Shannon entropy (H) for the crab's display repertoire. Since H is an average, all display types belonging to that repertoire will then have the same value of H, irrespective of their content. In other words, any two display types with different information (content) will have the same information (H). Since colloquial information and H can become separated in this way, they cannot be identical.

In other respects, however, the relation between the colloquial and mathematical sense of information remains unclear. For example, "technical" or "Shannon" information is often described as a reduction in uncertainty (e.g. Halliday, 1983; Krebs & Davies, 1993; Seyfarth *et al.*, 2010), which is also how the acquisition of knowledge by receivers is described (content 1; e.g. Quastler,

1958; Wiley, 1983; Seyfarth & Cheney, 2003; Bergstrom & Rosvall, 2011; Wheeler *et al.*, 2011). These practices suggest that for many researchers there is still some continuity between quantitative and colloquial information. To complicate matters, work in statistical decision theory offers a different yet explicitly quantitative approach to understanding information. A key quantity in this context is the change in the probability of a predicted event upon perceiving a signal (for similar measures see McNamara & Dall, 2010; Skyrms, 2010; Bradbury & Vehrencamp, 2011b).

The next section looks at manipulation, persuasion and influence (see also Chapters 2, 6–7, 9–10, 16, 18). These notions tend to be used synonymously and are often advanced as alternatives to information.

Manipulation and influence

Richard Dawkins and John Krebs (1978) were among the first to advocate an explicitly non-informational approach to animal communication. Signals, they argued, do not evolve to convey information, but rather to manipulate or persuade (Box 3). Manipulation does not imply (malevolent) intentions on the part of senders. It only implies that signals evolve in order to prompt receivers to behave in ways beneficial to the sender, even if the behavioural response comes at the receivers' expense. The latter part of this claim, i.e. that signalling may disadvantage receivers, continues to draw particular attention (and criticism; see 'Arguments concerning manipulation' below). Indeed, manipulation is often understood as an interaction whose *key feature* is the fitness cost to receivers (e.g. Smith, 1986; Searcy & Nowicki, 2005; Seyfarth *et al.*, 2010; Bradbury & Vehrencamp, 2011b; Wheeler *et al.*, 2011).

However, proponents of manipulation insist that receivers need not necessarily suffer fitness costs when being manipulated (Owren, Rendall & Ryan, 2010). This point has been illustrated with the mating calls of *Engystomops* frogs (Rendall *et al.*, 2009). *Engystomops* frogs are a closely related group of species in which the males emit species-specific calls ('whines') to court females. The males of some species have evolved the ability to (sometimes) add a distinct call component ('chucks') to their whines, which makes the resulting calls more attractive to females. Female preference for chucks is a sensory bias that predates the evolution of chucks (Figure 4). Females find them hard to avoid because they affect highly conserved neural features. The chucks therefore 'manipulate' females without females suffering fitness costs by responding more strongly to calls with chucks (reviewed in Ryan & Rand, 2003; but see Bradbury & Vehrencamp, 2011b; see also Ch. 9).

Box 3 Signal evolution

Among the key tasks in understanding the evolution of animal signals is specifying the selection pressures that shape signal design. Several sources of selection pressures have been identified, chief among them the physical environment and the sensory and neural capacities of receivers. Signals are selected for properties that make them detectable by the intended receivers in a given environment (reviewed in Bradbury & Vehrencamp, 2011a).

The way selection operates raises a fundamental puzzle for the view that signals evolve to convey information (cf. Markl, 1985). Many modelling studies have their origin in responses to this puzzle. If signals evolve in order to convey information, then senders should benefit from conveying information. But senders do not always benefit from revealing their intentions (Krebs & Dawkins, 1984). In addition, an honest signalling system in which all convey true information about themselves can be invaded by "cheaters" (e.g. Maynard Smith, 1976). Cheaters are animals that signal the presence of features they do not possess, e.g. aggressive intentions. Since cheaters benefit from misguiding receivers, their genes spread. Receivers eventually evolve to ignore the 'deceiving' signals, and this creates pressure on senders to cease signalling. How then could signals ever evolve to convey information?

Dawkins and Krebs' (1978) conclusion was that they do not evolve to convey information in the first place; they evolve to manipulate receivers instead (a view itself criticised as being evolutionarily implausible; see main text). Other theorists responded to this puzzle by seeking to identify evolutionary mechanisms that would allow signals to function as information transmitters. One of the most influential suggestions was that the production of signals about the features of senders must be so costly as to be restricted to senders that actually possess the features ("handicap" signals, Zahavi, 1975). Zahavi's suggestion initially met with skepticism, but over time a consensus emerged that some forms of costs can lead to honest or reliable signals (reviewed in Searcy & Nowicki, 2005). Since the 1970s, five additional mechanisms ensuring signal reliability have been identified (Searcy & Nowicki, 2005). The present consensus is that most signals are reliable on average, and that they must be reliable in order to evolve (Searcy & Nowicki, 2005; Seyfarth *et al.*, 2010; but see Rendall *et al.*, 2009). Evolutionary perspectives are further explored in Chapters 15 and 16.

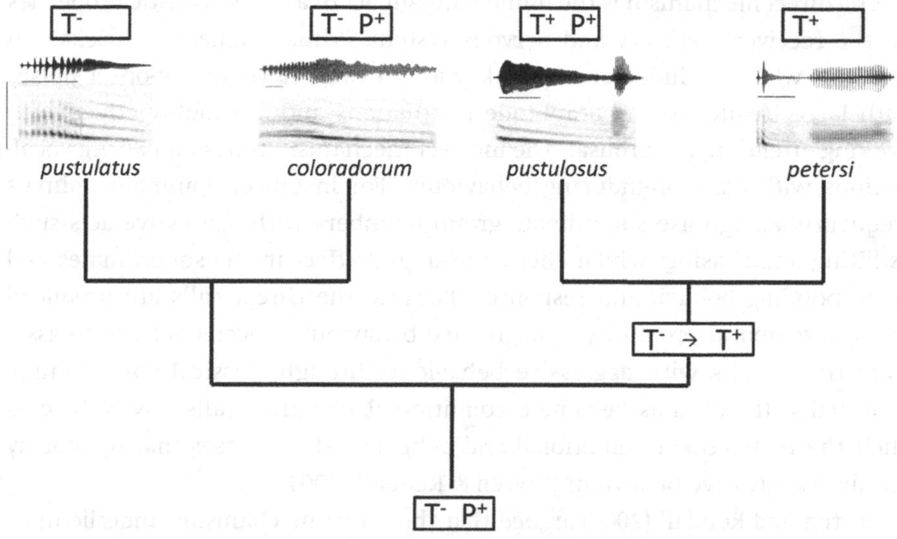

Figure 4 The evolution of male mating calls and female preferences of four species in the *Engystomops* (= *Physalaemus*) *pustulosus* species group. Each call is represented by a waveform (top) and a spectrogram (bottom; horizontal bar = 100 ms, vertical bar = 0–5000 Hz; all to the same vertical scale, but different horizontal scales). T^- indicates the absence of the terminal chuck, in both *E. pustulatus* and *E. coloradorum*, while T^+ indicates the presence of the chuck in both *E. pustulosus* and *E. petersi*. P^+ indicates that both *E. coloradorum* and *E. pustulosus* exhibit a preference for calls with chucks, despite the fact that the natural *E. coloradorum* call lacks a chuck; the preference was shown for an *E. coloradorum* call with *E. pustulosus* chucks appended to it. Analysis of the entire species group and several outgroup species (not shown) suggests that the ancestral condition of the species group is T^- and P^+ (lower box) and that chucks evolved prior to the separation of *E. pustulosus* and *E. petersi* (box $T^- \rightarrow T^+$). The trait distributions on this cladogram therefore suggest that the evolution of chucks exploited a preexisting sensory bias in females (Kirkpatrick & Ryan, 1991). Subsequent work has considerably added to this picture (e.g. Ryan & Rand, 2003), but also challenged it (Ron, 2008). Redrawn by Michael Ryan from Kirkpatrick and Ryan (1991).

Affect induction

For contemporary proponents of the manipulation view, manipulation is primarily characterised in terms of the proximate mechanisms that elicit receiver responses. A prominent example is the "affect-conditioning model" of non-human primate vocalisations (Owren & Rendall, 1997; later extended to other mammals in Owren & Rendall, 2001). According to this model, primate vocalisations employ two basic mechanisms for influencing receiver behaviour, a direct and an indirect mechanism.

The direct mechanism is the immediate impact of a call's acoustic properties on the receiver's sensory and nervous system. Primate squeaks, shrieks and screams, which include vervet monkey alarm calls, have abrupt-onset pulses with large frequency and amplitude fluctuations and are highly effective in evoking attention and arousal. The indirect mechanism relies on pairing vocalisations with emotion-inducing behaviours. For instance, dominant animals frequently antagonise subordinate group members with aggressive acts such as biting and chasing, which elicit arousal and affect in the subordinates and corresponding behavioural responses. Because the threat calls are produced in close temporal proximity to aggressive behaviours, receivers learn to associate threat calls with aggressive behaviour through classical conditioning. Eventually, threat calls become a conditioned stimulus: calls now suffice to elicit the motivational, emotional and behavioural responses that previously required aggressive behaviour (Owren & Rendall, 2001).

Owren and Rendall (2001) argued that these two mechanisms underlie most primate vocalisations and concluded that "a great deal of primate vocal signalling may be quite unsophisticated, functioning merely to draw another individual's attention, change its arousal level, induce affect, or serendipitously pair the caller's voice with some positive or negative state in the listener" (p. 69). In other words, the reason that primate vocalisations are said to lack information is the unsophisticated nature of signal processing in receivers (not the fitness costs to receivers). Interestingly, this way of drawing the line between information and manipulation parallels the approach taken by some proponents of information, who regard informational communication as a matter of evoking mental representations in receivers and who contrast this kind of signal processing with automatic, reflexive reactions which they count as non-informational forms of interaction (see 'Colloquial information').

Assessment/management

Initially, Dawkins and Krebs (1978) portrayed communication as the process by which senders manipulate receivers. They later revised this view, conceding that information does play an important role in communication after all (Krebs & Dawkins, 1984). They argued that receivers should evolve "mind-reading" capabilities (not merely "sales-resistance", i.e. the ability to withstand sender manipulation). Mind-reading is the ability to use statistical regularities in order to "predict" an animal's future behaviour (an ability acquired through individual learning or evolution) or, as they saw it, the ability to gather information about senders. Mind-reading does not demand complex cognitive capacities, let alone the ability to attribute mental states to other animals (theory of mind).

Krebs and Dawkins' (1984) view has found support (e.g. Johnstone, 1997; Carazo & Font, 2010). Donald Owings and Eugene Morton (1998) further developed this view into the assessment/management approach, according to which animal communication is the interplay between management on the part of senders ("managers") and assessment on the part of receivers ("assessors"). Management consists in influencing the behaviour of assessors in ways that benefit the manager: "from the perspective of management, signals do not refer to anything; they are pragmatic acts emitted to produce an effect of variable specificity" (Owings & Morton, 1997, p. 379). However, receivers are not merely passively used by managers. Assessors seek for cues that allow them to adjust their behaviour to prevailing circumstances. Assessment is the "active extraction of the cues needed for adaptive decision-making" (Owings & Morton, 1998, p. 72). Importantly, since assessors learn something from attending to cues or signals, assessment is thought to yield information (see also Ch. 8).

While Owings and Morton endorse information as one aspect of communication, they emphasise that cognitive or "information-processing" mechanisms are only one of four types of mechanisms of assessment. The three others are motivational, perceptual and emotional mechanisms. One of Owings and Morton's (1997) examples for a motivational mechanism is the effect of songbird vocalisations on hormone levels. In simulated territorial intrusion (STI) experiments, a caged male (or artificial dupe) is placed into the established territory of another male together with a loudspeaker, which plays the song of a conspecific male. In some species, STI increases the blood levels of testosterone and luteinising hormone in the territory owner, in addition to causing aggressive behaviour (Figure 5; e.g. Wingfield & Wada, 1989; McGlothlin *et al.*, 2008; but see Apfelbeck & Goymann, 2011). The call (signal) therefore influences the owner's neuroendocrine system (at least in conjunction with non-auditory cues, Wingfield & Wada, 1989). Owings and Morton concluded that this is a communicative effect which can hardly be described as information transfer. Note that information is, again, tied to the proximate mechanisms by which signals have their effects on receivers.

Evaluating informational and non-informational explanations of animal communication

So far we have explored how the concepts of information and manipulation are understood and how they are employed in order to explain animal communication. Both informational and non-informational approaches have their proponents and critics. Doubts about the legitimacy of informational explanations have been raised repeatedly (e.g. Dawkins & Krebs, 1978;

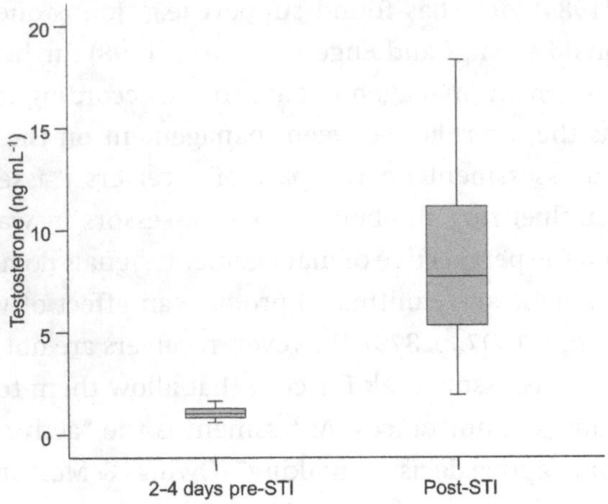

Figure 5 Testosterone levels in response to a simulated territorial intrusion in dark-eyed juncos (*Junco hyemalis*). In a simulated territorial intrusion (STI), a caged male was placed inside the territory of another male and pre-recorded junco songs were played from a loudspeaker. After 10 minutes the territory owner was captured and a blood sample taken. Males presented with an STI displayed significantly elevated testosterone levels following the intrusion (horizontal line: median; shaded box: interquartile range; bars: range). Reproduced with permission from McGlothlin *et al.* (2008).

Owings & Morton, 1997; Owren & Rendall, 2001) and they have received a moderate degree of attention (e.g. Philips & Austad, 1996; Seyfarth & Cheney, 2003; Scott-Phillips, 2008; Carazo & Font, 2010). An article by Rendall, Owren and Ryan (2009) brought these doubts to the forefront of ethological research, eliciting further responses (e.g. Font & Carazo, 2010; Scarantino, 2010; Seyfarth *et al.*, 2010; Bradbury & Vehrencamp, 2011b; Ruxton & Schaefer, 2011; Wheeler *et al.*, 2011). The purpose of the following three sections is to introduce a few of the central arguments that have been proposed on either side. These sections are not intended to adjudicate or to provide a comprehensive survey.

Arguments in favour of information

Empirical support

The most straightforward argument for the appropriateness of information is empirical evidence (Seyfarth *et al.*, 2010). Many studies now document structures or behaviours that (1) correlate with features of the sender or the environment and (2) elicit suitable responses in other animals (i.e. responses appropriate to the features with which the structures or behaviours correlate). One of the earliest studies to meet these criteria was Seyfarth, Cheney and Marler's (1980) seminal work on vervet monkeys described above. The three types of alarm calls are emitted specifically in response to three different types of predators (criterion 1). Furthermore, calls in the absence of non-acoustic cues are sufficient to prompt a behavioural response in receivers, and the response is appropriate for the type of predator that elicits a call (criterion 2). Alarm calls therefore enable vervets to 'predict' that a predator is approaching (at least if 'prediction' is understood in an undemanding sense; see 'Colloquial information'). And since signals are taken to carry information when they enable receivers to predict things from their occurrence, it follows that alarm calls carry information about specific types of predators.

Theoretical appeal

Another argument in support of the informational approach is its theoretical appeal (Seyfarth *et al.*, 2010). The informational view is in line with cognitive approaches to learning theory, according to which learning is a matter of acquiring information, which in turn involves mental representations (Box 2). Furthermore, the approach has great explanatory scope. Explaining receiver behaviour in terms of information content abstracts away from the physical properties of signals, especially their modality. This renders mathematical models of signal evolution applicable across taxa and modalities (Box 3). Critics object, however, that abstracting away from the physical structures has contributed to a neglect of research into signal production and design (Owings & Morton, 1997; Rendall *et al.*, 2009).

A good heuristic

For decades the informational framework has driven behavioural research on animal communication. It proves to be a fruitful strategy in other fields as well (Seyfarth *et al.*, 2010). With respect to the study of human language evolution, for instance, the framework has elucidated language evolution

Box 4 Animal signals and human language

Is animal signalling a kind of language? What is the relation between signalling systems and human language more generally? For a long time language was regarded as the gap separating humans from other animals. Of course, other animals lack a language insofar as they do not share any of our culturally specific communication systems (English, Chinese and so on). But 'language' also refers to the internal (neural and psychological) faculty that allows humans to learn and employ such systems (Hauser, Chomsky & Fitch, 2002). And with respect to that faculty a nuanced view about the relation between animal signals and human language has emerged. Following the linguist David Hockett, many contemporary theorists

Table 2 *Some components of the human language faculty and their presence in non-human animals.*

Humans (Fitch, 2010)	Non-human animals
Ability to learn the production of large vocabulary	Absent (Fitch, 2010; Fedurek & Slocombe, 2011)
Voluntary signal production	Mostly absent, but some species have degrees of control over signal production (e.g. audience effect) (Seyfarth & Cheney, 2003; Fedurek & Slocombe, 2011)
Discrete infinity[a]/recursion	Absent (Hauser *et al.*, 2002)
Reference (providing information about external states)	Present in some species (Cheney & Seyfarth, 2007)
Senders intend to provide information (Gricean maxims)	Absent (Seyfarth & Cheney, 2003; Fedurek & Slocombe, 2011)
Theory of mind (attributing mental states to others)	No attribution of beliefs; in some species attribution of intentions, goals and visual experience (Rosati *et al.*, 2010; Fedurek & Slocombe, 2011)
Listeners engage in pragmatic inferences	Present (Seyfarth & Cheney, 2003; Fitch, 2010)

[a] Discrete infinity is the ability to construct and understand an infinite number of linguistic expressions where the expressions are composed from a finite set of components.

advocate a multi-component view of the language faculty: language is composed of several partly independent subsystems with their own functions and neural implementations (e.g. Hauser *et al.*, 2002; Christiansen & Kirby, 2003; Hurford, 2007; Fitch, 2010). A select few of these components are listed in Table 2. Only some of the components are found in non-human animal species, and some are at the centre of controversies. For instance, Hauser *et al.*'s (2002) hypothesis that recursion (the ability to understand and produce recursive structures, such as embedded clauses) is the uniquely human language component reinvigorated interest in syntactic features of animal signals (e.g. Arnold & Zuberbühler, 2006; Gentner *et al.*, 2006; Van Heijningen *et al.*, 2009; Wheeler *et al.*, 2011).

Are animal signals evolutionary precursors of human language? It has been argued that at least some features of primate vocalisations are precursors of linguistic abilities, e.g. functional reference and the ordering of call types into sequences (Fedurek & Slocombe, 2011). According to an early view, language evolved from innate affective expressions such as sighs and screams, which were regarded as similar to animal signals. This idea is mostly rejected nowadays (Fitch, 2010; but see Bar-On & Green, 2010). Most contemporary theories of language evolution are concerned with the evolution of our 'proto-language', i.e. with the order in which the various components of our language faculty evolved in the hominid lineage that descended from our last common ancestor with chimpanzees (including its initial modality). The theories fall into three broad groups, proposing lexical, gestural and musical proto-languages, respectively (reviewed in Fitch, 2010; Wheeler *et al.*, 2011). Some theorists emphasise the extent to which the evolution of human language (as communication systems) depended on prior conditions, such as social interactions, context of use and capabilities like a theory of mind (Sperber & Origgi, 2010). (The relation between animal signalling and human language is further explored in Chapters 17 and 18.)

by identifying a number of striking similarities to and differences from non-human primate vocalisations (Fedurek & Slocombe, 2011; see also Box 4 and Chapters 17 and 18). Some of the similarities and differences concern the neural basis of language production and processing (Ch. 14). Such questions have in turn inspired research in primate neurophysiology (e.g. Platt & Ghazanfar, 2010).

Arguments against information

The classic objection against information concerns evolution: given how selection operates, signals simply could not evolve in order to convey information (Box 3). This objection was subsequently refuted. But new concerns took its place. Here I mention two lines of argument.

Problems surrounding the core concepts

One line of argument is that central concepts such as information are poorly understood and mired in difficulties. Often information is defined vaguely or not at all (Rendall *et al.*, 2009), and consequently it is unclear how something so vague and abstract can be reconciled with causal concepts like function and mechanism (Owren & Rendall, 2001). A related worry is that informational concepts are merely metaphors. For instance, 'information transfer' evokes some kind of concrete entity which senders hand over to receivers like a parcel, but there is no such thing, of course (Owren & Rendall, 2001; Rendall *et al.*, 2009). It is worth noting that proponents of information have acknowledged difficulties with their key concepts but regarded them as solvable (e.g. Burghardt, 1970; Markl, 1985; Hasson, 1994; Dawkins, 1995; Maynard Smith & Harper, 1995; Philips & Austad, 1996; Evans, 1997; Seyfarth *et al.*, 2010).

A bad heuristic

As a specifically linguistic metaphor (Owren & Rendall, 2001; Owren *et al.*, 2010), information is anthropomorphic (Owings & Morton, 1997) and strongly biases our perspective on animal communication (Rendall *et al.*, 2009): the informational view highlights whatever is similar to human language and neglects the rest. For example, our understanding of signal processing is skewed in favour of cognitive mechanisms (Owings & Morton, 1997; Owren & Rendall, 1997), especially in favour of cortical processing of the sort familiar from conceptual representation and language comprehension in humans (Owren & Rendall, 2001). The significance of non-cortical signal processing is downplayed (e.g. motivational effects in songbirds; see 'Assessment/management' above). Seyfarth *et al.* (2010) reject these criticisms. Information, they argue, is a non-linguistic concept, simply referring to the idea that the correlations between signals and conditions enable predictions (see 'Colloquial information'). Furthermore, information has not biased our view because, for instance, it underpinned the discovery of *dis*similarities between human and non-human primate vocalisations (Box 4).

The chapters in this volume explore these and other arguments both in favour of information (Chapters 1, 2, 4, 11–13, 15–17) and against it (Chapters 6–9). But it is time to consider arguments surrounding manipulation.

Arguments concerning manipulation

The overall argument advanced in favour of influence views is that they do not suffer the difficulties of informational approaches. In particular, explanations in terms of manipulation are thought to be neither metaphoric nor biased against non-cognitive signal processing (e.g. Owings & Morton, 1998; Rendall *et al.*, 2009). But influence models have seen their share of criticism. The following two difficulties stand out.

The rarity of direct impact

The affect induction model predicts that many primate calls have a direct impact on conserved, subcortical systems (see 'Affect induction' above). Therefore, calls with similar acoustic properties should elicit similar reactions, whereas calls with different properties should not. But neither prediction is well supported (Seyfarth *et al.*, 2010). First, calls with similar acoustic properties can often elicit different reactions depending on context. For instance, vervets hearing an eagle alarm call run into bushes; but if they are already there, they usually do not show any overt behavioural response (Seyfarth *et al.*, 1980). Second, vocalisations with very different acoustic properties can nonetheless elicit the same response (Box 2).

Inconsistency with evolutionary theory

Manipulation is often interpreted as implying a disadvantage to receivers (see 'Manipulation and influence' above). Disadvantaged receivers will be selected to decrease their responsiveness to manipulative signals until they ignore them. At that point senders cease to benefit from signalling (Box 3). Senders will then be selected for reducing their signalling costs, until eventually the signalling system disappears altogether (Searcy & Nowicki, 2005). But signal systems are ubiquitous, so the influence model must be wrong (Seyfarth *et al.*, 2010). Defenders of manipulation theories concede that receivers will evolve defence mechanisms against manipulation. But they argue that, owing to trade-offs and the dynamics of arms races, counter-selection need not always lead to the elimination of signalling systems (Rendall *et al.*, 2009; but see Bradbury & Vehrencamp, 2011b).

This section has sketched some of the major lines of conflict in the debate about informational and non-informational approaches to animal communication. We have seen that both sides have advanced powerful arguments. This may explain why the two approaches are sometimes seen as complementary rather than incompatible (e.g. Krebs & Dawkins, 1984; Owings & Morton, 1998; Carazo & Font, 2010). The following section moves beyond the to-and-fro within animal communication studies. It takes a broader and more abstract look at key concepts of the information view, some of which come with heavy philosophical baggage. Unpacking some of the baggage, if ever so cursorily, can shed light on theoretical commitments and opportunities.

Philosophical perspectives

Scientific realism

We can bring the information debate into sharper focus by situating it in the wider debate about scientific realism. Local scientific realists hold that at least some of our best scientific theories are (approximately) true and that some of their central terms refer to things in the world. At first blush, the claim that signals convey information is a local realist claim about a specific theoretical entity, information. It seems to imply that there is something in the world to which 'conveying information' refers, for example a capacity to enable predictions, and that signals do in fact have this capacity. By contrast, the claim that information is a metaphor denies that the word 'information' picks out anything in the world. The metaphor view is thus an anti-realist position about information.

However, informational views are not committed to realism about information. Proponents of information sometimes emphasise the heuristic value of concepts such as information and mental states while remaining neutral about any mechanistic implications (certain passages in Cheney and Seyfarth,1990, and Seyfarth and Cheney, 2003). This approach echoes Dennett's (1983) 'intentional stance'. The intentional stance recommends attributing mental states (goals, beliefs, desires) to animals in order to explain and predict their behaviour. It involves no assumptions about the internal, neural structure of these states; it does not even presuppose that animals possess any belief- or desire-like states at all. Treating animals as if they possessed mental states is justified simply to the extent that such practices increase explanatory and predictive power. By analogy, an 'informational stance' would recommend attributing information to signals in order to explain and predict behaviour without assuming anything about the nature or existence of information. The intentional (and informational) stance regards scientific and theoretical concepts primarily as tools for explanation. This is a form of instrumentalism, and adopting this version of instrumentalism with respect to information radically changes how we ought to assess informational claims. Rather than asking whether it is true that signals carry information we should ask whether such a claim is useful. However, this approach to information would still be vulnerable against arguments targeting its heuristic value (cf. Barret & Rendall, 2010).

A family of information concepts

Attempts to define the key notions of the informational view are sometimes dismissed as semantic squabbles. The point of definitions sometimes *is* semantic, e.g. when attempting to fix the meaning of a word like 'communication'. And disputes about which term to use for a given phenomenon can indeed be fruitless (although unifying language use can reduce misunderstandings). But sometimes it is not so clear what sorts of phenomena there are in the first place, and then definitions can be an important means of tracking distinguishing features (Maynard Smith & Harper, 2003). For instance, the goal of distinguishing between "cost-added signals" and "indices" was not to regiment language use, but to acknowledge that signals can differ markedly in the evolutionary mechanisms securing their reliability (Maynard Smith & Harper, 2003).

In philosophical jargon, definitions that aim to identify the key features of some phenomenon *X* are usually called 'theories of *X*' or 'accounts of *X*'. Philosophers have developed numerous theories of phenomena such as communication, information, representation, meaning and reference. This section sketches some of the insights most relevant to animal communication (although it can do no more than scratch the surface).

(1) Information

For many philosophers, information is simply a relation between two facts or events, something requiring no receivers, no minds, cognition or knowledge. Dretske (1981) was among the first to suggest that information is an 'objective commodity', a mind-independent relation in the world. He held that some state or event *A* carries the information that another state or event *B* obtains if there is a probabilistic relation between them, i.e. if *A* makes *B* certain (specifically, if *A*'s occurrence increases the probability of *B*'s occurrence to 1, and if that probability is less than 1 otherwise). One of the most attractive features of Dretske's theory is that information consists in a non-mysterious, probabilistic relation between states (it is 'naturalistic'). One of the arguably less attractive features is that it requires *A* to raise *B*'s probability to 1: which events are ever so tightly linked? Several philosophers have therefore turned to weaker notions of information (e.g. Millikan, 2004; Shea, 2007; Scarantino & Piccinini, 2010; see also Chapters 2 and 5).

(2) Representation

Philosophers usually distinguish sharply between information and representation. Carrying information about *B* implies that *B* exists (see above); whereas representing something as being *B* does not imply that it is *B*. Consider the philosophers' paradigm of representational entities, beliefs and desires. My belief that the sky is blue is a mental state that represents the sky as being blue (i.e. that the sky is blue is the belief's representational content). My belief may be false; just believing the sky is blue does not make it so. Hence, mental states can be about states that may or may not obtain (or be about things that may or may not exist). This remarkable property of mental states of being directed at things is also known as *intentionality*[2] and has nothing to do with having intentions (for related issues see Box 5).

[2] Intentionality (with a 't') must be distinguished from intensionality (with an 's'). The former is a property of mental states, i.e. their 'aboutness'. The latter is a property of languages rather than mental states, and it is defined in terms of certain inferential principles (see also Box 5).

Box 5 Referential opacity and indeterminacy of translation

Referential opacity and indeterminacy of translation are two philosophical ideas which must be mentioned because they have made their way into the ethological literature. But their value for ethology is doubtful.

Referential opacity

Suppose the statement "Susan believes that Bob Dylan is a musician" is true (i.e. she believes Dylan is a musician); now replace 'Bob Dylan' with his birth name 'Robert Allen Zimmerman'. The new sentence "Susan believes that Robert Allen Zimmerman is a musician" may well be false, for example if Susan does not know that both names refer to the same man. A sentence is said to create a 'referentially opaque' context for an expression if one can change the sentence's truth value by replacing the expression with a different term that refers to the same thing. Sentences about mental states such as beliefs and desires are referentially opaque. For this reason, referential opacity (or the broader notion of intensionality; see footnote 2) is sometimes taken to indicate the presence of intentionality (e.g. Chisholm, 1957; Dennett, 1983). But this is highly controversial (e.g. Allen, 1995; Crane, 2001).

Indeterminacy of translation

An anthropologist tries to translate into English the words of a newly discovered tribe. Quine (1960) argued that the difficulties in translating, say, 'gavagai' as 'rabbit' show that there is no fact of the matter about which translation is correct; indeed, there is no fact of the matter about what 'gavagai' means, or even 'rabbit'. Quine's point is much more radical than usually interpreted: it is not that identifying word meanings is difficult (cf. Hauser, 1996; Cheney & Seyfarth, 2007), but rather that words lack (determinate) meanings. Quine's meaning scepticism is now widely rejected (reviewed in Miller, 2006).

Some philosophers maintain that intentionality and representational content consist in physical and biological relations that are as non-mysterious as the relations constituting information. Dretske (1988) argued, for instance, that any state or event *A* represents a state or event *B* if *A* has the biological function to carry the information that *B* obtains. Dretske's proposal is relevant for present purposes because it implies that representational content is not the privilege of mental states alone: animal signals have representational content simply by virtue of having evolved in order to carry information; receivers do not need to mentally represent referents. Talk of 'false' animal signals is then not metaphoric, but expresses the idea that signals can represent what does not exist (but see Ch. 17). More recent accounts of representation deviate in various ways from Dretske's proposal, but accept that animal signals can represent states and events (e.g. Millikan, 1984, 2004; Bekoff & Allen, 1992; Stegmann, 2009).

(3) Communication

On the informational view, animal communication involves conveying information from senders to receivers. The cognitively most demanding view of conveying information requires signals to elicit mental representations in receivers (see 'Colloquial information' above). But even this considerable degree of cognitive complexity pales in comparison with the complexity normally associated with human communication.

The orthodox view of human communication is due to Grice (but see Millikan, 1984; Green, 2007). For Grice, speakers communicate when they utter sentences with certain "communicative intentions" (reviewed in Neale, 1992). The simplest of these intentions is that listeners believe that *p* (where *p* is the proposition the speaker intends to communicate, e.g. "the tree is green"). In order to meet even this basic condition of communication, speakers need to have at least one kind of mental state: intentions. More importantly, they need to be able to attribute to listeners the belief that *p*. Gricean communication requires still more complex mental state attributions, e.g. that listeners recognise that the speaker intends them to believe that *p*. Despite decades of research, there is little evidence that non-human primates attribute even simple beliefs, let alone false ones, to others (Cheney & Seyfarth, 2007; Rosati *et al.*, 2010). To the contrary, there is evidence that primates fail to reason about the beliefs of others (although some species attribute mental states such as intentions, goals and visual experience and therefore have a 'theory of mind' of sorts, reviewed in Rosati, Santos & Hare, 2010).

(4) Meaning

What speakers communicate is what they intend to convey by uttering a sentence. But the sentences employed to convey the intended meaning possess their own conventional or linguistic meanings, i.e. meanings which are independent of what speakers intend to convey by uttering the sentences. Perhaps the most influential theory of linguistic meaning holds that a sentence's meaning is its truth condition (e.g. Davidson, 1967). On this view, the meaning of the sentence "the tree is green" is the state of the world that makes this sentence true: the fact that the tree is green.

Critics of information concepts allege that comparing animal signals with human words is bound to skew our explanations of behaviour in terms of linguistic meaning analogues. But comparisons with human language can also include pragmatic aspects of communication. Horn (1997) suggested, for instance, that animal signals are analogous to speech acts. Speech acts are actions performed by uttering sentences, and they are effective primarily because of social rules, not because of the linguistic meaning attached to the sentences we utter (Austin, 1962). Note that there are other approaches in philosophy of language that minimise the role of linguistic meanings and that have been applied to animal signals (McAninsh *et al.*, 2009; Bar-On & Green, 2010).

(5) Reference

Names and general terms pick out (or refer to) particular individuals and kinds of things, respectively (e.g. 'Simon' picks out Simon, 'water' picks out water). Much philosophical work has focused on understanding the mechanism that secures the link between a term and what it picks out: why does 'water' refer to water rather than something else, and why does it pick out anything at all? The traditional answer points to the minds of speakers and listeners. A term like 'water' is associated with descriptions (or a set of concepts) that speakers have in their minds, for example "– is composed of H_2O molecules" or "– is transparent". The term 'water' refers to a particular body of fluid on the condition that this fluid exactly matches the descriptions. Ogden and Richards' (1923) "triangle of meaning" illustrates the descriptivist approach, which remains popular in the cognitive sciences. Crucially, descriptivism underlies much reasoning about referential signals: signals count as referential in a strong, word-like sense only if they elicit mental representations (see 'Colloquial information' above).

However, descriptivism in its classical form has been discredited in philosophy of language. Kripke (1980) and Putnam (1975) argued that reference depends on a term bearing the right kind of causal connection to a thing, not on the associations or concepts that a term evokes in speakers and in hearers. The causal-historical approach has its own problems. But the negative point, that reference is not determined by what speakers and hearers have in their minds ('semantic externalism'), is well supported.

Outlook

Perhaps the most obvious conclusion from this survey is that the suitability of information and/or manipulation for explaining animal communication is not simply an empirical matter. It also depends on which notions of information and manipulation one endorses.

Critics of information deserve credit for insisting that information concepts are still poorly understood. Several distinct notions of colloquial information are in use (a fact which largely has gone unnoticed), and it is unclear how they relate to one another. Moreover, each notion raises further questions which are seldom addressed rigorously: for example, on the view that carrying information consists in allowing predictions, should non-cognitive processes count as predictions? Furthermore, mathematical models of signal evolution use an information concept that appears to be distinct from the one used in applications of statistical decision theory (reliability versus changes to estimates of probability), and again it is unclear how they interrelate. However, in my view it is premature to conclude from these gaps that information concepts are inappropriate. First, it is not obvious that the gaps need to be filled, because tools such as statistical decision theory have proven fruitful without a unified, clear-cut concept of information. Second, it is likely that the gaps can be filled eventually, e.g. by integrating philosophical research on information concepts.

The concept of manipulation faces similar challenges. The costs-to-receivers interpretation, on which the opponents of manipulation have focused almost exclusively, should be more clearly distinguished from proximate interpretations. One proximate interpretation is that signals manipulate when receivers process signals by non-cognitive mechanisms. Since signals can affect receivers through either cognitive or non-cognitive mechanisms (or both, depending on the species), manipulation should play a role in any comprehensive account of signal processing. As far as I can see, this is the strongest argument for the importance of manipulation. And it should carry some weight with those who identify informational communication with a certain type of proximate mechanism of signal processing by receivers (i.e. a mechanism involving representations of referents). Such a proximate interpretation exacts its price, however. It ignores the uses of information in, for instance, evolutionary models; it undermines any outright rejection of information, because some receivers do process signals cognitively (and, hence, informationally); and it seems to requires a firm distinction between cognitive and non-cognitive mechanisms of signal processing.

I wish to resist characterising information in proximate terms. I believe that the informational approach is valuable, not because it captures a kind of proximate mechanism of signal processing, but because it provides ultimate (etiological) explanations of receiver responses (Stegmann, 2005, 2009). Let us return to the fireflies. The disposition of male fireflies to approach certain light pulses is explained, on the informational approach, by the signal's information that there is a receptive female. The presence of a receptive female at the source of a certain light pulse is, plausibly, the reason why males were selected to approach the light source. In other words, the information content of the light pulses specifies the reason by virtue of which males acquired their response dispositions over evolutionary time. This idea can be generalised as follows. Asserting that a receiver responds with *R* to a signal because (1) the signal carries the information that *p* is another way of saying that the receiver responds with *R* because (1*) *p* caused receivers to evolve/learn the disposition to do *R*. In other words, citing the information content *p* explains *R* by identifying the reason that caused receivers to evolve/learn the *R*-disposition in the first place. The information content therefore provides an ultimate explanation of *R*. The approach just sketched is compatible with requiring that full explanations of *R* ought to include *R*'s proximate mechanisms, as well. However, whether or not the mechanisms involve mental representations would be irrelevant to whether or not the signal carries information.

Acknowledgements

I am very grateful to Jack Bradbury, Andrew Horn and Robert Seyfarth for their feedback on the draft version. Richard Coss, Joel McGlothlin, Michael Ryan, Robert Seyfarth, Ron Swaisgood, Richard Wrangham and Klaus Zuberbühler were enormously helpful in providing drawings, diagrams and photographs. I thank Bartolomeu Bastos for being such a reliable and efficient research assistant. The work in preparation for this introduction was generously supported by two grants from the British Academy (PDF/2006/306 and SG-51996).

References

Allen, C. (1995). Intentionality: natural and artificial. In H. L. Roitblat & J. Meyer, eds., *Comparative Approaches to Cognitive Science*. Cambridge, MA: MIT Press, pp. 93–110.

Apfelbeck, B. & Goymann, W. (2011). Ignoring the challenge? Male black redstarts (*Phoenicurus ochruros*) do not increase testosterone levels during territorial conflicts but they do so in response to gonadotropin-releasing hormone. *Proceedings of the Royal Society of London Series B: Biological Sciences*, **278**, 3233.

Arnold, K. & Zuberbühler, K. (2006). Language evolution: Semantic combinations in primate calls. *Nature*, **106**, 303–303.

Austin, J. L. (1962). *How to Do Things with Words*, 2nd edn. Cambridge, MA: Harvard University Press.

Bar-On, D. & Green, M. (2010). Lionspeak: communication, expression and meaning. In J. O'Shea & E. Rubenstein, eds., *Self, Language, and World: Problems from Kant, Sellars, and Rosenberg: in Memory of Jay F. Rosenberg*. Atascadero, CA: Ridgeview Publishing Co.

Barret, L. & Rendall, D. (2010). Out of our minds: the neuroethology of primate strategic behavior. In M. L. Platt & A. A. Ghazanfar, eds., *Primate Neuroethology*. Oxford: Oxford University Press.

Bekoff, M. & Allen, C. (1992). Intentional icons: towards an evolutionary cognitive ethology. *Ethology*, **91**, 1–16.

Bergstrom, C. T. & Rosvall, M. (2011). The transmission sense of information. *Biology and Philosophy*, **26**, 159–176.

Bradbury, J. W. & Vehrencamp, S. L. (2011a). *Principles of Animal Communication*, 2nd edn. Sunderland, MA: Sinauer Associates.

Bradbury, J. W. & Vehrencamp, S. L. (2011b). *Web Topic 1.2: Information and Communication. Principles of Animal Communication*, 2nd edn companion website. http://sites.sinauer.com/animalcommunication2e

Bradbury, J. W. & Vehrencamp, S. L. (2011c). *Web Topic 8.7: Brains and Decision Making. Principles of Animal Communication*, 2nd edn companion website. http://sites.sinauer.com/animalcommunication2e

Burghardt, G. M. (1970). Defining 'communication'. In J. W. Johnston, D. G. Moulton & A. Turk, eds., *Communication by Chemical Signals*. New York: Appleton-Century Crofts, pp. 5–18.

Carazo, P. & Font, E. (2010). Putting information back into biological communication. *Journal of Evolutionary Biology*, **23**, 661–669.

Cheney, D. L. & Seyfarth, R. M. (1990). *How Monkeys See the World*. Chicago, IL: University of Chicago Press.

Cheney, D. L. & Seyfarth, R. M. (2007). *Baboon Metaphysics*. Chicago, IL: University of Chicago Press.

Chisholm, R. (1957). *Perceiving: A Philosophical Study*. Ithaca, NY: Cornell University Press.

Christiansen, M. & Kirby, S. (2003). *Language Evolution*. Oxford: Oxford University Press.

Clutton-Brock, T. & Albon, S. D. (1979). The roaring of red deer and the evolution of honest advertisement. *Behaviour*, **69**, 145–170.

Crane, T. (2001). *Elements of Mind: An Introduction to the Philosophy of Mind*. Oxford: Oxford University Press.

Danchin, E., Giraldeau, L. A., Valone, T. J. & Wagner, R. H. (2004). Public information: from nosy neighbors to cultural evolution. *Science*, **305**(5683), 487–491.

Davidson, D. (1967). Truth and meaning. *Synthese*, **17**, 304–323.

Dawkins, M. S. (1995). *Unravelling Animal Behaviour*. Harlow: Longman.

Dawkins, R. & Krebs, J. R. (1978). Animal signals: information or manipulation. In J. R. Krebs & N. B. Davies, eds., *Behavioural Ecology: An Evolutionary Approach*, 1st edn. Oxford: Blackwell, pp. 282–309.

Dennett, D. C. (1983). Intentional systems in cognitive ethology: the 'Panglossian Paradigm' defended. *Behavioral and Brain Sciences*, **6**, 343–390.

Dingle, H. (1969). A statistical and information analysis of aggressive communication in the mantis shrimp *Gonodactylus bredini* Manning (Crustacea: Stomatopoda). *Animal Behaviour*, **17**, 567–581.

Dretske, F. (1981). *Knowledge and the Flow of Information.* Cambridge, MA: MIT Press.

Dretske, F. (1988). *Explaining Behavior: Reasons in a World of Causes.* Cambridge, MA: MIT Press.

Dyer, F. C. (2002). The biology of the dance language. *Annual Review of Entomology*, **47**, 917–949.

Evans, C. S. (1997). Referential signals. In D. H. Owings, M. D. Beecher & N. Thompson, eds., *Communication. Perspectives in Ecology*, Vol. 12. New York: Plenum Press, pp. 99–143.

Evans, C. S. & Evans, L. (1999). Chicken food calls are functionally referential. *Animal Behaviour*, **58**, 307–319.

Evans, C. S. & Evans, L. (2007). Representational signalling in birds. *Biology Letters*, **3**, 8–11.

Fedurek, P. & Slocombe, K. E. (2011). Primate vocal communication: a useful tool for understanding human speech and language evolution? *Human Biology*, **82**, 153–173.

Fischer, J., Hammerschmidt, K. & Todt, D. (1995). Factors affecting acoustic variation in Barbary macaque (*Macaca sylvanus*) disturbance calls. *Ethology*, **101**, 51–66.

Fitch, W. T. (2010). *The Evolution of Language.* Cambridge: Cambridge University Press.

Font, E. & Carazo, P. (2010). Animals in translation: why there is meaning (but probably no message) in animal communication. *Animal Behaviour*, **80**, e1–e6.

Gallistel, C. R. (2008). Learning and representation. In R. Menzel, ed., *Learning Theory and Behavior. Learning and Memory: A Comprehensive Reference*, Vol. 1. Oxford: Elsevier, pp. 227–242.

Gentner, T. Q., Fenn, K. M., Margoliash, D. & Nusbaum, H. C. (2006). Recursive syntactic pattern learning by songbirds. *Nature*, **440**, 1204–1207.

Gil-da-Costa, R., Braun, A., Lopes, M. *et al.* (2004). Towards an evolutionary perspective on conceptual representation: species-specific calls activate visual and affective processing systems in the macaque. *Proceedings of the National Academy of Sciences, Biological Sciences (Neurosciences)*, **101**, 50.

Giraldeau, L. A. (1997). The ecology of information use. In J. R. Krebs & N. B. Davies, eds., *Behavioural Ecology: An Evolutionary Approach.* Oxford: Blackwell, pp. 42–68.

Green, M. (2007). *Self-expression.* Oxford: Oxford University Press.

Halliday, T. (1983). Information and communication. In T. Halliday & P. J. B. Slater, eds., *Communication. Animal Behaviour*, Vol. 2. Oxford: Blackwell Scientific, pp. 43–81.

Hasson, O. (1994). Cheating signals. *Journal of Theoretical Biology*, **167**, 223–238.

Hauser, M. D. (1996). *The Evolution of Communication.* Cambridge, MA: MIT Press.

Hauser, M. D. (1998). Functional referents and acoustic similarity: field playback experiments with rhesus monkeys. *Animal Behaviour*, **55**, 1647–1658.

Hauser, M. D., Chomsky, N. & Fitch, W. T. (2002). The faculty of language: what is it, who has it, and how did it evolve? *Science*, **298**, 1569–1579.

Hazlett, B. A. & Bossert, W. H. (1965). A statistical analysis of the aggressive communications systems of some hermit crabs. *Animal Behaviour*, **13**, 357–373.

Horn, A. G. (1997). Speech acts and animal signals. In D. H. Owings, M. D. Beecher & N. S. Thompson, eds., *Communication. Perspectives in Ethology*, Vol. 12. New York: Plenum Press.

Hurford, J. (2007). *The Origins of Meaning*. Oxford: Oxford University Press.

Johnstone, R. A. (1997). The evolution of animal signals. In J. R. Krebs & N. B. Davies, eds., *Behavioural Ecology: An Evolutionary Approach*, 4th edn. Oxford: Blackwell, pp. 155–178.

Kirkpatrick, M. & Ryan, M. J. (1991). The evolution of mating preferences and the paradox of the lek. *Nature*, **350**, 33–38.

Krebs, J. R. & Davies, N. B. (1993). *An Introduction to Behavioural Ecology*. Oxford: Blackwell Scientific Publications.

Krebs, J. R. & Dawkins, R. (1984). Animal signals: mind-reading and manipulation. In J. R. Krebs & N. B. Davies, eds., *Behavioural Ecology: An Evolutionary Approach*, 2nd edn. Oxford: Blackwell, pp. 380–402.

Kripke, S. (1980). *Naming and Necessity*. Cambridge, MA: Harvard University Press.

Laidre, M. E. (2009). How often do animals lie about their intentions? An experimental test. *American Naturalist*, **173**, 337–346.

Lee, D. (2010). Neuroethology of decision making. In M. L. Platt & A. A. Ghazanfar, eds., *Primate Neuroethology*. New York: Oxford University Press, pp. 550–569.

Lewis, S. M. & Cratsley, C. K. (2008). Flash signal evolution, mate choice, and predation in fireflies. *Annual Review of Entomology*, **53**, 293–321.

Lieberman, D. A. (2003). *Learning and Memory: An Integrative Approach*. New York: Wadsworth Publishing.

Lloyd, J. E. (1966). Studies on the flash communication system in Photinus fireflies. *Miscellaneous Publications, Museum of Zoology, University of Michigan*, **130**, 1–95.

Macedonia, J. M. & Evans, C. S. (1993). Variation among mammalian alrm call systems and the problem of meaning in animal signals. *Ethology*, **93**, 177–197.

Manser, M. B., Bell, M. B. & Fletcher, L. B. (2001). The information that receivers extract from alarm calls in suricates. *Proceedings of the Royal Society of London Series B: Biological Sciences*, **268**, 2485–2491.

Markl, H. (1985). Manipulation, modulation, information, cognition: some of the riddles of communication. In B. Hölldobler & M. Lindauer, eds., *Experimental Behavioral Ecology and Sociobiology*. Stuttgart: G. Fischer Verlag, pp. 163–194.

Marler, P. (1961). The logical analysis of animal communication. *Journal of Theoretical Biology*, **7**, 295–317.

Marler, P., Evans, C. S. & Hauser, M. D. (1992). Animal signals? Reference, motivation or both? In H. Papoucek, U. Jürgens & M. Papoucek, eds., *Nonverbal Vocal Communication: Comparative and Developmental Approaches*. Cambridge: Cambridge University Press, pp. 66–86.

Maynard Smith, J. (1976). Sexual selection and the handicap principle. *Journal of Theoretical Biology*, **57**, 239–242.

Maynard Smith, J. & Harper, D. G. C. (1995). Animal signals: models and terminology. *Journal of Theoretical Biology*, **177**(3), 305–311.

Maynard Smith, J. & Harper, D. (2003). *Animal Signals*. Oxford: Oxford University Press.

McAninsh, A., Goodrich, G. & Allen, C. (2009). Animal communication and neo-expressivism. In R. W. Lurz, ed., *Philosophy of Animal Minds: New Essays on Animal Thought and Conciousness*. Cambridge: Cambridge University Press, pp. 128–144.

McGlothlin, J. W., Jawor, J. M., Greives, T. J., Phillips, J. L. & Ketterson, E. D. (2008). Hormones and honest signals: males with larger ornaments elevate testosterone more when challenged. *Journal of Evolutionary Biology*, **21**, 39–48.

McGregor, P. K. (1993). Signalling in territorial systems: a context for individual identification, ranging and eavesdropping. *Philosophical Transactions of the Royal Society of London Series B*, **340**, 237–244.

McNamara, J. M. & Dall, S. R. X. (2010). Information is a fitness enhancing resource. *Oikos*, **119**(2), 231–236.

Miller, A. (2006). Meaning scepticism. In M. Devitt & R. Hanley, eds., *The Blackwell Guide to the Philosophy of Language*. Oxford: Blackwell, pp. 91–113.

Millikan, R. G. (1984). *Language, Thought and Other Biological Categories*. Cambridge, MA: MIT Press.

Millikan, R. G. (2004). *The Varieties of Meaning*. Cambridge, MA: MIT Press.

Munz, T. (2005). The bee battles: Karl von Frisch, Adrian Wenner and the honey bee dance language controversy. *Journal of the History of Biology*, **38**(3), 535–570.

Neale, S. (1992). Paul Grice and the philosophy of language. *Linguistics and Philosophy*, **15**(5), 509–559.

Ogden, C. K. & Richard, I. A. (1923). *The Meaning of Meaning: A Study of the Influence of Language upon Thought and of the Science of Symbolism*, 8th edn. New York: Harcourt, Brace &; World, Inc.

Otte, D. (1974). Effects and functions in the evolution of signaling systems. *Annual Review of Ecology and Systematics*, **5**, 385–417.

Owings, D. H. & Morton, E. S. (1997). The role of information and communication: an assessment/management approach. In D. H. Owings, M. D. Beecher & N. S. Thompson, eds., *Communication. Perspectives in Ecology*, Vol. 12. New York: Plenum Press, pp. 359–390.

Owings, D. H. & Morton, E. S. (1998). *Animal Vocal Communication: A New Approach*. Cambridge: Cambridge University Press.

Owren, M. J. & Rendall, D. (1997). An affect-conditioning model of non-human primate vocal signaling. In D. H. Owings, M. D. Beecher & N. S. Thompson, eds., *Communication. Perspectives in Ethology*, Vol. 12. New York: Plenum Press, pp. 299–346.

Owren, M. J. & Rendall, D. (2001). Sound on the rebound: bringing form and function back to the forefront in understanding non-human primate vocal signaling. *Evolutionary Anthropology*, **10**, 58–71.

Owren, M. J., Rendall, D. & Ryan, M. J. (2010). Redefining animal signaling: influence versus information in communication. *Biology and Philosophy*, **25**, 755–780.

Philips, M. & Austad, S. N. (1996). Animal communication and social evolution. In M. Bekoff & D. Jamieson, eds., *Readings in Animal Cognition*. Cambridge, MA: MIT Press, pp. 257–267.

Platt, M. L. & Ghazanfar, A. A. (eds.) (2010). *Primate Neuroethology*. Oxford: Oxford University Press.

Putnam, H. (1975). The meaning of 'meaning'. In K. Gunderson, ed., *Language, Mind, and Knowledge. Minnesota Studies in the Philosophy of Science*, Vol. 8. Minneapolis, MN: University of Minnesota Press, pp. 131–193.

Quastler, H. (1958). A primer on information theory. In H. P. Yockey, R. L. Platzman & H. Quastler, eds., *Symposium on Information Theory in Biology. Gatlinburg, Tennessee, October 29–31, 1956*. London: Pergamon Press, pp. 3–49.

Quine, W. V. O. (1960). *Word and Object*. Cambridge, MA: MIT Press.

Radick, G. (2007). *The Simian Tongue: The Long Debate about Animal Language*. Chicago, IL: University of Chicago Press.

Reby, D., McComb, K., Cargnelutti, B. *et al.* (2005). Red deer stags use formants as assessment cues during intrasexual agonistic interactions. *Proceedings of the Royal Society of London Series B: Biological Sciences*, **272**, 941–947.

Rendall, D., Owren, M. J. & Ryan, M. J. (2009). What do animal signals mean? *Animal Behaviour*, **78**(2), 233–240.

Romanski, L. M. & Ghazanfar, A. A. (2010). The primate frontal and temporal lobes and their role in multisensory vocal communication. In M. L. Platt & A. A. Ghazanfar, eds., *Primate Neuroethology*. Oxford: Oxford University Press, pp. 500–524.

Ron, S. R. (2008). The evolution of female mate choice for complex calls in túngara frogs. *Animal Behaviour*, **76**, 1783–1794.

Rosati, A. G., Santos, L. R. & Hare, B. (2010). Primate social cognition: thirty years after Premack and Woodruff. In M. L. Platt & A. A. Ghazanfar, eds., *Primate Neuroethology*. Oxford: Oxford University Press.

Rowe, M. P. & Owings, D. H. (1990). Probing, assessment, and management during interactions between ground squirrels and rattlesnakes. *Ethology*, **86**(3), 237–249.

Ruxton, G. D. & Schaefer, H. M. (2011). Resolving current disagreements and ambiguities in the terminology of animal communication. *Journal of Evolutionary Biology*, **24**(12), 2574–2585.

Ryan, M. J. & Rand, A. S. (2003). Mate recognition in túngara frogs: a review of some studies of brain, behavior, and evolution. *Acta Zoologica Sinica*, **49**, 713–726.

Scarantino, A. (2010). Animal communication between information and influence. *Animal Behaviour*, **79**(6), e1–e5.

Scarantino, A. & Piccinini, G. (2010). Information without truth. *Metaphilosophy*, **41**, 313–330.

Scott-Phillips, T. C. (2008). Defining biological communication. *Journal of Evolutionary Biology*, **21**, 387–395.

Searcy, W. & Nowicki, S. (2005). *The Evolution of Animal Communication*. Princeton, NJ: Princeton University Press.

Seyfarth, R. M. & Cheney, D. L. (2003). Signalers and receivers in animal communication. *Annual Review of Psychology*, **54**, 145–173.

Seyfarth, R. M., Cheney, D. L., Bergman, T. *et al.* (2010). The central importance of information in studies of animal communication. *Animal Behaviour*, **80**, 3–8.

Seyfarth, R. M., Cheney, D. L. & Marler, P. (1980). Vervet monkey alarm calls: semantic communication in a free-ranging primate. *Animal Behaviour*, **28**, 1070–1094.

Shannon, C. E. (1948). The mathematical theory of communication, I and II. *Bell System Technical Journal*, **27**, 379–423, 623–656.

Shea, N. (2007). Consumers need information: supplementing teleosemantics with an input condition. *Philosophy and Phenomenological Research*, **75**, 404–435.

Shettleworth, S. J. (2001). Animal cognition and animal behaviour. *Animal Behaviour*, **61**, 277–286.

Shettleworth, S. J. (2010). *Cognition, Evolution, and Behaviour*, 2nd edn. Oxford: Oxford University Press.

Skyrms, B. (2010). *Signals: Evolution, Learning, and Information*. Oxford: Oxford University Press.

Slocombe, K. E. & Zuberbühler, K. (2005). Functionally referential communication in a chimpanzee. *Current Biology*, **15**(19), 1779–1784.

Smith, W. J. (1965). Message, meaning, and context in ethology. *American Naturalist*, **99**, 405–409.

Smith, W. J. (1986). An 'informational' perspective on manipulation. In R. W. Mitchell & N. S. Thompson, eds., *Deception: Perspectives on Human and Non-human Deceit*. Albany, NY: State University of New York Press, pp. 71–86.

Smith, W. J. (1997). The behavior of communicating, after twenty years. In D. H. Owings, M. D. Beecher & N. S. Thompson, eds., *Communication. Perspectives in Ethology*, Vol. 12. New York: Plenum Press, pp. 7–53.

Sperber, D. & Origgi, G. (2010). A pragmatic perspective on the evolution of language. In R. K. Larson, V. Déprez & H. Yamakido, eds., *The Evolution of Human Language: Biolinguistic Perspectives*. Cambridge: Cambridge University Press, pp. 124–132.

Stegmann, U. E. (2005). John Maynard Smith's notion of animal signals. *Biology and Philosophy*, **20**, 1011–1025.

Stegmann, U. E. (2009). A consumer-based teleosemantics for animal signals. *Philosophy of Science*, **76**, 864–875.

Stephens, D. W. (2007). Models of information use. In D. W. Stephens, J. S. Brown & R. C. Ydenberg, eds., *Foraging: Behaviour and Ecology*. Chicago, IL: University of Chicago Press, pp. 48–75.

Swaisgood, R. R., Rowe, M. P. & Owings, D. H. (1999). Assessment of rattlesnake dangerousness by California ground squirrels: exploitation of cues from rattling sounds. *Animal Behaviour*, **57**, 1301–1310.

Templeton, J. J. & Giraldeau, L. A. (1996). Vicarious sampling: The use of personal and public information by starlings foraging in a simple patchy environment. *Behavioral Ecology and Sociobiology*, **38**, 105–114.

Valone, T. J. (1989). Group foraging, public information, and patch estimation. *Oikos*, **56**, 357–363.

Van Heijningen, C. A. A., De Visser, J., Zuidema, W. & Ten Cate, C. (2009). Simple rules can explain discrimination of putative recursive syntactic structures by a songbird species. *Proceedings of the National Academy of Sciences USA*, **106**, 20538–20543.

von Frisch, K. (1967). *The Dance Language and Orientation of Bees*. Cambridge, MA: Harvard University Press.

Wagner, R. H. & Danchin, E. (2010). A taxonomy of biological information. *Oikos*, **119**(2), 203–209.

Wheeler, B. C., Searcy, W. A., Christiansen, M. H. *et al.* (2011). Communication. In R. Menzel & J. Fischer, eds., *Animal Thinking: Contemporary Issues in Comparative Cognition*. Cambridge, MA: MIT Press, pp. 187–205.

Wiley, R. H. (1983). The evolution of communication: Information and manipulation. In T. R. Halliday & P. J. B. Slater, eds., *Communication. Animal Behaviour*, Vol. 2. Oxford: Blackwell, pp. 156–189.

Wilson, E. O. (1975). *Sociobiology: The New Synthesis*. Cambridge, MA: Harvard University Press.

Wingfield, J. C. & Wada, M. (1989). Changes in plasma levels of testosterone during male–male interactions in the song sparrow, *Melospiza melodia*: time course and specificity of response. *Journal of Comparative Physiology A*, **166**, 189–194.

Zahavi, A. (1975). Mate selection – a selection for a handicap. *Journal of Theoretical Biology*, **53**, 205–259.

Zuberbühler, K., Cheney, D. L. & Seyfarth, R. M. (1999). Conceptual semantics in a non-human primate. *Journal of Comparative Psychology*, **113**, 33–42.

Zuberbühler, K., Ouattara, K., Bitty, A., Lemasson, A. & Noë, R. (2009). The primate roots of human language: Primate vocal behaviour and cognition in the wild. In F. d'Errico & J. Hombert, eds., *Becoming Eloquent: Advances in the Emergence of Language, Human Cognition, and Modern Cultures*. Amsterdam: John Benjamins Publishing Company, pp. 235–266.

PART I VARIETIES OF INFORMATION

1

Influence and information in communication networks

ANDREW G. HORN AND PETER K. MCGREGOR

1.1 Introduction

In the cold Canadian dawn, from a nest hole in a punky birch, a female black-capped chickadee, *Poecile atricapillus*, listens to the males that sing from widely spaced song posts in the forest all around her. They shift the frequency and timing of their songs in response to one another, according to rules of engagement that the female is attuned to but that researchers are only starting to tease apart (Foote *et al.*, 2010). She shifts her attention from one male to another, as they engage in a ritual that serves partly to sort out their territorial boundaries, and partly as a performance for her and other conspecific listeners scattered through the woods.

This dawn chorus of the chickadees illustrates the natural context in which most communication occurs: not in the bare-bones dyad of one signaller, one receiver, but rather in a network of communicators – signaller receivers that exchange signals all within receiving range of one another (McGregor, 2005). The complications introduced by such networks can be daunting, but if we are to understand animal communication, we have to understand what is going on in this, its most common context and its evolutionary foundation (Wisenden & Stacey, 2005). The purpose of this chapter is to show how the concept of information is indispensable for these efforts. Specifically, we will show that viewing signalling interactions in the context of a communication network operationalises three problematic but useful concepts: information transfer, information gathering and information flow.

Animal Communication Theory: Information and Influence, ed. Ulrich Stegmann. Published by Cambridge University Press.

1.2 The problem: the role of information in communication

Such concepts have come under fire recently, with renewed criticisms of the view that animals communicate by exchanging information (Rendall, Owren & Ryan, 2009, and commentaries thereafter). To illustrate the problems with the informational approach, we will use its most extreme caricature, the conduit metaphor, which presents communication as a flow of information from sender[1] to receiver, like water flowing down a pipe or electricity through a conduit (Reddy, 1979; Rendall *et al.*, 2009). According to the metaphor, communication starts with encoding, in which a sender transfers information into a signal, which then carries that message to a receiver, and this receiver decodes the meaning of the signal.

At first sight, nothing seems wrong with this picture of communication, as the key concepts it represents – encoding, decoding and information flow – are so heavily ingrained in how most of us think about communication. Nevertheless, critics of the informational approach see problems in each step.

First, the encoding step implies that senders actively encode information, whereas, in fact (the critics argue), senders usually simply produce signals at times when, on average, it is adaptive to do so. Usually this criticism is levelled at the view that encoding requires the sender to have a mental construct, perhaps including an intention and/or belief, that somehow mirrors either the construct that the signal is to produce in the receiver or the receiver's response. Even without some such mental constructs, however, if senders have no alternative in sending one signal over another, or no signal at all, then, so the critics say, there is no sense in which they can be said to be encoding information, except perhaps in the same passive sense that clouds mean rain (Font & Carazo, 2010).

A second criticism is that the decoding step, too, implies that receivers actively decode signals, whereas in fact receivers do not decode signals; they are manipulated by them. Granted, there may be selection on receivers only to respond to signals when the response is adaptive, but it is a stretch to call such a response 'decoding'. Instead, decoding should involve comparing a signal against an array of possible signals, then selecting the response that corresponds appropriately to the signal. If receivers instead react to signals passively like struck billiard balls, without an intervening step of selecting a response, we can dispense with the concept of decoding.

Third, as presented in the conduit metaphor, "encoded information is afforded a material form that exists independently of the individuals that are communicating" (Rendall *et al.*, 2009, p. 240), even though "it is simply not

[1] We consider the terms sender and signaller to be equivalent.

correct to think of communication as information flowing from sender to receiver" (Font & Carazo, 2010, p. e3, paraphrasing Rendall *et al.*, 2009).

For us, these statements take the metaphor too literally; the metaphor's encoding and decoding steps clearly imply that information, if it is physical at all, starts and stops in the head of the sender and starts and stops again in the head of the receiver. Nonetheless, the metaphor does imply a broad overlap between the information that is sent and received. It may allow for some differences between the encoded and decoded information, between broadcast and transmitted information (Wiley, 1983), and between message (evidence the sender has actively made available in signalling) and meaning (upshot of that evidence as interpreted by the receiver; Smith, 1977). For the information-based view of communication to work, however, there must be a strong commonality between what starts the signalling chain and what ends it, usually conceived of as some kind of match between how the sender is selected to signal and how the receiver is selected to respond.

Thus critics of the informational approach make three main claims: senders do not actively encode information, receivers do not parse through information to select an adaptive response, and information does not flow from sender to receiver. In making a strong case for each of these points, others view communication as a one-way exchange between one sender and one receiver – the dyadic view of animal communication. This view approaches animal communication from the wrong direction, however, by building it up from rudimentary dyadic interactions, rather than by starting with the broader perspective of the social interactions that signalling interactions are part of. When we take the latter, top-down approach, the concept of information becomes more accurate, less vague and more useful (Horn, 1997; Scott-Phillips, 2010). In the next section, we will walk through such an approach, as a prelude to the main part of our chapter, which shows how studying signalling interactions in their natural context addresses each of the above criticisms, and supports an informational approach to animal communication.

1.3 Our approach to information

One's approach to animal communication of course depends on what one finds most interesting. We are behavioural ecologists, and so study the function and evolution of behaviour. Our studies of signals and signalling behaviours focus on how they were shaped by natural selection to have the forms and usage that they do. When we say behaviours are shaped by natural selection, we are of course using the usual shorthand of evolutionary biologists, which is understood to mean that the behaviours are not designed per se, but are the product of a history of selection against variants that are maladaptive. Of particular interest to us is identifying the targets and agents of selection (Endler, 1986): the features of traits that have been 'designed' in this way and the selective pressures, i.e. the hard facts of life, that those features are an evolutionary response to.

Our approach to signals is no different from our approach to any other social behaviour, or non-social behaviour such as foraging, for that matter. To emphasise this, and to try to avoid any misunderstandings about the role that information plays in our approach, we start with the simple example of two rams, *Ovis canadensis*, fighting. When one ram hits the other with its horns, the effectiveness of that action and its adaptive consequences are relatively easy to explain. Horns are hard physical objects, so hitting a conspecific with them is clearly an effective method for getting a rival out of the way. The agent of selection – i.e. the evolutionary pressure that accounts for hefty horns – is the displacement of rivals, and the target of selection – i.e. what aspect of the trait has been selected for – is the hardness of the horns and how they are used.

Now imagine a horn that is only used as a signal. For instance, perhaps a ram deters rivals just by holding its horns high. Here, the horns are effective not because they exert a physical force, but because of the psychological force they exert on receivers; they serve as a stimulus for the receiver to go away. What is it now about the horns that makes them effective and has thus been selected for – the target of selection? It is no longer their hardness and thrust, which were so obviously the targets of selection when they were used as weapons. Identifying the target requires more observation and experimentation than it did for fighting, but it is doable. One likely conclusion of such work may be that animals that avoid big-horned conspecifics succeed because they are less likely to have their heads bashed in, increasingly so the larger the horn size.

Since this research suggests that horn displays are just surrogate fights, we might quite reasonably identify the target and agent of selection in this case the same way we did for horns that served as weapons: the target is horn size and the agent is displacement of rivals. That might work for some purposes, but does not work for ours, because the horns achieve their effect not through the direct action of their size on the receiver, as they would if one ram hit another, but through the receiver's perception of horn size. Thus the target of selection is whatever features receivers respond to in this situation that serve as an indicator of horn size. Similarly, the agent of selection is not displacement directly, because the ram has not physically pushed the other aside. Instead, the horn's effect is mediated through some decision process, whether simple as a reflex or complex as contemplation. In the black box that is the psychology of the receiver, a decision process has been selected for through generations of rams avoiding situations in which there is a high probability of getting bashed on the head. The agent of selection is not actually displacing (for senders) or being displaced (for receivers), but the increased likelihood of getting bashed that comes with being around rams with big horns.

That is all a long-winded answer to what these large horns are for, so how should we behavioural ecologists describe, in a nutshell, what these horns are for? If we said they are used to coax receivers into avoidance (Rendall *et al.*, 2009), that would be safely true, but it would not capture the evolutionary rationale for their design, because it would miss the key reason why they are effective, the agent of selection on horns: that they correlate with the brawn of the signalling ram. Thus it is far better for our purposes, and far clearer, to say that rams display their horns to advertise horn size, and other rams get information about their chances in a fight from the horn display. This approach also makes more sense of the rams' responses to the display, which are not just direct consequences of seeing the display, but depend on context, such as their internal states and the presence of onlookers.

Note that when we say "other rams get information about their chances in a fight", we are not attributing information processing to the animals themselves. The approach does depend on the fact that both the signalling and the response are conditional on many factors, even in the simplest forms of signalling, so it entails the weighing of information of the sort a neuroendocrinologist might call perceptual or physiological information, a cognitive ethologist might call conceptual information, and so on. This is not how we as behavioural ecologists are invoking information here, however. Instead, for us, the information is the functional foundation of the signalling interaction, our interpretation of the interaction in a way that makes evolutionary sense, in that it makes explicit the adaptive value of the sender's signalling and the receiver's responding. In the proximate timeframe of any given signalling interaction, the give and take of signals can be carried on without the intercession of this kind of information at all, a mere tossing back and forth of stimuli that is somewhere between saying and doing (Brandom, 2008); far less than a conversation but far more than just leaving tracks in the snow.

Having said that, many organisms are indeed able to process signals more abstractly, whether by simply having probabilistic responses that weigh stimulation from a variety of stimuli before selecting a response, like tyrant flycatchers (Tyrannidae) (Smith, 1986), by having such abilities as judgements about intentions that rely upon a theory of mind, like monkeys (Cheney & Seyfarth, 1990), or by accessing information still more directly through the giving and asking for reasons (Brandom, 1997), like us. But in all these cases, the 'hard facts' that signals 'stand for', though real, are absent from the interactions themselves.

1.4 Information transfer, gathering and flow in communication networks

We can now return to the problems with the informational approach to animal communication as seen in the conduit metaphor, and see how very different they look when signalling is viewed within the natural context of a communication network. Again, the three criticisms are:

(1) Senders do not actively encode information;
(2) Receivers do not actively decode information;
(3) There is no such thing as information flow.

Our responses to each point stem from the view of information exchange that we outlined above:

(1) Encoding is the adaptive presentation of stimuli by senders;
(2) Decoding is the adaptive parsing and weighting of that evidence by receivers;
(3) The adaptive upshot of (1) and (2) is that information flows through a community of signallers.

1.4.1 *Encoding as adaptive information transfer*

According to some critics of the informational approach to animal communication, senders do not actively encode information. Receivers respond only to behaviours by senders when it is useful for receivers to do so, and this is what selects for those sender behaviours to be shaped into signals. Beyond that, senders play no active role in communication. If this is true, then signals have a meaning for receivers in the same way as clouds naturally mean rain, but no 'non-natural' meaning, in the way that words and other truly communicative signals have. Receiver meaning alone drives signalling. Even if animal communication involves meanings in the way any stimulus–response behaviours do, it certainly does not involve messages (Font & Carazo, 2010).

We see many good reasons to contest this view, some of which are nicely laid out by Seyfarth *et al.* (2010). Here, however, we will restrict ourselves to showing how this criticism breaks down as soon as one considers communication as occurring within a network of senders and receivers. Specifically, doing so challenges the crux of the above argument, which is that senders do not adaptively select among alternative signals when signalling. On the contrary, when signallers are faced with multiple receivers, as senders are in a network, there is a selective advantage to directing signals at particular receivers and withholding them from others. Indeed, there is good evidence that senders do both, in the form of selective addressing and audience effects (for withholding information, see for example Dabelsteen *et al.*, 1998; Grinnell & McComb, 2001).

Selective addressing occurs when senders direct signals at particular receivers. This can be done in many ways, most simply by signalling only in the presence of particular receivers. The most interesting cases, however, occur when senders are signalling in the presence of multiple signallers, but the way that they signal or the types of signals they deliver selectively addresses their signals to particular individuals in the network. Songbirds show the clearest examples of selective addressing, directing their songs to particular signallers by physically facing them, timing or changing their signals in near-synchrony with the bird that is addressed, or, most strikingly, by matching the song that the other individual is singing or at least is able to sing and thus can recognise (e.g. Todt & Naguib, 2000; Brumm & Todt, 2003), a strategy that bottlenose dolphins, *Tursiops truncatus*, use to hail individuals up to half a kilometre away (Janik, 2000).

Audience effects are a second phenomenon that communication networks make possible, and that shows that senders actively signal, in this case by signalling differently depending on what particular individuals are present. They thus adaptively adjust their influence over particular receivers. Audience effects have now been shown in a broad range of species, from fish to primates (Matos & Schlupp, 2005). A simple example comes from fighting fish, *Betta splendens*, in which two males will display at each other more vigorously, as measured by the duration of particularly energetic displays, when there is a third male in a neighbouring tank than when there is a female, and more vigorously when there is a female than when there is a heterospecific or an empty tank (Matos & Schlupp, 2005).

Since animals are nothing more or less than their physiology, one could of course explain selective addressing and audience effects from a causal, physiological point of view, or in terms of manipulation or influence. For example, in the case of fighting fish, seeing a male beforehand primes males for more vigorous combat, probably via an increase in androgen levels (Matos & Schlupp, 2005). Nonetheless, at a functional level this hormonal mechanism is a way for senders to choose, physiologically if not intentionally, which signals are appropriate for any given situation.

On this account, the encoding step in animal communication need not involve anything more complex than the sender singling out a particular receiver(s) in an adaptive way, and filling part of that receiver's perceptual field in an adaptive way. Such a view of encoding need not involve intentionality or similar mental operations (although it can), concepts that one is more tempted to resort to when senders are imagined to be in a dyadic relation with one receiver, rather than embedded in a network amid multiple receivers where they naturally occur. Of course, for this directed tossing out of signals to be effective, there must be uptake on the part of the receiver, which is the topic of subsection 1.4.2 below.

1.4.2 *Decoding as adaptive information gathering*

In the dyadic view of animal communication, it is easy to view the receiver as a passive dupe to the behaviours of the signaller. By setting the receiver inescapably opposite one sender at the other end of the conduit, the dyadic view presents the receiver as an audience captive to the sender's manipulation, influence or management. In most signalling situations, however, receivers have access to not just one but multiple signallers (as well as to non-signalling conspecifics). Thus receivers have a choice of which signallers to attend to and which to ignore. While on the one hand they must work at extracting useful signals from the cacophony before them, on the other hand they have the opportunity to tap into information made available by multiple signalling interactions.

There is a huge body of evidence showing how receivers actively parse useful signals from irrelevant input, i.e. 'noise' (see Wiley, Ch. 4 of this volume). However, as Seyfarth *et al.* (2010) note, it is the phenomenon of social eavesdropping that delivers perhaps the most damaging salvo against a naïve influence approach to animal communication. Social eavesdropping occurs when receivers base their responses not on the signal of a particular sender, as in the dyadic model of communication, but rather on the structure of signalling interactions between other senders and receivers (Peake, 2005). Note the specific usage of the term here. 'Eavesdropping' has also been used to describe the overhearing of signals by 'unintended' recipients, particularly by predators or parasites. Apart from the nature of the relationship between sender and receiver, however, this kind of 'eavesdropping' is no different, in principle, from dyadic signalling. It is the fact that social eavesdropping is based on signalling interactions, rather than signals themselves, that makes them reliant on the network situation, and makes them so interesting and compelling for an information view of communication (Peake, 2005).

Social eavesdropping has now been demonstrated in a broad array of organisms (Peake, 2005; Bonnie & Earley, 2007); we will illustrate it using an example from playback experiments on great tits, *Parus major*, which suggest that females eavesdrop on song interactions between males to decide which males to mate with. Male great tits defend territories with short, repeated songs, and females, while mainly staying on a particular male's territory (their social mate), do often enter neighbouring territories to solicit extra-pair matings. Studies of song interactions show that males lengthen their songs and overlap their songs when they are likely to escalate a singing interaction, whereas they shorten and alternate their songs when they are likely to de-escalate (Dabelsteen *et al.*, 1996). In effect, the two patterns show whether a male is 'winning' or 'losing' an interaction. On average, after playbacks of a recording in which a female's social mate 'loses' an interaction, and his neighbour 'wins' one (against the same simulated opponent), a female is more likely to venture into that neighbour's territory than when her social mate is a winner (Otter *et al.*, 1999). Similar experiments on black-capped chickadees show that females do indeed obtain extra-pair copulations on these sorties (Mennill, Ratcliffe & Boag, 2002).

Such social eavesdropping is not just a response to signals, but a response to an exchange of signals. This added layer of complexity to eavesdropping in a network, compared with signal reception in a dyadic interaction, makes an informational approach still more preferable to an influence approach. While, in a dyadic interaction, it is easy to imagine that a great tit male's song woos females towards or repulses them from his territory, in social eavesdropping it is much more awkward to construe females as being blindly manipulated by a complex pattern of signal exchange. Indeed, rather than seeing them as responding directly to the signalling interaction, it seems far more parsimonious to see them as responding to the upshot of the interaction. Whether a male is a winner or loser, not whether it sings leading or following songs, is the agent of selection in this case, an agent whose target is the ability to integrate what is more easily referred to as information from several sources – including not just the signalling interaction, but also its context, past territorial encounters and so on – so that a receiver can select an appropriate response.

Thus we can see that, when they are viewed in a communication network, receivers actively parse and selectively respond to signals, in ways that are adaptive because of what those signals, on average, correlate with. That is all we mean when we say that receivers attend to and interpret the messages of signals, to decode their meaning. Decoding is indeed a form of inference (Sperber & Wilson, 1995), but a brute form that, like encoding, need not involve complex mental constructs, such as intentions or perceptions of intentions, nor indeed any sort of match between the state of the receiver and that of the sender (whose roles are probably overstated for humans, too; e.g. Arundale, 2008). The fact that receivers are embedded in a context of multiple inputs highlights this interpretive labour – inference, decoding, call it what you will – that is required even for very simple animal communication.

1.4.3 *The adaptive upshot of signalling is information flow*

Perhaps the most damning criticism of the informational approach to communication is that, at least when communication is seen as a dyad, as in the conduit metaphor, it implies that information flows from sender to receiver like water down a pipe. With multiple senders and receivers within signalling range, however, signal transactions can pass through many links in many directions, throughout the network. Trying to capture these connections in terms such as influence and manipulation is ponderous; they are much more easily and accurately captured in terms of information flow.

Consider a wide expanse of prairie inhabited by western meadowlarks, *Sturnella neglecta*, on regularly spaced, large territories. A northern harrier, *Circus cyaneus*, flies near one male at his songpost, who gives the whistled hawk alarm call, which is taken up by the neighbouring male, who does not perceive the hawk, but only the call, and whose call in turn stimulates calling by the next male, and so on across several territories. One way to describe this situation is to say that the hawk stimulates a whistle, which stimulates a chain of whistles across neighbouring territories. But the functional import of the situation is so much clearer if we instead say that information about the hawk's arrival was passed along across several territories. Doing so not only simplifies things from the point of view of description, but also better captures the functional significance of this signalling among territory holders – that a direct perception of the hawk triggers a domino effect in which the hawk's direction and speed is indirectly conveyed via the pattern of signals spreading through the neighbourhood (McGregor & Dabelsteen, 1996).

Studies of aerial alarm calling in communities of Australian woodland birds are an illustration of the success of an informational, rather than an influence, approach. The calls that passerine birds give when they see a hawk, aerial alarm calls, were initially considered to be very similar across species: thin, high-pitched calls with a steady pitch and gradual start and finish (Marler, 1955). As is well known among naturalists, but only recently tested experimentally (Magrath, Pitcher & Gardner, 2007), birds will often head for cover when they hear another species' aerial alarm call. Originally interpreted as a consequence of the universally adaptive acoustics of the calls – readily recognised but hard for predators to localise – this would seem to make the calls fit perfectly into a view of communication that favours "concrete explanations grounded in the influence that specific acoustic properties of the calls have on broadly conserved neural, sensory, affective and learning systems in listeners" (Rendall *et al.*, 2009).

Observations of responses to predators and playback experiments of alarm calls show, however, that different species do not respond to each other's calls universally, but asymmetrically, depending on how reliable particular signalling species are for particular receiving species. Among three species studied, New Holland honeyeaters, *Phylidonyris novaehollandiae*, only called when predators were present, and all species fled for cover in response to their calls. The honeyeaters themselves, however, only fled in response to white-browed scrubwren, *Sericornis frontalis*, calls, which reliably indicated a predator 82% of the time, but not to superb fairy-wrens, *Malurus splendens*, which were reliable only 48% of the time. In contrast, scrubwrens fled in response to fairy-wren calls, but that is most likely because the calls that fairy-wrens did give to non-predators were to red wattlebirds, *Anthochaera carunculata*, a species strongly aggressive to scrubwrens (fairy-wrens responded to all calls; Magrath, Pitcher & Gardner, 2009).

Furthermore, this study system also provides evidence that response to aerial alarm calls has a learned component in fairy-wrens. Fallow, Gardner and McGrath (2011) show that fairy-wrens only respond to aerial alarm calls of species with which they are unfamiliar if the calls of these rarely encountered species are very similar in acoustic structure to their own fairy-wren calls. Also, fairy-wrens ignore aerial alarm calls from noisy miners, *Manorina melanocephala*, unless miners are common in their area (Magrath & Bennett, 2012).

What this example shows is that the functionally relevant behavioural relationships among these three species and the role of learning are better described by the information they correlate with, and its reliability, than by physical influence through signal–response chains. Moreover, conceiving of communication in this way (i.e. as information flowing through a community just as energy flows through the trophic structure of an ecological community) yields a more richly informative conception of behavioural dependencies among different species, identifying, for example, which species are reliable 'keystone' species that may be particularly important targets for conservation efforts (Goodale *et al.*, 2010). The flow of information through such communities, or indeed any communication network, can be mapped in ways that give insight into social structure not accessible through broadcast of signals per se (Matessi, Matos & Dabelsteen, 2008), especially given that individual receivers may not elect, or may not be able, to respond to signals that, physically, are broadcast widely across many nodes in the network.

This higher-level concept of information flow is accessible, and valuable, for communication networks in a way that is inconceivable for single sender–receiver dyads. Indeed, there is emerging evidence that animals themselves are attuned to this higher order of signal exchange; Richardson's ground squirrels, *Spermophilus richardsonii*, for example, can track the direction of movement of a predator through a communication network through the 'wave' of calls travelling across widely spaced callers (Thompson & Hare, 2010; see also

Dabelsteen & McGregor, 1996). Again, one could argue that this is a case of signal flow, not information flow, although the timing and location of the signals would have to be included in the account. But even then, it seems hard to imagine that the agent of selection in this case is some aspect of the signal per se, rather than the elevated risk of being eaten if a receiving squirrel does not heed the pattern of signalling.

1.4.4 *Summary*

When animal communication is viewed in its commonest and most likely evolutionary context, i.e. as a communication network, animals can be seen to be actively singling out receivers to show them particular perceptual stimuli (encoding), actively parsing out and seeking perceptual input that enables them to select adaptive responses (decoding), and, as these two processes spread through a net of interactants, creating a higher order of social structure that is succinctly captured by the concept of information flow through the communication network. Considering animal communication as whispers conveyed between two cans through a string misses the ubiquitous network aspect of communication and with it the integration of social and non-signal sources of information that more accurately reflect the spectrum of information available to animals.

1.5 Conclusion

We have argued that viewing communication in the wider context of its natural occurrence and evolutionary history – a communication network – operationalises concepts of information transfer, gathering and flow. Whether the informational approach really is supported by this broader perspective can be evaluated in two ways. First, does the information approach reflect what is really going on when animals communicate within a communication network? Second, is the information approach useful?

Does the approach accurately reflect what is really going on?

We believe that the approach does reflect reality. Animals respond adaptively to the world around them, and to do so they should base their responses on what is happening – if food is nearby, if a predator is approaching and so on. To do so, they must necessarily rely on information identifying things of functional relevance, and one such set are the signals sent by other animals. Similarly, if animals are to affect each other's behaviour, it makes sense for them to provide information on which those other animals can base their responses. There may be a mismatch between the two sorts of information and the correspondence to functional relevance – i.e. the information they convey – but that just makes the situation more interesting.

Is the approach useful for empirical studies?

Our experience is that the information view has utility. As explained above, animals must assess (albeit indirectly) reality in order to behave adaptively. This does not require that some vitalistic entity is passed from the world or from senders to them, nor do they need to have images or any mental constructs in their heads (although it may be easier if they have). But the concept of information does allow us to discuss communication in a network in a fruitful way and to postulate the existence of effects such as eavesdropping and audiences that can be, and have been, experimentally verified.

An appeal for signals to be studied in the wider context in which they occur is not a new idea. In ethology, the main theme of Smith's (1977) magnum opus, *The Behavior of Communicating*, was not his oft-cited (oft-undeservedly) informational approach to communication, but rather the overriding importance of context in interpreting the meaning of animal signals, for which his book still repays close study. In sociology, Goffman (1959), too, emphasised how social settings framed human interactions in ways that had to be understood for interpreting signals. In psychology, relevance theory (Sperber & Wilson, 1995), and in philosophy, pragmatics (Bernstein, 2010) have situated the meaning of speech in everyday interactions rather than inside people's heads. Nonetheless, in the intervening four decades, studies of animal communication are still catching up to this broader perspective, a situation that, we believe, has left disputes over various aspects of animal communication, most recently information, smouldering ever since. It's time to catch up.

References

Arundale, R. B. (2008). Against (Gricean) intentions at the heart of human interaction. *Intercultural Pragmatics*, **5**, 229–258.

Bernstein, R. J. (2010). *The Pragmatic Turn*. Cambridge: Polity Press.

Bonnie, K. E. & Earley, R. L. (2007). Expanding the scope for social information use. *Animal Behaviour*, **74**, 171–181.

Brandom, R. B. (1997). *Making It Explicit*. Cambridge, MA: Harvard University Press.

Brandom, R. B. (2008). *Between Saying and Doing: Towards an Analytical Pragmatism*. Oxford: Oxford University Press.

Brumm, H. & Todt, D. (2003). Facing the rival: directional singing behaviour in nightingales. *Behaviour*, **140**, 43–53.

Cheney, D. L. & Seyfarth, R. M. (1990). *How Monkeys See the World*. Chicago, IL: University of Chicago Press.

Dabelsteen, T., McGregor, P. K., Lampe, H. M., Langmore, N. E. & Holland, J. (1998). Quiet song in song birds: an overlooked phenomenon. *Bioacoustics*, **9**, 89–106.

Dabelsteen, T., McGregor, P. K., Shepherd, M., Whittaker, X. & Pedersen, S. B. (1996). Is the signal value of overlapping different from that of alternating during matched singing in great tits? *Journal of Avian Biology*, **27**, 189–194.

Endler, J. A. (1986). *Natural Selection in the Wild*. Princeton: Princeton University Press.

Fallow, P. M., Gardner, J. L. & Magrath, R. M. (2011). Sound familiar? Acoustic similarity provokes responses to unfamiliar heterospecific alarm calls. *Behavioural Ecology*, **22**, 401–410.

Font, E. & Carazo, P. (2010). Animals in translation: why there is meaning (but probably no message) in animal communication. *Animal Behaviour*, **2010**, e1–e6.

Foote, J. R., Fitzsimmons, L. P., Mennill, D. J. & Ratcliffe, L. M. (2010). Black-capped chickadee dawn choruses are interactive communication networks. *Behaviour*, **147**, 1219–1248.

Goffman, E. (1959). *The Presentation of Self in Everyday Life*. New York: Doubleday Anchor.

Goodale, E., Beauchamp, G., Magrath, R. D., Nieh, J. C. & Ruxton, G. D. (2010). Interspecific information transfer influences animal community structure. *Trends in Ecology and Evolution*, **25**, 354–361.

Grinnell, J. & McComb, K. (2001). Roaring and social communication in African lions: the limitations imposed by listeners. *Animal Behaviour*, **62**, 93–98.

Horn, A. G. (1997). Speech acts and animal signals. In D. W. Owings, M. D. Beecher & N. Thompson, eds., *Communication. Perspectives in Ethology*, Vol. 12. New York: Plenum Press, pp. 347–358.

Janik, V. M. (2000). Whistle matching in wild bottlenose dolphins (*Tursiops truncatus*). *Science*, **289**, 1355–1357.

Magrath, R. D. & Bennett, T. H. (2012). A micro-geography of fear: learning to eavesdrop on alarm calls of neighbouring heterospecifics. *Proceedings of the Royal Society of London Series B*, **279**, 902–909.

Magrath, R. D., Pitcher, B. J. & Gardner, J. L. (2007). A mutual understanding? Interspecific responses by birds to each other's aerial alarm calls. *Behavioural Ecology*, **18**, 944–951.

Magrath, R. D., Pitcher, B. J. & Gardner, J. L. (2009). An avian eavesdropping network: alarm signal reliability and heterospecific response. *Behavioural Ecology*, **20**, 745–752.

Marler, P. (1955). Characteristics of some animal calls. *Nature*, **176**, 6–8.

Matessi, G., Matos, R. J. & Dabelsteen, T. (2008). Communication in social networks of territorial animals: networking at different levels in birds and other systems. In P. d'Ettorre & D. P. Hughes, eds., *Sociobiology of Communication: An Interdisciplinary Perspective*. Oxford: Oxford University Press, pp. 33–53.

Matos, R. J. & Schlupp, I. (2005). Performing in front of an audience: signalers and the social environment. In P. K. McGregor, ed., *Animal Communication Networks*. Cambridge: Cambridge University Press, pp. 63–83.

McGregor, P. K. (ed.) (2005). *Animal Communication Networks*. Cambridge: Cambridge University Press.

McGregor, P. K. & Dabelsteen, T. (1996). Communication networks. In D. E. Kroodsma & E. H. Miller, eds., *Ecology and Evolution of Acoustic Communication in Birds*. Ithaca, NY: Cornell University Press, pp. 409–425.

Mennill, D. J., Ratcliffe, L. M. & Boag, P. T. (2002). Female eavesdropping on male song contests in songbirds. *Science*, **296**, 873.

Otter, K., McGregor, P. K., Terry, A. M. R. *et al.* (1999). Do female great tits (*Parus major*) assess males by eavesdropping? A field study using interactive song playback. *Proceedings of the Royal Society of London Series B*, **266**, 1305–1309.

Peake, T. M. (2005). Eavesdropping in communication networks. In P. K. McGregor, ed., *Animal Communication Networks*. Cambridge: Cambridge University Press, pp. 13–37.

Reddy, M. J. (1979). The conduit metaphor: a case of frame conflict in our language about language. In A. Ortony, ed., *Metaphor and Thought*. Cambridge: Cambridge University Press, pp. 284–324.

Rendall, D., Owren, M. J. & Ryan, M. J. (2009). What do animal signals mean? *Animal Behaviour*, **78**, 233–240.

Scott-Phillips, T. C. (2010). Animal communication: insights from linguistic pragmatics. *Animal Behaviour*, **79**, e1–e4.

Seyfarth, R. M., Cheney, D. L., Bergman, T. *et al.* (2010). The central importance of information in studies of animal communication. *Animal Behaviour*, **80**, 3–8.

Smith, W. J. (1977). *The Behavior of Communicating*. Cambridge, MA: Harvard University Press.

Smith, W. J. (1986). Signaling behavior: contributions of different repertoires. In R. J. Schusterman, J. A. Thomas & F. G. Wood, eds., *Dolphin Cognition and Behavior: A Comparative Approach*. Hillsdale, NJ: Erlbaum, pp. 315–330.

Sperber, D. & Wilson, D. (1995). *Relevance: Communication and Cognition*, 2nd edn. Oxford: Blackwell.

Thompson, A. B. & Hare, J. F. (2010). Neighbourhood watch: multiple alarm callers communicate directional predator movement in Richardson's ground squirrels, *Spermophilus richardsonii*. *Animal Behaviour*, **80**, 269–275.

Todt, D. & Naguib, M. (2000). Vocal interactions in birds: the use of song as a model in communication. *Advances in the Study of Behavior*, **29**, 247–296.

Wiley, R. H. (1983). The evolution of communication: information and manipulation. In T. R. Halliday & P. J. B. Slater, eds., *Communication. Animal Behaviour*, Vol. 2. Oxford: Blackwell, pp. 156–189.

Wisenden, B. D. & Stacey, N. E. (2005). Fish semiochemicals and the evolution of communication networks. In P. K. McGregor, ed., *Animal Communication Networks*. Cambridge: Cambridge University Press, pp. 540–567.

Commentaries

We applaud the pioneering efforts of Horn and McGregor to highlight important aspects of non-dyadic communication. But do such higher-level interactions necessitate incorporating transmitted information, as we describe this in our chapter? Is it not the perceiver that drives the evolution of communication? Yes, there are complex interactions with social eavesdropping but this does not change the idea that information emerges from the perception of others, not from something transmitted. We would like to see these authors try to formulate their discussion from the standpoint of perceiver control, which they seem to agree is important. We do not see the need to use the information metaphor even though they describe its use as "more accurate, less vague and more useful". The functional foundation of a signalling interaction is the signal's structure and assessment without the need to invoke information as its foundation.

Eugene S. Morton and Richard G. Coss

Say what you mean, mean what you say. Horn and McGregor focus in part on the critical question of whether *information* should remain a central idea in animal communication. Like Adams and Beighley, however, their understanding of this construct is quite flexible. Sometimes information is a physical entity, other times it is psychological. Information may also be a pure abstraction – "the functional foundation of the signalling interaction". We have to question the value of any construct that is so pliable and underspecified. Normative scientific explanation is grounded in the material, not in ephemeral constructs that can take whatever form or meaning is convenient in the moment. Horn and McGregor suggest the allied concepts of information *encoding* and *decoding* are also best understood in an abstract, functional way, where encoding simply refers only to signallers selecting among multiple possible signals, and decoding conversely being perceivers selecting among multiple possible responses. We agree that animals can show active selection of signals and responses. However, both encoding and decoding are centred on the notion of *coding* – meaning converting a signal from one form to an alternative, but corresponding form. Coding thus requires symbolic representation – there is, to our knowledge, no sense in which a code can be non-symbolic. Coding is thus a heavily freighted term, and using it requires specific explanation of its rich connotations. If the authors are not endorsing these connotations, retaining coding-based terminology is inevitably confusing and counterproductive.

Michael J. Owren and Drew Rendall

Response

Morton and Coss are after similar form/function answers as we are; our disagreement is mainly over terminology. To us, information is the elephant in the room when one tries to talk only of management and assessment. If the abstract, metaphorical aspects of information talk can be paid out by the kinds of explications that we advanced in our chapter, and that the philosophers in this volume have done much more skilfully, then perhaps our contrasting views can be bridged.

One remaining substantive difference, however, is their overemphasis on the perceiver side. True, if signals are stimuli, they are nothing without the perceiver. But isn't it interesting that there are some signals where senders give receivers what they want, and others where receivers are being duped by their own perceptual rules? Talk of information allows us to distinguish the cases where they coincide from cases where they don't, in terms that express what each party gains or loses. Indeed, we cannot conceive of how one could formulate a discussion of any signalling interaction solely "from the standpoint of perceiver control"; sender control (or lack thereof) is equally important, as is most dramatically obvious in a network of multiple signallers.

This brings us to what, if anything, it is about networks per se that makes an informational approach particularly important. This is a work in progress, but here are two points that we can make in these early stages. The first is logistical. Trying to avoid such talk seems to us a form of overzealous verbal purity that quickly gets unwieldy (strongly reminiscent of the 'Voldemort' versus 'He Who Must Not Be Named' stricture in the *Harry Potter* novels), as can be readily appreciated from our alarm signalling example. The second point is empirical. Higher order signalling lifts communication out of the sender–receiver dyad, where information exchange is confounded with stimulus–response. Networks make it all the more obvious that what is functionally relevant – what senders are selected to show or hide, and what receivers are selected to extract – is not the signal per se, but what that signalling exchange 'says' about the interactants and their circumstances.

Owren and Rendall: No one could disagree with the dictum "Say what you mean, mean what you say". The trouble is, certainty is not a feature of science. None of us always knows exactly what we mean, or how to say it; we discover it through argument and, ultimately, through that unyielding test that makes all of our talk "grounded in the material": the test of experience.

That is the pragmatist's view of both communication and science, a view that we endorsed in our chapter and that we thought Owren and Rendall endorsed in theirs. Information and meaning is not about images encoded in the head, but is about selecting and rejecting practical consequences. Science works the same way. So we are surprised to read in their commentary:

> Normative scientific explanation is grounded in the material, not in ephemeral constructs that can take whatever form or meaning is convenient in the moment.

On the face of it, again, who could disagree? Scientific constructs should not be vague or wishy-washy, nor held so briefly as to be "ephemeral". But they are constructs all the same. True, they are grounded in the material, because our use of them commits us to certain stances about the world, but those stances are only tested against hard facts through a cycle of hypothesis, test and readjustment. Thus a certain amount of pliability and sensitivity to what works at our current state of knowledge (close to what "is convenient in the moment") is not only inevitable, but essential, for science to evolve.

As with science, so too with animal signals. A rooster's crow is his commitment – to his fighting ability and his health. Just as a scientist's use of the word 'information' is tested through observation and experiment, so too the rooster's commitment, signalled by his crow, is tested by combat and disease. Other roosters accept that commitment just as if they had been physically struck, but they only do so because the commitment is underwritten by a history of selection – "grounded in the material", as Owren and Rendall might put it.

Sorting out what we mean by 'information', 'encoding' and even 'function', for that matter, is admittedly a messy business. Animals are not perfectly adapted, so the information they perceive is less than ideal, not least because of phylogenetic constraints and trade-offs. But if a stickleback responds so fiercely to the red of rivals that it will attack the reflection of a passing post van, that need not prevent us from saying that the red carries information, perhaps about readiness to attack. Sure, it is messy, but what is good enough, in evolutionary terms, for the stickleback should be good enough, in interpretive terms, for us.

In the end, these are arguments over words. They should not be dismissed as 'mere' semantic arguments, though, because testing semantic arguments against material experience is what science is all about. In the end, our explanations should indeed be "grounded in the material". Contra Owren and Rendall's stance that everyone is dodging this responsibility, the animal communication literature is in fact very much engaged in giving our emerging groping terminology real bite (as elegantly summarised by Bradbury and Vehrencamp, 2011).

Again, since we agree so whole heartedly with so much of Owren and Rendall's approach, especially their emphasis on context, we will agree to disagree on their terminological recommendations, and test our own ways of saying the same things against a research approach that is really not all that far from the very one they advocate.

Bradbury, J. W. & Vehrencamp, S. L. (2011). *Web Topic 1.2: Information and Communication. Principles of Animal Communication*, 2nd edn companion website. http://sites.sinauer.com/animalcommunication2e (Accessed 18 March 2012).

Andrew G. Horn and Peter K. McGregor

2

Animal communication as information-mediated influence

ANDREA SCARANTINO[1]

2.1 Introduction

Two main approaches to the definition of animal communication or signalling are generally contrasted. One is the *information-based* approach championed by theorists who think that communication should be defined in terms of information transfer between signaller and recipient. Proponents of this approach include Otte (1974), Zahavi (1987), Bradbury and Vehrencamp (1998), Hauser (1996), Seyfarth, Cheney and Marler (1980) and others. The other is the *influence-based* approach championed by theorists who think that communication should be defined in terms of influence on a recipient by a signaller. Proponents of this approach include Dawkins and Krebs (1978), Owings and Morton (1998), Maynard-Smith and Harper (2003), Owren, Randall and Ryan (2010) and others.

In this chapter I argue that animal communication should be defined neither exclusively in terms of information nor exclusively in terms of influence. Defining communication exclusively in terms of information wrongly suggests that what drives the selection of signals is the information that signals carry, rather than the fitness benefits that signals earn for their producers. Defining communication exclusively in terms of influence, on the other hand, amounts to leaving in the background precisely what must be emphasised, namely that what distinguishes communication from other forms of influence is that signals earn benefits to their producers by carrying information to signal recipients. The take-home message of this chapter is that influence-based and information-based

[1] I want to thank Eddy Nahmias, Ulrich Stegmann and especially an anonymous referee for their helpful comments on a previous draft.

Animal Communication Theory: Information and Influence, ed. Ulrich Stegmann. Published by Cambridge University Press.

definitions of communication should not be contrasted but rather combined into a theoretically richer hybrid.

2.2 Communication as information transfer

Theorists of animal communication tend to agree on what count as paradigm cases of animal signals: alarm calls, food calls, begging calls, mating calls, threat displays, dominance displays, status badges, facial, vocal and postural expressions and so on. What is still fiercely debated is how animal communication as a whole should be defined. According to a still dominant but increasingly besieged view, animal communication should be defined in terms of information transfer.

In a popular textbook, Bradbury and Vehrencamp (1998, p. 2) argue that "[n]early all authors agree that communication involves the provision of information by a sender to a receiver". They add that the "vehicle that provides the information is called the signal" (p. 2). Hauser (1996, p. 6) similarly states that "[t]he concepts of information and signal form integral components of most definitions of communication". But what is information?

No single answer to this question can be provided. As I have argued elsewhere (Scarantino & Piccinini, 2010; Piccinini & Scarantino, 2011), information is a mongrel concept comprising a variety of different phenomena under the same heading. This being said, one species of the genus strikes me as capturing a large portion of information talk in the animal communication literature. This is the species of what I call *predictive information*. Roughly speaking, a bearer of predictive information (henceforth, information *simpliciter*) is something that can be used by someone to predict something else.[2] Since organisms live in an uncertain world, what bearers of information generally do is to change the probabilities of various states of affairs.

Thus, a signal carries information about every state of affairs the probability (*P*) of which it changes. Formally, *X* carries information about *Y* if and only if $P(Y \text{ given } X) \neq P(Y)$.[3] This notion of information can be quantified by taking a

[2] A second notion of information often conflated with predictive information is that of referential information or representation (I designated it as non-natural information in previous publications, and contrasted it with natural or predictive information; cf. Scarantino & Piccinini, 2010). Roughly speaking, a bearer of referential information is something that is taken by someone to stand for something else. I will not further discuss the notion of referential information in what follows.

[3] I discuss this notion in more detail in Scarantino and Piccinini (2010). Similar theories of information are articulated, in somewhat different terms, by Millikan (2000, 2004), Shea (2007), Skyrms (2010) and several other authors.

suitable function of $P(Y \text{ given } X)$ and $P(Y)$.[4] A common, but by no means unique, measure of the information carried by X about Y is the so-called *difference measure*: $d = P(Y \text{ given } X) - P(Y)$. The higher the difference, the more information X carries about Y.[5]

An example may help. Consider a female bird who must decide which male bird to mate with. Suppose that before receiving a mating call the prior probability that a male is healthy is $p(\text{male is healthy}) = 0.5$. If call M increases or decreases such probability, M carries information about health. Assume that the posterior probability is $p(\text{male is healthy given call M}) = 0.9$. In such a case, M would significantly reduce uncertainty about the male's health, shifting it from 0.5 (equal odds that the male is healthy or unhealthy) to 0.9 (high likelihood that the male is healthy). This in turn would allow the female to reliably predict that the courting male is healthy.[6]

The ability to transfer information is considered by many animal communication theorists to be a necessary property of signals, but not a sufficient one. An additional requirement is that a signal must be *shaped by natural selection*. This

[4] As I explain in my answers to commentators, the probabilities involved in information transmission are assigned relative to background knowledge. Such background knowledge determines which possibilities exist at the source, but it is often left implicit in ordinary information talk.

[5] A complicated question I cannot fully address in this chapter is how probabilities should be interpreted in the context of informational ascriptions. The short answer is that they should be interpreted in an objectivist fashion, roughly along the lines of what Carnap (1950) labelled *inductive probability*. This is the sort of probability ascribed to a state of affairs given another state of affairs taken as evidence, and a set of further states of affairs taken as background. For informational purposes, the background is the *knowledge state* of the signal recipient, the evidence is the *signal* and the state of affairs whose probability is being investigated is *what the information is about*. Subjective probabilities and inductive probabilities are normatively related, in the sense that the inductive probability of a state of affairs given a certain evidence and background knowledge is the degree of belief that is epistemically rational to have for someone with that evidence and background knowledge.

[6] The predictive information about health clearly does not exhaust the informational content of the mating call. For example, the mating call will also raise the probability that the male is ready for sexual intercourse, that the male is not being chased by a predator, that the male is awake, that the female is at a less-than-five-mile distance from the caller and so on. For this reason, we should think of the informational content of a signal as a *vector* which specifies how the signal changes the probabilities of various states of affairs (cf. Skyrms, 2010). Most entries of the vector will not matter to the signal recipient, either because the probabilities have not been changed to a sufficient degree to make a reliable prediction, or because the states of affairs whose probability has changed to a sufficient degree are irrelevant to the recipient's decision. Some entries, on the other hand, will matter a great deal, because they represent an ecologically significant change in the probability of a state of affairs that affects the recipient's evolutionary interests.

grounds the common distinction between *signals* and *cues*. Information bearers that carry information, but did not evolve for that reason, are considered *cues* rather than *signals* (Hasson, 1994).[7]

The following definition embodies as well as any the dominant, information-based view on animal signalling:

> [Animal signals are] behavioural, physiological, or morphological characteristics fashioned or maintained by natural selection because they convey information to other organisms. (Otte, 1974, p. 385)

A key feature of this definition is that conveying information is presented as the reason why signals are fashioned or maintained by natural selection. As Zahavi (1987) makes explicit, "a signal is defined as a character which has evolved *in order* to transmit information to other individuals" (1987, p. 306; emphasis added). On this view, the evolutionary point of signalling is to transfer information.

2.3 Communication as influence

In an influential paper, Dawkins and Krebs (1978) rejected the assumption that the evolutionary point of signalling is to transfer information – an assumption they associated with the "classical ethological view" of animal communication. This assumption presupposes that signaller and recipient are engaged in a *cooperative* interaction, whereas many cases of signalling occur in *competitive* interactions. In competitive interactions, transferring information about features such as, say, one's low reproductive quality may put the signaller at a disadvantage, so it cannot be assumed that signals evolved in order to transfer such information.

Consider an unhealthy male bird that is trying to reproduce. It is not in his interest to signal that he is unhealthy, since females tend to prefer mating with healthy males. Consequently, if the type of mating call he produces is selected for, it will not be *in order* to make information about his actual reproductive quality available, but rather because it leads females to mate with him *despite* his

[7] For instance, the dark colour of a morsel of meat may carry information about the meat being rotten, but it did not evolve in order to carry such information, so it would qualify as a cue rather than a signal. Similarly, having a large size may carry information about fighting ability, but it would qualify as a cue rather than a signal because it presumably did not evolve in order to carry such information. On the other hand, the roar of a male whose acoustic properties were shaped by natural selection for the purpose of carrying information about having a large size would qualify as a signal.

low quality. Perhaps he can achieve this objective by reproducing the calls of healthy males and being mistaken for one of them.

The evolutionary point of sending signals, Dawkins and Krebs concluded, is not to transfer information to recipients, but to get recipients to *do things that are advantageous to the signaller*. The appropriate metaphor for signalling is therefore *manipulating* rather than *informing*.[8] This led them to offer a new, influence-based definition of communication:

> Communication is said to occur when an animal, the actor [henceforth, the signaller], does something which appears to be the result of selection to influence the sense organs of another animal, the reactor [henceforth, the recipient], so that the reactors' behaviour changes to the advantage of the actor. (Dawkins and Krebs, 1978, p. 283; my additions in brackets)

This definition preserves the idea that signals are fashioned or maintained by natural selection, but it replaces the assumption that they are selected because of the information they carry with the assumption that they are selected because of the fitness benefits they earn for signallers.[9] An objection quickly comes to mind. In some cases, the signaller does not gain any benefit from signalling, as when an alarm call leads the signaller to be located and eaten by the predator. But it certainly does not follow that the alarm call is not a signal. If so, asking that "reactors' behaviour changes to the advantage of the actor" seems to be asking too much.

Dawkins and Krebs dealt with this problem by arguing that the signaller's advantage must be understood as an *average advantage* over all instances of signalling of the same type. The requirement is that producers of alarm calls benefit on average from their calls thus leading to signal selection. This is compatible with tokens of the type not leading to any advantage, or even leading to detrimental consequences. From here on, when I write that the

[8] This shift of focus took place against the background of the so-called *selfish gene* theory of evolution (Dawkins, 1976), according to which animals are machines built by genes whose only evolutionary objective is self-preservation by whatever means necessary.

[9] Even though both information-based and influence-based accounts assume that a signal is by definition an adaptation, compelling empirical evidence about a history of selection is rarely provided. This leads the whole field of animal communication to sound remarkably Panglossian with respect to the origin of signals, with potentially negative effects on the field's ability to consider mechanisms for the emergence of signals other than adaptation (cf. Gould & Lewontin, 1978). I will disregard this limitation in what follows.

signaller *benefits* from signalling, I will mean that the signaller benefits on average.[10]

Dawkins and Krebs' critique unveiled a serious problem. The assumption that signals are selected in order to transfer information suggests that transferring information is an end in itself, whereas it is quite clearly a means to an end. What drives signal selection, just as what drives the selection of other traits, is the fitness benefit associated with signalling.[11] Furthermore, in some circumstances transferring information about one's actual features will *not* lead the recipient to do what is in the evolutionary interest of the signaller, so evolutionary pressures will be at work to *avoid* transferring such information if at all possible.

This being said, we should not conclude that information is dispensable in understanding communication. Dawkins and Krebs (1978) are largely responsible for the anti-informational turn taken by the influence approach. This is because, at least initially, they presented it as an *alternative* to the information view, suggesting that it is "reasonable to eschew the ideas of information and of meaning and to think instead of the caller as 'manipulating' the behaviour of its companions" (p. 287). The implication here is that thinking of the caller as manipulating the recipient does not require positing information (and meaning) at all.

Many proponents of the influence view have echoed this anti-informational spirit. Owings and Morton (1998) write that "[t]he information concept has ... become too central, deflecting our attention from the more fundamental idea of regulation" (p. 11). This passage also suggests that focusing on information takes attention away from regulation (another label for influence), and that, when picking between the two, the focus should be on regulation.

Rendall, Owren and Ryan (2009) have been especially explicit in their opposition to the information concept, suggesting that questions such as "What information do animal signals convey?" are "ill-posed" (p. 238). They have argued that the informational approach has three fatal flaws. First, it presupposes cooperation

[10] The commonly used expression "benefits on average" is infelicitous, because there may be cases of signalling in which the benefits are very rare, but so significant from an evolutionary point of view that signalling is still selected for. Consider a signal that leads to neither beneficial nor harmful consequences in 80% of the cases, but that leads to saving the life of the signaller in 20% of the cases. Even though 'on average' the signaller does not benefit from signalling, this signal would still be selected for. I will disregard this complication in what follows.

[11] This fact was most likely clear to proponents of the information-based view. Their mistake was not to make it explicit in their definition. This omission allowed Dawkins and Krebs (1978) to mount their case against the information-based view.

between signaller and recipient.[12] Second, it relies on a concept – information – that is systematically invoked but rarely defined, thereby creating "a conceptual vacuum at the heart of the field" (p. 240). Third, the informational approach wrongly models animal signals on linguistic signals, disregarding the important differences that exist between them.

In Scarantino (2010), I discussed the arguments of Rendall *et al.* (2009) to the effect that the information concept is poorly defined and covertly linguistic, concluding that lack of definitional clarity is not a good reason to get rid of the information concept altogether, and that suitable, non-linguistic definitions of information are both necessary and possible. In what follows, I will explain why information is crucial for understanding animal communication.

2.4 Why information is crucial for communication

Dawkins and Krebs' (1978) conclusion was that signals evolve for "effective manipulation" rather than for "effective information transfer". This view was soon criticised for neglecting the role played by recipients in signal evolution (Hinde, 1981). If signals are selected because they efficiently manipulate recipients, recipients appear to take on the role of "automata that can be manipulated to respond in ways beneficial to the signaler" (Seyfarth *et al.*, 2010, p. 4).

But recipients are selected to behave in ways that are beneficial to themselves, not to the signaller. Seyfarth *et al.* (2010) pointed out that even signals that produce a direct influence on recipients by exploiting their pre-existing sensory and neural biases (Rendall *et al.*, 2009) – e.g. courtship calls directly producing sexual receptivity, or alarm signals directly producing preparatory flight responses – must generate benefits for their recipients in order to explain why nervous systems that are directly affected by such signals are selected for.

Furthermore, most animal signals influence the nervous system of their recipients only indirectly, by affecting the decisions they make upon receiving the signal. Upon hearing a courtship call, a sexually receptive female must decide which male to pick for reproductive purposes. Upon hearing an

[12] According to Rendall *et al.* (2009), the assumption of cooperation is revealed not only by the fact that the evolutionary point of signalling is taken to be transferring information, but also by the fact that information is often described as being 'encoded' by signallers and 'decoded' by recipients. This "implies an initial, cooperative stage of signal evolution during which signallers and perceivers converge on a common code" (Owren *et al.*, 2010, p. 764). I share the view that the coding and encoding metaphors are inappropriate. The notion of (predictive) information I have discussed in Section 2.2 does not involve any encoding and decoding operations.

alarm call, a vervet monkey primed for escape must decide which escape behaviour to choose. It is to explain these decisions that the information construct is key.

What affects the decisions of a sexually receptive female bird or an alarmed vervet monkey is the information signals transfer about, respectively, reproductive quality and predator type. As Searcy and Nowicki (2005) have emphasised, if signals did not carry any useful information, recipients would stop responding to them, and signallers would not earn any benefits from signalling, ultimately leading to the collapse of the signalling system.

In an updated version of their paper, Krebs and Dawkins (1984) seemed receptive to this line of reasoning. They acknowledged that, as signallers have an evolutionary interest in influencing recipients to their advantage, recipients have an evolutionary interest in using signals to gain information to their advantage. As they put it, recipients are *mind-readers*, where "mind-reading" is a "catch-word to describe what we are doing when we use statistical laws to predict what an animal will do next" (Krebs & Dawkins, 1984, p. 386).

The caveat introduced with respect to signallers' benefits applies here as well: not every token of a signal type will lead to a response that is beneficial to the recipient. For instance, a bird may take flight upon hearing an alarm call only to realise that the call was produced deceptively by a signaller as a means to eliminating competitors for a morsel of food (Møller, 1988). What must be the case is that recipients benefit on average from responding to signals, just like signallers must benefit on average from signalling.

Now, which mechanisms see to it that signals are informative? One mechanism is cooperation. Even on a selfish gene view, cooperative contexts emerge by means of kinship, reciprocity or possibly other evolutionary mechanisms (see West, Griffin & Gardner, 2007). When they do, the interest of the signaller to influence and the interest of the recipient to be informed coincide. In such cases, Krebs and Dawkins (1984, pp. 391–392) remarked, signallers will show "an active 'willingness' to be mind-read", and signals will resemble "conspiratorial whispers" between willing partners.

Alas, not all contexts are cooperative. In non-cooperative contexts, signalling has to be understood as emerging from a co-evolutionary race between manipulators and mind-readers. Krebs and Dawkins (1984) suggested that, in competitive contexts, signals will be shaped by effective advertising techniques, and will consequently include "redundancy, rhythm repetition, bright packaging and supernormal stimuli" (p. 386). Several mechanisms have been proposed to explain how the informational content of signals can be preserved in non-cooperative contexts (see Maynard-Smith & Harper, 2003; Searcy & Nowicki, 2005).

I conclude that even if we accept that the evolutionary point of signalling is to influence a recipient to one's advantage, it is not a good idea to eschew information altogether. Doing so prevents us from understanding the central role information plays in competitive and cooperative signalling. But should information be part of the *definition* of animal communication?

2.5 Defining animal communication

Good definitions of scientific concepts should be extensionally adequate and fruitful. Definitions can be extensionally inadequate because they are too broad – they apply to non-instances of the concept – and/or because they are too narrow – they do not apply to instances of the concept. If we defined 'animal communication' as 'animal communication', we would have produced a counterexample-proof, extensionally adequate definition. However, we would not have produced a fruitful definition on account of its patent circularity.

Fruitful definitions should non-circularly make explicit what all and only the essential properties of a given concept are, and productively embed such a concept into a network of other scientific concepts and empirically supported generalisations. A fruitful definition of 'animal communication' should tell us what animal communication essentially is, and it should lead to scientifically interesting and empirically testable predictions and explanations about the items that satisfy the definition.

Influence theorists are right to point out that any definition of animal communication presupposing that signals are selected for in order to carry information will not be fruitful, because it contradicts, or at least fails to make explicit, a central evolutionary principle according to which traits are selected because of the benefits they confer to their owners. But they have gone too far by trying to define animal communication in an information-free fashion. Definitions of animal communication framed solely in terms of influence are both unfruitful and extensionally inadequate. They are unfruitful because they neglect to make explicit what is essential about communication, namely that it is a form of advantageous influence that relies on information transfer rather than other means. They are extensionally inadequate because they count as signals things we should not count as signals, and they do not count as signals things we should count as signals.

2.5.1 *Defining communication without information*

I will make my case by focusing on the most sophisticated influence-based definition of animal communication currently on offer. This is the definition formulated by Maynard-Smith and Harper (henceforth MSH; 2003).

It should be emphasised that MSH, unlike many proponents of the influence approach, are clear about the importance of information in the signalling process. They explicitly argue that "the signal must carry information . . . that is of interest to the receiver" (p. 3), devoting a large part of their book to unveiling the mechanisms underlying signal reliability.

Yet, their definition of signal is information-free:

> We define a 'signal' as any act or structure which alters the behaviour of other organisms, which evolved because of that effect, and which is effective because the receiver's response has also evolved. (MSH, 2003, p. 3)

According to this definition, a signal is an adaptation for altering the *behaviour* of another such that the response to the signal is itself an adaptation. But what does it mean to alter the behaviour of another? At first blush, anything an animal *does* counts as behaviour, understood as a goal-oriented production of a sequence of bodily movements (or lack thereof). A predator chasing its prey engages in a behaviour driven by the goal of eating the prey. A prey animal that hides motionless behind a tree engages in a behaviour driven by the goal of avoiding being eaten by the predator.[13]

Behaviours must be contrasted with *happenings*, namely things that occur to an organism without resulting from the selection of a goal on the organism's part. Happenings can be positive, negative or neutral. Positive happenings include being groomed, being fed, being protected etc. Negative happenings include being eaten, being hit, being pushed etc. Neutral happenings include being looked at, being passed by, being flown over etc.

To influence the behaviour of another individual, then, is to change what such an individual will do next. For example, an alarm call influences the behaviour of a recipient insofar as it leads the recipient to adopt an escape behaviour rather than, say, a grooming behaviour. MSH's proposal is that a signal is an act or structure evolved specifically for changing what another individual will do next (*specialised behaviour influencing requirement*), and such that what another individual will do next also evolved (*selected response requirement*).

From the *specialised behaviour influencing requirement* it follows that influencing the behaviour of another to the benefit of the actor does not make an act or structure a signal, unless it has features specifically adapted to have that effect on the behaviour of another. For example, suppose a predator chases a prey that

[13] Some behaviours are goal-oriented and reflex-like, such as the recoiling behaviours produced by a suddenly looming object. Other behaviours are goal-oriented but not reflex-like, as the escape behaviours of a vervet monkey upon hearing an alarm call.

runs faster, eventually leading the slower predator to stop chasing (Hasson, 1994). Running faster than a predator, however, is not a signal the prey sends to the predator.

The reason is that, although running faster than a predator is adaptive and influences the predator's behaviour to the benefit of the prey, it did not evolve in order to influence the behaviour of the predator. As clarified by Stegmann (2005), what is selected for is outrunning the predator rather than leading him to abandon the chase (even though outrunning him does lead him to abandon the chase). The point is that the adaptiveness of outrunning a predator does not hinge on changing the predator's behaviour: it would be selected for even if the predator continued running.

The specialised behaviour influencing requirement also explains why having a large size is not a signal. Even though it is an adaptation and it influences the behaviour of others in beneficial ways (e.g. it leads them to submit without a fight), it presumably did not evolve in order to influence such behaviour, and so it would not qualify as a signal according to MSH's definition.

MSH initially thought that the specialised behaviour influencing requirement sufficed for defining animal communication.[14] In 1995, they defined a signal as any "action or structure that increases the fitness of an individual by altering the behaviour of other organisms detecting it, and that has characteristics that have evolved because they have that effect" (MSH, 1995, p. 306). They then realised that this definition does not distinguish between coercion and communication, and amended it by adding the *selected response requirement*.

2.5.2 *Three counterexamples: coercion, reciprocity and deception*

Coercion is widely considered not to be a form of signalling. This was clear to Dawkins and Krebs (1978, p. 604), who cited approvingly Cullen's claim that "to a man the command 'Go jump in the lake' is a signal [whereas] the push which precipitates him is not". But how is a push different from a signal? According to Dawkins and Krebs, whereas the coercer only relies on his own "physical power" to achieve advantageous influence, the signaller "can exploit the senses and muscles of the animal it is trying to control" (p. 282). Communication is then "a means by which one animal makes use of another animal's muscle power" (p. 283).

[14] In a recent paper, Owren *et al.* (2010) have re proposed a definition of animal communication that exclusively relies on the requirement that signals are adaptations for changing the behaviour of another. I will not discuss such definitions in this chapter owing to space limitations.

MSH's (2003) definition aims to exclude coercive behaviours from the domain of signals by requiring that a signal is effective in altering the behaviour of another because the recipient's response has also evolved (selected response requirement). The effectiveness of coercive behaviours, MSH thought, does not depend on the presence of an evolved response. Thus, coercive behaviours are not signals.

I agree that coercive behaviours are not signals, but I will argue that they are diagnosed as such by MSH's (2003) definition. Let us distinguish two ways in which a coercive behaviour such as pushing can influence another. On the one hand, there is the *being pushed* component of the influence, which is not a behaviour but a happening. On the other hand, there is the *response to being pushed* component of the influence, which is instead a behaviour. What an animal does as a result of being pushed (or hit, or bitten etc.) may be to give up on a certain contested resource.

According to the *specialised behaviour influencing requirement*, signals are specialised for altering the behaviour of a recipient. So if we only focused on the first source of influence – the being pushed part – coercive behaviours would not qualify as signals not because there is no *evolved* response to them, but more simply because there is no response to them at all. Being pushed is not a behavioural response to pushing any more than dying is a behavioural response to being shot. As argued by Stegmann (2005), this would make the *selected response requirement* superfluous for explaining why pushing is not a signal. The specialised behaviour influencing requirement would suffice, because pushing would not qualify as an act that alters the behaviour of another organism (it only alters what happens to another organism).

The fact that MSH considered their 1995 definition incapable of excluding coercive behaviours suggests that their interpretation of the influence exerted by coercive behaviours included *behavioural responses* to being pushed. This broadening of the scope of the analysis is appropriate, because we are considering the proposal that signals are adaptations for influencing another, so all evolutionarily relevant aspects of the influence an act or structure has on another should be taken into account.

Our focus is now on the responses organisms display to being pushed, being hit, being bitten and so on. In order for coercive behaviours not to count as signals on MSH's definition, such responses must not have evolved. The problem is that responses to coercive behaviours are as likely to have evolved as coercive behaviours themselves. Let us consider what it would take for a receiver's response to have evolved. In some passages, MSH seemed to suggest that the response to a signal must have evolved *somehow*, but not necessarily as a response to the signal. Let us call this the *generalised response interpretation* of the selected response requirement.

This is the interpretation endorsed by Stegmann (2005, p. 1022), who argues that "Maynard Smith and Harper (2003) demand only that the reaction evolved as a response to some features, but not necessarily to the signal". Some remarks by MSH support this interpretation. For example, MSH (2003) wrote that if a stag "roars and the other stag retreats, it is a signal, because the response depends on evolved properties of the brain and sense organs of the receiver" (p. 3). Here, the behavioural response of retreating evolved only in the sense that retreating depends on properties of the brain and of the sensory system that evolved for other reasons.

In other places, MSH appeared to argue for a stricter requirement, demanding that the response evolved specifically as a response to the signal. Call this the *specialised response interpretation* of the selected response requirement. This is the interpretation endorsed by Scott-Phillips (2008), who argues that according to MSH's definition the act or structure that is the signal must have evolved to alter the behaviour of other organisms and be "effective because the effect (the response) has evolved to be affected by the act or structure" (p. 388).

Other remarks by MSH support this interpretation as well. They write that camouflage is not a signal because it lacks an evolved response (MSH, 2003, p. 5). Yet, there is an evolved response to being exposed to a camouflaged prey in the sense that there is a response that depends on evolved properties of the brain and sense organs of the predator. This is the response of *ignoring the camouflaged prey*, interpreted in light of stored sensory experiences as an inedible feature of the environment. What is missing in camouflage is a response evolved specifically with respect to the act of camouflage. Lack of specificity is due to the fact that camouflaged prey cannot be detected, and consequently cannot be responded to as camouflaged prey.

Keeping in mind that there are two possible interpretations of the selected response requirement, let us confront anew the question of whether responses to coercive signals evolved. Consider a confrontation between two stags over a contested resource. A weaker stag keeps being pushed backwards by a stronger stag. This goes on for a while, until the weaker stag adopts behavioural responses to the negative happening to which he is being subjected, namely being pushed. In the short term, the response may be to give up on the contested resource. In the medium and long term, the response may be to accept a more submissive position in the social hierarchy, and avoid further confrontations with the stronger stag.

These responses to being pushed probably explain why pushing was selected for: it is an effective means of getting contested resources, acquiring social dominance and avoiding future conflicts. These responses quite clearly depend on evolved properties of the brain and sense organs of the coerced, in the same sense in which retreating when faced by the roar of another male depends on evolved properties of the brain and sense organs of the signal recipient. Furthermore, they arguably are responses evolved *specifically* to the happening of being coerced. It seems reasonable to posit evolutionary pressures selecting in favour of organisms that take being coerced as a sign of a competitor's superior strength, and change their future behaviour towards that stronger competitor accordingly.

If this is right, coercive behaviours qualify as signals on both the generalised response interpretation and the specialised response interpretation. They alter what organisms do as a result of being coerced, they evolved at least in part because of that effect, and they are effective because the receiver's response has also evolved. But any definition of animal signalling that counts coercive behaviours as signals is too broad.

Coercion is not a solitary problem. As noted by West *et al.* (2007), MSH's "definition of a signal does not exclude actions that operate because of their substantive effects rather than their information content, so for example, it could include reciprocity, where cooperation is conditional upon the cooperative behaviour of others" (p. 419).

In cases of reciprocity, actors take turns in benefiting each other. In each interaction, the giver produces a positive happening for the receiver (e.g. being groomed). If we only looked at this aspect, reciprocal behaviours would not qualify as signals because they would fail the *specialised behaviour influencing requirement*. Being the recipient of a grooming behaviour is not something an organism *does*, any more than being pushed is something an organism does. But, as in the case of coercive behaviours, we need to broaden our focus to *behavioural responses* to being groomed. These include *reciprocating* the grooming act at a later time.

It follows that grooming behaviours alter the behaviour of another individual, and presumably evolved to influence the recipient's behaviour towards reciprocation, because this is the main expected payoff of an otherwise costly activity. Finally, grooming behaviours appear to be effective because the receiver's response to the behaviour has also evolved. This is true both in the sense that the response depends on evolved properties of the brain and sensory system of the groomed, and in the sense that the response – reciprocating a positive happening – evolved specifically as a response to earlier grooming behaviours.[15]

[15] Scott-Phillips (2008) has argued that the response to a cooperative act in a reciprocating interaction evolved, but not specifically as a response to the cooperative act. If so, the counterexample constituted by reciprocating behaviours would only apply to the generalised response interpretation of the selected response requirement. To illustrate Scott-Phillips' counterargument, let us consider the case of reciprocal grooming, in

The troubles with MSH's definition are not yet over. Besides being too broad, such definition is too narrow (at least under the specialised response interpretation). Consider a case of deception such as the one constituted by the dangling of lures by the anglerfish. These lures are worm-like objects designed to attract prey. The problem is that, even though the anglerfish lure alters the behaviour of other organisms and evolved because of that effect, what makes it effective is not that the receiver's response has evolved to be affected specifically by the lure. The receiver's response to the anglerfish lure, namely approaching it and trying to eat it, is maladaptive, as it leads to the receiver's death.

On the other hand, it is a response that depends on evolved properties of the brain and sense organs of the receiver. In light of stored sensory experiences, the prey responds to the anglerfish lure as an actual worm, from which it is visually indistinguishable. Since there are many fewer anglerfish lures than actual worms, evolutionary pressures preserve approaching responses to worm-like objects, which usually lead to the eating of worms. But, in the same way that the response to a camouflaged prey did not evolve specifically to the camouflaged prey, the response to an angler lure did not evolve specifically to the angler lure. It follows that angler lures are incorrectly diagnosed as non-signals on the specialised response interpretation, and correctly diagnosed as signals on the generalised response interpretation.

The three problem cases I have considered so far – coercion, reciprocation and deception – can be solved if we conceptualise signals as information-mediated influencers. On the view I am proposing, a signal must be specialised for *influencing recipients by carrying information to them.* Given my definition of predictive information, this boils down to influencing recipients by changing the probabilities of states of affairs relevant to their decision-making. Coercive

which two partners take turns in grooming each other. If my response to being groomed had evolved to be affected by the grooming, he claims, the response would have to be selected in order "to reward the other participant's cooperation" (p. 390). However, the response to the grooming is not selected for this reason, but rather "to induce the other participant into a further act of altruism" (p. 390). So my response to being groomed did not evolve "to be affected by the signal" (p. 390). This argument is not persuasive. It is an arbitrary assumption that my response to grooming would have to consist in a 'reward to cooperation' in order to properly count as having evolved to be affected by grooming. Even under the specialised response interpretation, MSH's definition only demands that my response evolved as a response to your act of grooming, rather than as a response to something else. No boundaries are set on the reasons why it was selected, as long as it was selected specifically as a response to the grooming. I conclude that my grooming you is a signal by the lights of MSH's definition also on the specialised response interpretation. It is an act that alters your behaviour by making you inclined to groom me in the future, it evolved because it has that effect, and it is effective because your response to my grooming has also specifically evolved as a way to alter my behaviour by making me inclined to groom you again in the future.

and reciprocal behaviours are instead specialised for influencing recipients by other means, namely the production of, respectively, negative and positive happenings through mechanical interaction.[16]

This distinction explains why communication is, as Dawkins and Krebs (1978) noted, a good energetic bargain. Instead of recruiting one's own muscle power to bring about positive or negative happenings, communicators exploit the muscle power of another to their advantage. For instance, instead of physically "roll[ing] a female along the ground and into his burrow" (coercion), a male cricket can deliver information through a song (signalling) and "the female comes to him under her own power" (p. 282).

Requiring that information transfer mediates influence solves the problem of deceptive predation as well. As we have seen, anglerfish lures do not count as signals on the specialised response interpretation of MSH's definition (they do on the generalised response interpretation). But they qualify as signals if signals are acts or structures specialised for influencing the behaviour of another individual by means of information transfer. This is because worm-like objects carry (predictive) information about the presence of worms.

As I have argued in Section 2.2, signals carry information by changing the probability of what they are about. Given the relative frequency of worm-like objects that are actual worms (many) and worm-like objects that are anglerfish lures (few), the appearance of a worm-like object significantly increases the probability that a worm is present. This is how angler lures manage to exert their influence on signal recipients: they affect their decisions by raising the probability that a worm is present.

A critic may object that worm-like objects do not carry information about worms unless worms are present, from which it follows that worm-like objects that are anglerfish lures do not carry information about worms. This would reveal a confusion about the concept of information. If the ability of a signal to carry information about a given state of affairs amounts to the ability of the signal to change the probability of that state of affairs, the signal carries such information whether or not the state of affairs obtains. An event's failure to obtain is compatible with the reception of information about its obtaining, just like the claim that the probability that o is G is high is compatible with the claim that o is not G. No valid inference rules take us from claims about

[16] Being subjected to a positive and negative happening also carries information (e.g. my opponent is stronger) that will be factored into the future decision-making process of the recipient. This information, however, is not what the coercive or reciprocating act is specialised in transferring, but a by-product of the happenings that the coercive or reciprocating act is specialised in producing through mechanical interaction. I thank an anonymous referee for raising this issue.

the transmission of information to claims about how things turn out to be (Scarantino & Piccinini, 2010).

I conclude that any extensionally adequate and scientifically fruitful definition of animal communication should conceptualise signalling as a specialised, information-mediated form of influencing. A systematic discussion of how a definition of this sort should be formulated, and a consideration of possible objections to it, will have to wait for another paper.

2.6 Conclusion

Information-based accounts have suggested that the evolutionary point of signalling is to transfer information. Influence theorists have rejected this view, arguing that the point of signalling must be to influence other organisms to one's advantage. However, they have assumed that it is possible to define signals in an information-free fashion, using only the notions of influence and selection. I have argued that even the most sophisticated information-free influence-based definition currently on offer faces significant counterexamples. The way to address them, I concluded, is not to fine-tune information-free accounts, but rather to conceptualise signals as acts or structures specialised for influencing by means of information transfer. This proposal combines information-based and influence-based approaches, which differ more in emphasis than in substance. Bringing both information and influence to the foreground in the definition of animal communication will allow us to combine the insights of the two research programmes into a theoretically richer hybrid.

References

Bradbury, J. W. & Vehrencamp, S. L. (1998). *Principles of Animal Communication.* Sunderland, MA: Sinauer.

Carnap, R. (1950). *Logical Foundations of Probability.* Chicago, IL: University of Chicago Press.

Dawkins, R. (1976). *The Selfish Gene.* Oxford: Oxford University Press.

Dawkins, R. & Krebs, J. R. (1978). Animal signals: information or manipulation. In J. R. Krebs & N. B. Davies, eds., *Behavioural Ecology: An Evolutionary Approach.* Oxford: Blackwell Scientific, pp. 282–309.

Dretske, F. (1981). *Knowledge and the Flow of Information.* Cambridge, MA: MIT Press.

Gould, S. J. & Lewontin, R. (1978). The Spandrels of San Marco and the Panglossian Paradig a critique of the adaptationist programme. *Proceedings of the Royal Society of London Series B*, **205**, 581–598.

Hasson, O. (1994). Cheating signals. *Journal of Theoretical Biology*, **167**, 223–238.

Hauser, M. D. (1996). *The Evolution of Communication.* Cambridge, MA: MIT Press.

Hinde, R. A. (1981). Animal signals: ethological and games-theory approaches are not incompatible. *Animal Behaviour*, **29**, 535–542.

Krebs, J. R. & Dawkins, R. (1984). Animal signals: mind-reading and manipulation. In J. R. Krebs & N. B. Davies, eds., *Behavioural Ecology: An Evolutionary Approach*, 2nd edn. Oxford: Blackwell, pp. 380–402.

Maynard Smith, J. & Harper, D. G. C. (1995). Animal signals: models and terminology. *Journal of Theoretical Biology*, **177**(3), 305–311.

Maynard Smith, J. & Harper, D. (2003). *Animal Signals*. Oxford: Oxford University Press.

Millikan, R. G. (2000). *On Clear and Confused Ideas: An Essay about Substance Concepts*. Cambridge and New York: Cambridge University Press.

Millikan, R. G. (2004). *Varieties of Meaning: The 2002 Jean Nicod Lectures*. Cambridge, MA: MIT Press.

Møller, A. P. (1988). False alarm calls as a means of resource usurpation in the great tit *Parus major*. *Ethology*, **79**, 25–30.

Otte, D. (1974). Effects and function in the evolution of signaling systems. *Annual Review of Ecological Systematics*, **5**, 385–417.

Owren, M., Rendall D. & Ryan, M. J. (2010). Redefining animal signaling: influence versus information in communication. *Biology and Philosophy*, **25**, 755–780.

Owings, D. H. & Morton, E. S. (1998). *Animal Vocal Communication: A New Approach*. Cambridge: Cambridge University Press.

Piccinini, G. & Scarantino, A. (2011). Information processing, computation and cognition. *Journal of Biological Physics*, **37**, 1–38.

Rendall, D., Owren, M. & Ryan, M. (2009). What do animal signals mean? *Animal Behaviour*, **78**, 233–240.

Scarantino, A. (2010). Animal communication between information and influence. *Animal Behaviour*, **79**(6), e1–e5.

Scarantino, A. & Piccinini, G. (2010). Information without truth. *Metaphilosophy*, **41**, 313–330.

Scott-Phillips, T. C. (2008). Defining biological communication. *Journal of Evolutionary Biology*, **21**, 387–395.

Searcy, W. & Nowicki, S. (2005). *The Evolution of Animal Communication*. Princeton, NJ: Princeton University Press.

Seyfarth, R. M., Cheney, D. L., Bergman, T. *et al.* (2010). The central importance of information in studies of animal communication. *Animal Behaviour*, **80**, 3–8.

Seyfarth, R. M., Cheney, D. L. & Marler, P. (1980). Monkey responses to three different alarm calls: evidence of predator classification and semantic communication. *Science*, **210**, 801–803.

Shea, N. (2007). Consumers need information: supplementing teleosemantics with an input condition. *Philosophy and Phenomenological Research*, **75**, 404–435.

Skyrms, B. (2010). *Signals: Evolution, Learning, and Information*. Oxford: Oxford University Press.

Stegmann, U. (2005). John Maynard Smith's notion of animal signals. *Biology and Philosophy*, **20**, 1011–1025.

West, S. A., Griffin, A. S. & Gardner, A. (2007). Social semantics: altruism, cooperation, mutualism and strong reciprocity. *Journal of Evolutionary Biology*, **20**, 415–432.

Zahavi, A. (1987). The theory of signal selection and some of its implications. In U. P. Delfino, ed., *International Symposium on Biology and Evolution*. Bari: Adriatica Editrice, pp. 294–327.

Commentaries

Signals may have predictive value, but only perceivers predict. Scarantino argues that 'information talk' is useful in animal communication, in the particular sense that signals have *predictive value*. We agree with his approach of understanding information as environmental regularity (similar to Scott-Phillips and Kirby's *indication function*). Importantly, however, that regularity exists independently of perceivers. A conceptual firewall is therefore needed between information as correlations in the world versus observer representations of those correlations. Furthermore, information-as-correlation exists only via the recurrence of events over time, and is not instantiated in any one occurrence. Signals thus have predictive value only to observers that have been previously exposed to the regularity involved – whether developmentally or through phylogeny. When signals are said to contain or transmit information, the firewall is critically breached – environmental regularity becomes conflated with observer knowledge of that regularity. Information talk is therefore harmful – in its current form – because it blurs a critical distinction that it should instead highlight and codify. For Scarantino, true communication occurs when signallers are specialised to influence others specifically through information transmission. Yet, that transmission is metaphorical, relying on notions of information being contained and conveyed. When a signal occurs, perceivers may respond *as if* information transmission has occurred, but such cannot be literally true. The metaphor 'works' only because the perceiver already has experience of relationships between signals and events – the correlation does not reside in the signal itself. While Scarantino's solution is to invoke a metaphorical characterisation, scientific explanation requires that we remain firmly in the material realm. To be useful, information talk should help keep us in that world, rather than separating us from it.

Michael J. Owren and Drew Rendall

Defending an effects-based definition of communication. Scarantino argues that influence-based definitions (IBDs) of animal communication are neither scientifically fruitful nor extensionally adequate. This commentary replies to both criticisms.

The first criticism is that IBDs exclude what is central to communication, namely information transfer. Two points should be made in response. First, the adoption of an IBD does not imply the rejection of information (Carazo & Font, 2010). The point made by IBDs is only that communication is, at bottom, a matter of effects. Information transfer is a consequence of this. IBDs are not claims that we should remove all talk of communication-as-information-transfer; only that we should be clear that such talk is coherent only if the criteria for an IBD are satisfied. Second, IBDs have informed several theoretical issues in animal signalling and in linguistic pragmatics, and as such are fruitful in their own right. (I briefly discuss these applications in my own contribution to this volume.) The reason it is fruitful is that it captures the functional interdependence of signal and response which lies at the heart of communication (Scott-Phillips *et al.*, 2012).

Scarantino discusses three types of interaction that, he argues, are extensionally problematic for IBDs. As Scarantino notes, IBDs typically include what he calls a *selected response requirement* (SRR) to address such cases. Scarantino shows that this requirement only excludes *happenings* – yet IBDs are typically expressed in terms of behaviours, and hence the SRR fails to achieve its purpose. Scarantino is correct in all of this. However, IBDs are easily saved if they are expressed in terms of happenings rather than behaviours. When IBDs are expressed this way, both coercion and reciprocity fall outside them. (I will not enter into the details of this argument here, for reasons of space.) At least for me, the idea that signals cause happenings has always been the spirit of IBDs; this is why I prefer to talk of *effects* rather than *influence*. However, Scarantino is right to draw attention to the lack of precision in present formulations of IBDs, and the distinction between behaviours and happenings is a useful one. But his comments do not fatally undermine either the utility or the extensional adequacy of IBDs.

Carazo, P. & Font, E. (2010). Putting information back into biological communication. *Journal of Evolutionary Biology*, **23**, 661–669.

Scott-Phillips, T. C., Blythe, R., Gardner, A. & West, S. A. (2012). How do communication systems emerge? *Proceedings of the Royal Society of London Series B*, **279**, 1943–1949.

Thomas C. Scott-Phillips

Can animals know things on Scarantino's account of information? Can the reason animal A chooses to mate with animal B be that signal 's' informs A about B's certain healthful properties if the signal 's' can happen without those properties being possessed by the animal B? On his view this should be possible, but it seems false.

Fred Adams and Steve M. Beighley

Response

The take-home message of my chapter is that any suitable definition of animal communication must include both influence and information in order to be scientifically fruitful and extensionally adequate. In his commentary, **Scott-Phillips** defended influence-based definitions from the charge of inadequacy. He pointed out that endorsing an influence-based definition of animal communication does not entail rejecting information, and that influence-based definitions have led to fruitful discoveries in animal communication and linguistic pragmatics.

I agree, which is why I proposed to preserve the insights of influence-based accounts in a new hybrid definition of animal communication. My charge was addressed to those influence theorists who believe that animal communication should be defined *exclusively* in terms of influence. This group includes Scott-Phillips (2008, p. 388), according to whom "if it is to be discussed at all information should be seen only as an emergent property of communication and certainly not as a defining quality".

As testified by this volume, many influence theorists still consider the thesis that signals carry information superfluous for definitional purposes, if not problematic in its own right. I replied that definitions of animal communication which fail to treat information as a "defining quality" miss the essential difference between communication and other forms of influence (they are not fruitful) and give the wrong verdict about what is and what is not a signal (they are not extensionally adequate).

In particular, some popular information-free influence-based definitions wrongly count coercion and reciprocation as signals, and wrongly exclude deception from the domain of signals. Scott-Phillips does not address the counterexample of deception, but argues that coercion and reciprocation would not count as signals if we expressed influence-based definitions in terms of *effects* rather than *behaviours*.

I argued that in cases of coercion and reciprocation two types of effects must be distinguished: effects that are happenings (e.g. being pushed, being groomed) and effects that are behaviours (e.g. giving up on a contested resource, grooming back). Scott-Phillips' proposal is not developed in any detail owing to space limitations, but I understand it roughly as follows. Signals should be re-defined as acts or structures that produce *effects* (rather then mere behaviours) in other organisms, that evolved because of such effects and that are effective because the effects evolved to be affected by the act or structure.

This shift from behaviours to effects, however, would not solve the extensional problem faced by the influence account. It would still be the case that the *behavioural effects* of being pushed by a stronger competitor or being groomed by a conspecific are as likely to have been selected as the pushing and grooming behaviours of the coercer and of the one who initiates reciprocation. If so, coercion and reciprocation continue to satisfy the definition of a signal: they are acts producing effects in recipients (happenings and behaviours), they evolved because of such effects and they are effective because at least some of such effects evolved to be affected by the coercive or reciprocating act.[1]

My commentators have also challenged my analysis of information. **Owren and Rendall** have defended the view that signals do not carry predictive information *in the literal sense*, from which it follows that information talk must be *metaphorical*. Since metaphorical claims lack straightforward truth conditions, information talk stands in the way of the scientific understanding of animal communication. I will now explain why my claim that signals carry predictive information is not metaphorical at all.

Owren and Rendall infer that signals do not carry predictive information in the literal sense from the recipient-relativity of predictive value. For instance, whereas a ringing bell has predictive value with respect to a foot shock relative to a fear-conditioned rat, it does not have such predictive value relative to a rat just placed into the conditioning box.

Owren and Rendall interpret this as indicating that predictive information is not *in* the signals themselves. If it were, they assume, any recipient would be able to pick it up. This supposedly distinguishes signals from sentences, in which information is encoded. We should first notice that in order for a sentence to have any informative value for a recipient, such recipient must be familiar with the language in which it is written/spoken. This is to say that the informative value of both linguistic and non-linguistic signals amounts to a dispositional property, namely the property of allowing a suitable recipient to learn something from the signal in suitable circumstances.[2]

This being said, there is an important difference between linguistic and non-linguistic signals. Whereas linguistic signals carry the same encoded information to all recipients familiar with the language, what predictive information a

[1] If anything, the shift from behaviours to effect would block a possible line of defence on the part of the influence theorist. Such a theorist may argue that coercion and reciprocation are not signals because the definition of a signal requires that what is affected by a signal is a behaviour, and the effects of coercion and reciprocation are happenings rather than behaviours. Replacing behaviours with effects in the definition of animal communication would effectively block this line of reply. It is a reply worth rejecting anyway, because when considering the proposal that signals are adaptations for influencing another, all evolutionarily relevant aspects of the influence an act or structure has must be taken into account, whether they consist of happenings or behaviours.

[2] The way we learn from sentences is different from the way we learn from non-linguistic signals in ways I cannot explore in this reply.

signal carries changes depending on what the recipient already knows. This is a central property of predictive information, but not one that supports the conclusion that signals carry predictive information only in a metaphorical sense.

Rather, it supports the conclusion that signals *literally speaking* carry predictive information in a recipient-dependent fashion. On this view, the information relation is a *three-place relation* between signals, states of affairs and the states of background knowledge of recipients. For example, a ringing bell carries predictive information about a foot shock relative to the background knowledge of a fear-conditioned rat, but it does not carry such information relative to the background knowledge of a rat just introduced into the conditioning box.

When fully spelled out, the predictive information relation takes the following form: X carries information about Y relative to background knowledge k when $P(Y \text{ given } X \ \& \ k) \neq P(Y \text{ given } k)$. This inequality provides a non-metaphorical definition of information, clearly spelling out the conditions under which X carries predictive information about Y relative to k. If $P(Y \text{ given } X \ \& \ k)$ is larger (smaller) than $P(Y \text{ given } k)$, we will say that the signal and what the signal is about are positively (negatively) correlated.

A corollary of this analysis is that, contra Owren and Rendall, no "conceptual firewall" is needed between "correlations in the world" and "observer representations of those correlations". For purposes of transmission of predictive information, the only correlations that matter are those defined relative to the background knowledge of observers, namely those defined relative to the conditional probabilities $P(Y \text{ given } X \ \& \ k)$ and $P(Y \text{ given } k)$.

A final challenge to my analysis comes from **Adams and Beighley**, who wonder whether "animals can know things on [my] account of information", and whether "the reason animal A chooses to mate with animal B [can] be that signal 's' informs A about B's ... healthful properties ... if the signal 's' can happen without those properties being possessed by the animal B." My reply is that what animals come to know from receiving predictive information is simply that the probabilities of various states of affairs have changed. This generally falls short of knowing what states of affairs have occurred, so the reception of predictive information does not generate knowledge in the traditional sense.

For example, a signal s may carry predictive information to animal A about animal B being healthy because s – e.g. a courtship call – raises significantly the probability of B being healthy. But receiving this sort of information is *not* coming to know that B is healthy, and it is compatible with B *not* being healthy. Adams and Beighley find this objectionable, but I consider it an asset of my theory. Following Dretske (1981), Adams and Beighley assume that a single theory of information can reduce knowledge to information and explain the behaviour of creatures in natural environments. My view is that two distinct theories are required to fulfil these two tasks.

This is because what explains why A chooses to mate with B is not that A received knowledge-producing information that B is healthy (real-world courtship calls do not conclusively settle such matters) but that A received probabilistic confirmation that B is healthy. So, while I concede that knowledge is not gained from the reception of predictive information, I hold that it is the reception of predictive information that explains the behaviour of animals in natural environments.

Dretske, F. (1981). *Knowledge and the Flow of Information*. Cambridge, MA: MIT Press.

Andrea Scarantino

3

Communication as information use: insights from statistical decision theory

CAITLIN R. KIGHT, JOHN M. MCNAMARA, DAVID W. STEPHENS AND SASHA R. X. DALL

3.1 Introduction

Uncertainty is an unavoidable product of any encounter between two or more animals. Although the level of uncertainty may vary as a function of many factors – including species, sex, age and condition – even at its minimum it still presents a challenge that must be overcome over the course of every animal's life (Dall, 2010). This process is facilitated by the use of socially acquired information, which one animal gleans by observing the behaviour of another (Danchin *et al.*, 2004; Dall *et al.*, 2005), thereby reducing its prior uncertainty before taking definitive action (Dall, 2010). Socially acquired information may be produced inadvertently (i.e. 'public information' and 'social cues'), or actively broadcast by one individual in order to influence the behaviour of others (i.e. a 'signal') (Danchin *et al.*, 2004; Dall *et al.*, 2005). This chapter focuses on the latter, which forms the basis of animal communication.

Animal communication has been observed in both terrestrial and aquatic habitats and, so far as we are aware, in all taxa in which it has been investigated (Lishak, 1984; Lugli, Yan & Fine, 2003; Marler & Slabbekoorn, 2004; Belanger & Corkum, 2009; Caro, 2009; Houck, 2009; Mäthger *et al.*, 2009; Bruschini, Cervo & Turillazzi, 2010; Costa-Leonardo & Haifig, 2010; Haddock, Moline & Case, 2010; Wyatt, 2010; Thiel & Breithaupt, 2011). Communication occurs between both con- and heterospecifics (Rabin *et al.*, 2003; Magrath, Pitcher & Gardner, 2007;

Animal Communication Theory: Information and Influence, ed. Ulrich Stegmann. Published by Cambridge University Press.

Lea *et al.*, 2008; Pope & Haney, 2008; Touhara, 2008; Shabani, Kamio & Derby, 2009; Bruschini *et al.*, 2010) and, if one relaxes the definition of 'animal communication' to include any information transfer where either the signaller or receiver is an animal, it also occurs across phyla (Schaefer, Schaefer & Levey, 2004; Gera & Srivastava, 2006; Raguso, 2008).

Cumulatively, animals broadcast signals using nearly every known sensory modality. Chemical signals are the most common, in part because of the widespread – perhaps even ubiquitous – use of pheromones and signature mixtures (Wyatt, 2010) throughout the animal kingdom, in both aquatic (Belanger & Corkum, 2009; Houck, 2009; Thiel & Breithaupt, 2011; Zhang *et al.*, 2011) and terrestrial (Ayasse, Paxton & Tengö, 2001; Houck, 2009; Harder & Jackson, 2010) environments. Visual signals make use of variations in light (both reflected and generated), patterning, symmetry, size and coordinated movements (Rosenthal, 2007); some animals have specialised structures that appear to serve no purpose other than delivering a visual message to other animals (as in stalk-eyed flies; Wilkinson & Dodson, 1997). In many cases, extended phenotypes, such as the bowers and hoods built by bowerbirds (Borgia, 1985; Patricelli, Uy & Borgia, 2003) and fiddler crabs (Christy *et al.*, 2002), respectively, may also be thought of as visual signals (Schaedelin & Taborsky, 2009). The category of vibratory signals comprises both near- and far-field signals, which may be produced with dedicated acoustic apparati (e.g. the larynx in mammals and the syrinx in birds), or other, multipurpose, morphological features (e.g. beaks or feet; Wilkins & Ritchison, 1999; Rose *et al.*, 2006; Delaney *et al.*, 2007). Comparatively little is known about electrical and tactile signalling. Although the primary purpose of electrogenesis appears to be predation, it has also been shown to play a role in dominance interactions, as observed in *Sternarchorhynchus* spp. (Fugere, Ortega & Krahe, 2011), suggesting that this signalling method may be important in other electrogenic species as well. Tactile signalling remains the least well understood of all five categories. Reception of tactile stimuli has been documented in diverse species, such as captive deermice (*Peromyscus maniculatus bairdii*) (Terman, 1980), emigrating ants (*Temnothorax albipennis*) (Pratt, 2005) and client reef fish that are groomed by cleaner wrasses (Bshary & Würth, 2001), but it is not clear whether these events represent active transfer of information or merely cues.

Many animals maximise the diversity of their potential signal catalogue by employing 'complex signals', or those that incorporate multiple individual signals (Hebets & Papaj, 2005). The components of complex signals may be delivered simultaneously or sequentially, may occur in the same or different sensory modalities and may or may not elicit independent behavioural responses if delivered individually (McCowan, Doyle & Hanser, 2002;

Candolin, 2003; Hebets & Papaj, 2005; Kulahci, Dornhans & Papaj, 2008; Gordon & Uetz, 2011). Given the potential complexity of the signalling process, it is unsurprising that many animals require a learning period during which they perfect signal performance or delivery. However, a signal's simplicity or complexity is not necessarily correlated with whether it is learned or innate (Rosenthal, 2007).

The most important characteristic of a signal is conspicuousness against the background, since it cannot be perceived, interpreted and reacted to without first being detected (Bradbury & Vehrencamp, 2011). This appears to be one of the factors driving the use of complex signal displays – particularly those that involve components in multiple modalities. While much attention is (often rightly) focused on the behaviours and structures that signallers use to optimise signal delivery, receiver characteristics also play a vital role in determining whether, and under what circumstances, signals are detected. Morphological features such as antennae, eyes, ears and vomeronasal organs are sensitive across a given range of stimulus strengths and types, such that receivers will only be able to perceive signals that achieve a minimum signal-to-noise ratio (SNR). Over evolutionary time, many receivers have developed extreme sensitivity within the range over which 'their' signallers produce stimuli, allowing the perception of signals with remarkably low SNR.

Following signal reception, higher-level cognitive processing ultimately determines a receiver's response. Comparatively little is known about this stage of the communication process, although it is clear that individual differences in processing and/or decision-making stem from variations in a number of receiver traits, including sex, age, physical condition and prior experience (Nowicki, Peters & Podos, 1998; Janik, 2000; Bailey & Zuk, 2008; Beckers & Schul, 2008; Dyakonova & Krushinsky, 2008; Groot *et al.*, 2010). Even less is understood about the genetics underpinning many of these relationships, and, indeed, the bulk of characteristics, behaviours and preferences vital to the process of communication as a whole. What *is* known is that communication mediates a variety of interactions between animals, including, but not limited to, mate choice, resource competition, predator–prey encounters, parent–offspring dynamics and social group cohesion (Bradbury & Vehrencamp, 1998).

3.2 Animal communication and statistical decision theory

As detailed in our brief overview, the process of animal communication involves a number of clearly identifiable components: signallers, signals, environments through which signals propagate and receivers. Despite claims to the contrary (e.g. Rendall, Owven & Ryan, 2009), this structure, and the way these components are thought to interact, both fit very comfortably within modern frameworks for thinking about information use in evolutionary ecology (e.g. Wiley, 1994, 2006; Wiley & Richards, 1981; Dall *et al.*, 2005; McNamara, Green & Olsson, 2006). Indeed, such structural properties fit particularly well into an explicit framework based on statistical decision theory (McNamara & Houston, 1980), which is increasingly being employed to generate quantitative predictions, from a functional (ultimate) perspective, about information use by animals in a wide range of contexts (Dall *et al.* 2005; McNamara *et al.*, 2006; Schmidt, Dall & Eils, 2010).

The approach of statistical decision theory (referred to here as SDT and not to be confused with the acronym for 'signal detection theory') involves three main elements (Dall *et al.*, 2005) within which the key features of animal communication can be incorporated:

- **Receiver priors and posteriors**. The prior distribution represents what is knowable about the world to an animal without specific experience. From a communication perspective, this can be thought of as the receiver's expectation of the state of a signaller before a signal has been detected. Such a prior might be genetically determined (set by the selective 'experience' of a lineage) or based on acquired experience, and may be either static or updated during the animal's lifetime (continuously or at 'sensitive' periods during development). When it observes something about a particular aspect of its environment (e.g. perceives a signal from a conspecific), this discovery transforms the prior distribution into a posterior distribution via Bayes' theorem (McNamara & Houston, 1980). Although the ideas of prior and posterior distributions are very general, specifying them can be quite parochial. In practice, we have to make 'educated' guesses as to what specific priors and updating functions seem biologically plausible in any specific context since measuring them directly is often impractical for even the simplest scenarios.
- **Sampling information and information channels**. For an information problem to exist, an animal needs some way of discovering things that will update the prior to a posterior. Most combinations of sensory, cognitive and physiological processes can be involved: any environmental change that induces a change in a receiver can generate a posterior. SDT assumes that current communication systems are functional (i.e. have reached an equilibrium), because selection has acted to shape changes in signaller phenotype to facilitate the updating

of receiver priors – or, in other words, to make it easier for receivers to understand the signaller's message and respond appropriately. Therefore, key factors include the environment in which signals are elicited (e.g. signal detection problems) and the information-processing capacities (e.g. sensory and cognitive characteristics) of receivers.

- **Information and receiver action**. In SDT, the information that generates the posterior distribution (by updating the prior) is valuable because it influences the receiver's actions. In a well-formulated model, we can calculate the optimal action and the fitness consequences of any given posterior distribution; ultimately, for environmentally induced changes to have informational value, the posterior must change the functioning of an organism in an evolutionarily relevant manner (Stephens, 1989; McNamara & Dall, 2010). For animal communication, this emphasises the importance of signals' being shaped by their ability to change (or even manipulate) receiver behaviour (Maynard Smith & Harper, 2003).

When we have clearly specified these three components of the communication system, we can use SDT to ask several sorts of questions – for instance, if the animal can receive or elicit signals via multiple modalities, which is better? How much would the receiver pay to detect a signal? Is there an optimal strategy for signal assessment? Moreover, SDT offers a natural framework within which to integrate approaches to animal communication that emphasise the information content of signals (reviewed in Scott-Phillips, 2008) with those that focus on how signallers influence receiver behaviour (e.g. Maynard Smith & Harper, 2003). The former is specified in the way in which signal detection updates receiver priors, while the latter can be quantified when the changes in behaviour resulting from prior updating are specified. Thus, statistical decision theory is a framework for thinking about information problems within which communication and signalling fit naturally. Box 3.1 illustrates how SDT can be applied to signalling problems.

3.3 Issues in animal communication from a statistical decision theory perspective

The following subsections highlight how SDT can be used to re-frame several outstanding issues in the study of animal communication. This list is not intended to be exhaustive, but instead to indicate the variety of topics that can be addressed through an SDT approach.

3.3.1 *Identifying signals and receivers*

One of the most difficult tasks for animal communication researchers is identifying signals in the first place. Male eastern bluebirds (*Sialia sialis*), for instance, have (to human eyes) brilliant blue feathers on their heads, backs and wings, and deep orange feathers on their breasts and vents (Hubbard, 2008); they sing a complex and variable song (Huntsman & Ritchison, 2002; Kight, 2010); and they often use partially built nests as a sort of extended phenotype (Gowaty & Plissner, 1998). Which of these characteristics and behaviours, if any, is a signal? SDT suggests that the phenotypic traits with the strongest impacts on behaviour and fitness are those most likely to act as signals. This focus on signal variation is also helpful in determining which characteristics (e.g. time, frequency and/or amplitude of a vibrational signal; hue, brightness and/or chroma of a colour patch; Grill & Rush, 2000) encode information.

Even once a signal has been identified, human observers may have difficulty pinpointing the intended receiver. Some male cuttlefish, for example, may masquerade as females in order to gain matings (Norman, Finn & Tregenza, 1999). Is this signal intended more for the females who are eventually wooed, or for the males who fail to recognise a potential rival? Could there even be other advantages to this visual display, such as reducing visibility to certain types of predators or potential prey? In this and many other systems, there are likely to be multiple intended or possible receivers, each exerting different selection pressures on the signal and its display. It is not yet clear what the effects are of having a diverse audience. The relative strengths of selection pressures generated by each receiver should vary depending on the particulars of individual species' environments and life histories, but it is also likely that broad patterns may emerge that allow researchers to predict which signal features may have been shaped by which type of receiver, or whether different audience members are the primary or secondary target of a display. Such analyses fit naturally into an SDT framework, within which those types of individuals most affected by variations in influential phenotypic traits are best thought of as the evolved receivers. It is possible to determine the relative importance of multiple potential receivers (including 'unintended' receivers such as eavesdroppers, e.g. Johnstone, 2001), since SDT considers which of these have their behaviour changed in the most impactful way. This is done from the joint perspectives of both receiver and signaller fitness. In fact, a communication system will only be at evolutionary equilibrium (i.e. when we can sensibly identify evolved signallers and receivers) when the fitnesses of signallers and receivers are simultaneously maximised (i.e. cannot be improved by any party changing its behaviour unilaterally). This offers a powerful *a priori* means to hypothesise about components of such systems by deploying the array of formal techniques, such as evolutionary game theory, available to modern evolutionary theorists.

3.3.2 *Identifying or predicting relevant communication modalities*

A related question is what determines which modalities a species will use, or emphasise, when communicating. In some cases, the answer is obvious; for example, species that live in caves or in the deep sea are generally unlikely to rely on visual signals (but see Bush, Robison & Caldwell, 2009). But for an animal that is communicating with a receiver possessing, for instance, both eyes and ears, what factors determine whether the signaller utilises a visual, acoustic or complex signal? Current environmental conditions will have an important influence – acoustic signals may be more useful over long distances or in dark habitats, for instance, while visual signals might be superior over short distances and in well-lit habitats. Where these features are fairly equal, however, why might one modality be preferable to another? The SDT approach suggests that such issues will be resolved by determining the channel that maximises the reliability of signal impact on receiver behaviour over the range of environmental conditions typically experienced by the receivers in question; thus, SDT offers a way to structure research efforts, although in practice this may be challenging. Furthermore, the explicitly economic perspective enforced by SDT suggests that costs of using the different channels (e.g. energy, time, lost opportunity; Stephens & Krebs, 1986) will shape such aspects of animal communication systems.

3.3.3 *Understanding signal variety*

Seyfarth and Cheney (2003) recently asked why we find both 'general' and 'specific' stimuli, sometimes within the same species. Golden-marmots (*Marmota caudate*), for example, are known to produce 'situationally specific' vocalisations (Blumstein, 1995), whereas other species such as the putty-nosed monkey (*Cercopithecus nictitans martini*) apply a single type of alarm call to all situations (Arnold, Pohlner & Zuberbuehler, 2008). Does this merely reflect differences in cognitive abilities, or are there other reasons for these variations? Thinking about priors and how they are updated and then used may shed some light here. SDT states that it is crucial to identify the key elements that will influence receiver decisions and to determine when similar receiver responses will be adaptive in different contexts (Smith, 1965). If the same aspect of the signaller (e.g. its competitive ability) is crucial information for all receivers, or if the same response will suffice to cope within multiple signal contexts (e.g. one antipredator response will function well against many different predators), then the same signal is likely to be used in multiple contexts.

Over time, individual receivers may respond differently to the same signals, or shift their interest to a new type of signal. In bowerbirds, for example, young females seem to feel threatened when courting males perform their visual displays too vigorously; older females, however, prefer displays that are more intense (Coleman, Patricelli & Borgia, 2004). If a vigorous display is a reliable sign of quality, then a female might reasonably be expected to prefer that signal at all times of her life if she is interested in choosing the fittest mate. Why, then, should female responses to male displays differ over time, and, furthermore, why should females of different ages focus on different male signals? Such questions are best addressed in an SDT framework using state-dependent optimisation techniques (Houston & McNamara, 1999) to ascertain optimal responses and the information value of different types of signals when individuals are in different states (e.g. age or condition). Further, the features of adaptive information use specified by SDT will prove useful in understanding situations where, as with the bowerbirds, it might pay for a signaller to 'scale down' a particular signal, either to a specific level or below a given threshold. Investigations of these situations should focus on details of prior–posterior updating (Box 3.1), properties of information channels and the evolutionary utility of information obtained at different signal intensities. Such work might also shed some light on the concept of signaller 'self-images' – including how they are generated and how prior estimates of 'quality' (e.g. competitive ability) are updated over individual life histories.

3.3.4 *Understanding signal 'individuality'*

In some species, signal variety is so great that it can be used to identify particular individuals. In some singing species, for example, a male's song can provide information on identity, condition, whether the performer is native to the area and what his developmental conditions were (Marler & Tamura, 1962; Nowicki *et al.*, 1998; Holzer *et al.*, 2003). Individual-specific signals are likely to be most relevant in species where individuals encounter each other multiple times during the course of a single life cycle, and thus might find it useful to recognise other animals with which they share a history. So why, then, is individuality of signals not ubiquitous across such species? Under what circumstances was individuality likely to have evolved, and under what conditions should we expect it to be most common? Within systems where signallers have unique signals, which receivers are most likely to use that information? Again, the economics of information use encapsulated in SDT can be revealing in this context.

Box 3.1 Applying statistical decision theory to signalling

In order to examine how statistical decision theory can be applied to signalling, it is useful to work through a basic model describing receiver–signaller interactions in a hypothetical system where there are multiple potential responses to a received signal, as well as multiple potential receiver states. Imagine, for instance, that the receiver is a female bird looking for a potential mate during the breeding season. She uses males' songs to assess their quality and to decide which males to interact with.

A signalling male can exist in one of three states, each of which will elicit different reactions from the female: S_1 (high condition), S_2 (moderate condition) and S_3 (low condition). This is only one example of a suite of states; others might describe a male's size, the quality of his territory, where he is from and so on. Overall, the prior likelihoods of the three states are given by the distributions p_1, p_2 and p_3. The male will use prior knowledge of his own state to select the appropriate signal (S1, S2 or S3, respectively).

We can assume that it is to the receiver's advantage to adopt a different action appropriate to each state. In situations where the male is advertising high condition, S_1, the female should immediately engage him (a_1) in order to ensure that she procures the best mate available. On the other hand, when the male's song indicates that he is only of moderate (S_2) or low (S_3) condition, the female might be increasingly selective in her responses (a_2 and a_3, respectively), as she should be unwilling to mate with an individual with poor genes and/or an inability to compete for sufficient resources.

If the female does not have detailed information about the state of the environment (in this case, the correlation between a certain type of signal and a male's condition), she will use previous information, or priors, to decide upon the best course of action; this is equally true regardless of whether the receiver does not have information because she does not seek it (as shown in the top two boxes in Figure 3.1) or because she waits for a signal but does not receive one (as shown in the bottom left box). Under all three circumstances, she should adopt the action that is best on average (e.g. abandon mate choice and do something else, such as forage), which we will call a^*; this is associated with an expected gain of g^*. If, however, the receiver knows the current state of the male, she can adopt the appropriate action, a_i (where i indicates actions 1, 2 or 3, corresponding to states 1, 2 or 3, respectively; as shown in the bottom right box in Figure 3.1).

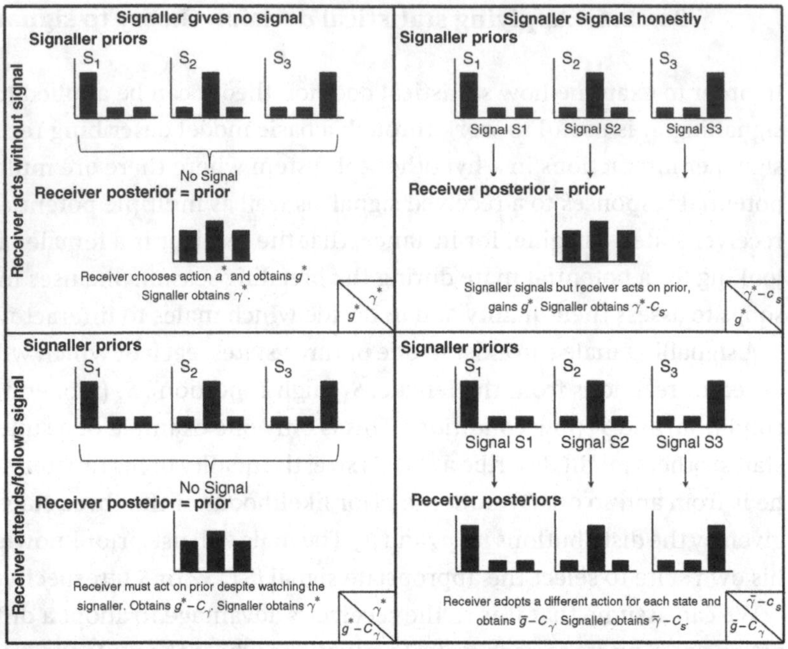

Figure 3.1 A diagrammatic representation of a signaller–receiver game matrix from a Bayesian perspective. The figure considers a situation in which a signaller 'knows' the underlying state of interest to the receiver and can choose to signal it or not; and the receiver, limited to prior information, can choose to act, or not, on 'more detailed' information provided by the signal. As described in more detail in the text, an example of this would be a female songbird listening to the singing display of a potential mate whose song indicates whether he is of high, moderate or low condition; depending on which of these three states is advertised, the female's potential appropriate responses might be immediately making contact with the male; waiting for a second vocal performance before making any mating decisions; or ignoring the male completely. **The combination 'Emit Signal/Use Signal' is in equilibrium (e.g. is an evolutionarily stable strategy, or ESS) if $\bar{\gamma} - c_s > \gamma^*$, and $\bar{g} - c_r > g^*$.** In other words, for the signalling system to persist, the signaller must, *on average*, benefit from the state-appropriate actions of the receiver, and the receiver must also experience improved performance by adopting an action appropriate to each state. The figure shows how the machinery of Bayesian inference can be used to characterise these quantities. In each cell, the upper row of histograms shows the signaller's information state. Within each histogram, bars represent the likelihoods of each state (from left to right, p_1, p_2 and p_3). The signaller's state can be determined by observing which bar is tallest; thus, the left histogram indicates a male in S_1 (or, keeping with the songbird example, high condition), while the middle and right histograms indicate males in S_2 and S_3 (or moderate and low condition), respectively. Note that it is possible for males to be classified as low, moderate or high condition even when there is a low probability associated with the other two states; this is

Thus, the expected payoff for a perfectly informed receiver is $\bar{g} = \Sigma p_i g_i$. In any given situation, we assume that the signaller (in this case, the singing male) knows his state (albeit with some degree of uncertainty) and can choose to emit a signal that accurately represents this state. The payoff that a signaller gains from this signal will vary according to both the receiver's actions and the current state. When the female immediately responds to a high-condition male (action a_1 in state S_1) the signaller's payoff is γ_1; likewise, payoffs are γ_2 and γ_3, respectively, when action a_2 occurs in S_2, and action a_3 occurs in S_3. It follows that the signaller's expected payoff from the actions of a well-informed receiver are $\bar{\gamma} = \Sigma p_i \gamma_i$. On the other hand, γ^* is the average benefit the signaller receives if the receiver adopts its default action a^*.

Both the receiver and the signaller must pay costs associated with this social transaction. In the case of the receiver, attending to the signal costs c_r units of benefit; this results from the time, energy and attention devoted to the communication process. This cost is paid even in the absence of a signal: the female songbird, for example, might forfeit potential feeding time in favour of sitting and listening for a male's vocalisation; alternatively, waiting to hear the song of a male who is absent from his territory might cost the female an opportunity to mate with a high-condition male elsewhere. These lost opportunities are responsible for the difference in payoffs between the top left and bottom left boxes in Figure 3.1. In the case of the signaller, emitting the signal costs c_s units; for a male songbird, this can be thought of as the calories burned while producing the vocalisation, or the danger of acoustic exposure to nearby predators.

Caption for Figure 3.1 (cont.)

because even a signaller's knowledge of its own condition (e.g. relative quality) may be somewhat uncertain. The lower histogram(s) in each cell shows the information that the receiver acts upon. In the top and bottom left cells, the receiver utilises only its priors; all three bars in the histogram are fairly equal, showing there is high uncertainty in these situations. In the bottom right cell, however, the receiver can take advantage of the signal in order to generate posteriors and generate a more situation-specific (appropriate) response. The box in the lower right corner of each cell shows, in traditional game matrix form, the payoffs for a given strategy combination; the variable or equation in the bottom half indicates the receiver's payoffs, while the signaller's payoffs are indicated in the top half.

For instance, formal analyses (e.g. Eliassen *et al.*, 2007) have revealed that the value of information varies with residual reproductive value; it may be less crucial for older individuals to know the detailed characteristics (e.g. exact individualised quality) of a mate or opponent, when it would suffice to simply know that the mate/opponent is in, say, the top half of the distribution of some relevant trait. This is because the high-grade information needed to establish individuality may require more time and energy than are worth expending given the number of reproductive opportunities available to a receiver.

3.3.5 *Explaining dishonesty and deception*

Researchers have long pondered how, and whether, a communication system could persist when it contained a disconnect between what an animal signalled and what was actually true – in other words, misinformative signalling, or 'dishonesty'[1] (Johnstone & Grafen, 1993; Rowell, Ellner & Reeve, 2006). Both empirical and theoretical studies have shown how dishonesty can be useful, as well as how it can endure (Bywater, Angilletta & Wilson, 2008; Hamblin & Hurd, 2009; Heinze & d'Ettorre, 2009; Laidre, 2009; Szalai & Szamado, 2009; Bro-Jorgensen & Pangle, 2010). SDT has been at the heart of this understanding: when a system is at a signalling equilibrium, where neither signaller nor receiver can gain by changing its behaviour unilaterally, signals are always informative on average. Nevertheless, receivers can be disadvantaged by responding to signals under some of the conditions at which the equilibrium persists (Johnstone & Grafen, 1993). This offers animals interesting possibilities for the strategic manipulation of social partners using information. The details behind the success of dishonesty, however, are less clear (Fitch & Hauser, 2002). For instance, what process leads to the use of dishonesty among signallers? How do receivers know when a signaller is being dishonest – do they learn to tell the difference between 'truth' and 'lies' and, if so, how? Are there consequences of being discovered as a dishonest signaller, and, if so, what are they and how long do they last? Continued use of the SDT framework (Box 3.2) should help to elucidate the answers to these questions by predicting the evolutionary and ecological circumstances under which deception-related communication behaviours might arise and persist.

3.3.6 *Understanding the role of learning in animal communication*

In some cases, individual differences in signalling may result from variations in the learning process, as observed in, for instance, birds (Brenowitz &

[1] This may also be referred to as 'unreliable' signalling, as found in Hurd and Enquist (2005).

Box 3.2 'Deception' from a statistical decision theory perspective

Problem: Signallers can be one of two types, Honest (informative) or Deceptive (un- or misinformative). If a receiver receives a signal x from a sender, should the receiver act on this signal?

Priors and posteriors: To answer this question, we first find the probability[2] that the sender is honest given the signal. Let ρ_H be the proportion of signallers that are honest. Let $f_H(x)$ and $f_D(x)$ be the (prior) probabilities that the signal is x, given the sender is Honest and Dishonest, respectively. Then the posterior probability that the sender is Honest given signal x is given by Bayes' theorem as:

$$p_H(x) = \frac{\rho_H f_H(x)}{\rho_H f_H(x) + (1-\rho_H) f_D(x)} \qquad (3.1)$$

To illustrate this analysis suppose that the signal received is a random variable X (e.g. an intensity at which it is produced). In this simple example, an Honest signaller produces X with a probability drawn from a normal distribution with a mean of 6 and a variance of 1, while a Dishonest signaller might produce X according to a normal distribution where the mean is 4 and the variance is 1 (Figure 3.2). Thus, there is overlap in the potential signals received from the two types of signallers, but for a given ρ_H it is easy to see from Equation (3.1) that the (posterior) probability that the signaller is honest increases with increasing signal x (Figure 3.2).

Optimal actions: Suppose that the benefit from responding to the signal if the sender is Honest is a and the cost of responding if sender is Deceptive is b. Under these circumstances, the mean payoff for acting on this signal is $p_H(x)a - (1 - p_H(x))b$. The receiver should respond if this mean payoff is positive; i.e.

$$p_H(x) > \frac{b}{a+b} \qquad (3.2)$$

In the case of a normally distributed signal this will hold provided $x > \hat{C}(\rho_H)$. Not surprisingly, the critical threshold $\hat{C}(\rho_H)$ increases as the proportion of Honest signallers, ρ_H, decreases; i.e. the receiver should be more choosy the more likely the signaller is to be Dishonest (Figures 3.2 and 3.3).

[2] A *probability* indicates the likelihood associated with a discrete event. In order to calculate likelihoods associated with a continuum of outcomes, however, it is necessary to use a *probability density function*, which measures the area under a curve describing all potential probabilities.

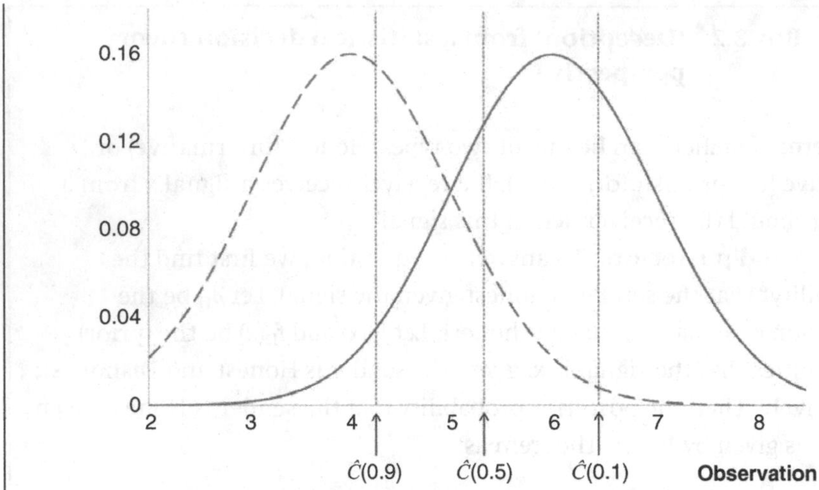

Figure 3.2 The probabilities, $f_H(x)$ and $f_D(x)$, that the signal is x given the sender is Honest (solid) and Dishonest (dashed), respectively. The probability density functions shown assume potential signals (e.g. display intensities) are drawn from normal distributions with means of 6 and 4, respectively (both with a variance of 1). Critical signalling thresholds, $\hat{C}(\rho_H)$, are shown for a range of proportions of signallers that are Honest (informative) in the population, $\rho_H = 0.1, 0.5, 0.9$. These are based on $a = 1$, $b = 2$ (critical posterior = 2/3: Equation (3.2)).

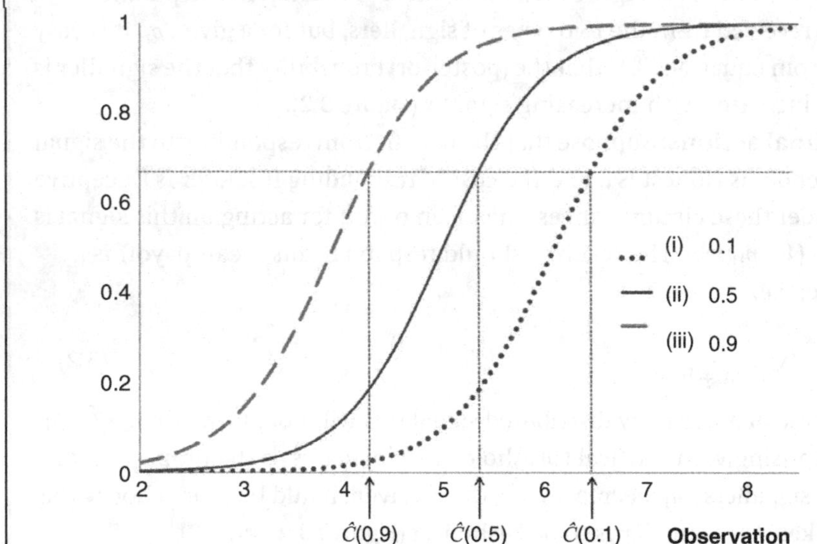

Figure 3.3 The posterior probabilities (calculated from Equation (3.1)) of being Honest (informative) given the signal (e.g. display intensity) observed for a range of proportions of signallers that are Honest in the population, $\rho_H = 0.1$ (dotted), 0.5 (solid), 0.9 (dashed). Critical signalling thresholds, $\hat{C}(\rho_H)$, are shown for each given $a = 1$, $b = 2$ (critical posterior = 2/3: Equation (3.2)).

The evolution of 'deception': To put this signalling problem into a wider biological context, suppose that genes determine whether a signaller is Honest or Dishonest, and that signals are costly to produce but advantageous to the sender if believed by the receiver (e.g. if the receiver uses this information to choose a mate). Under these circumstances, increases in the number of Dishonest signallers in the population will result in the evolution of increasingly choosy receivers. This will favour Honest signallers at the expense of Dishonest signallers, and hence reduce the proportion of the latter in the population. Thus, we expect an evolutionary equilibrium at which there are both Honest and Dishonest signallers in the population. At this equilibrium, receivers employ a threshold that performs best *on average*, although some Dishonest signallers will occasionally be believed. This explains how deception (i.e. un- or misinformative signalling) can evolve and persist in a population subject to Darwinian selection.

Beecher, 2005) and humans (Kuhl, 2004). Given that learning and flexibility are likely to improve an individual's ability to contend with both a changing audience and a variable environment, why are they not more ubiquitous within taxa (e.g. some bird species are 'open-ended' learners and continue learning new vocalisations throughout their lives, while other species are 'closed-ended learners', and do not; Brenowitz & Beecher, 2005) and among taxa? Learning has not generally been reported for other forms of signalling (but see Collis & Borgia, 1993), a dearth that probably stems not from its absence, but from the difficulty associated with quantifying it. In which systems might we expect learning, or at least phenotypic plasticity, to be most prevalent, and under what circumstances? A related question is why some animals use only innate signals, whereas others use a mixture of innate and learned. SDT-based analyses have formed the basis of many formal accounts of the evolution of learning (e.g. Stephens & Krebs, 1986; Stephens, 1991) and phenotypic plasticity (e.g. Leimar, Hammerstein & Van Dooren, 2006) and would therefore offer a natural framework within which to analyse the role of learning (and canalisation) in animal communication.

3.3.7 *Identifying genetic and morphological constraints on communication*

Variations in signalling among individuals may arise from differences in both genetic and morphological features. Although some genetic and molecular aspects of particular systems have been fairly well characterised (Shaw, 1996; Ferveur, 2005; Hubbard *et al.*, 2010), this is by no means a universal achievement; the most recent reviews of the communication literature are unanimous in urging more detailed mechanistic research in the future. Likewise, additional morphological and evolutionary work are needed in many systems to assess whether physical features have shaped signals, or vice versa (Podos, 2001). Because the SDT framework is ideal for evaluating the fitness value of signalling, it can offer insights into the communication-based selection pressures acting, at multiple biological levels, on the traits associated with signalling. Indeed, SDT has already been used to explore the role of heritable (genetically encoded) priors in non-communication animal information use (e.g. the use of socially inadvertent or abiotic cues; Leimar *et al.*, 2006; McNamara & Dall, 2011); similar analyses in a communication context are not only possible, but also should prove insightful.

3.4 Conclusions

Communication is influenced by a complex interplay of environment, learning, genes and the influences of social groups (Janik, 2000), and one of the major tasks of future research will be to tease apart the effects of these various pressures in order to determine how, when and to what extent they influence both signallers and receivers. In this chapter, we hope we have illustrated how statistical decision theory offers a natural framework within which to deal with such issues. For the most part, past research has focused overwhelmingly on signallers, with the result that we often only understand one end of the communication process in much detail. SDT emphasises the centrality of receivers in evolved information systems and so offers an opportunity to redress this balance. Among the signallers that have been studied, most are full-grown adults (though juvenile birds have been fairly well studied in this context); as a result, we have relatively little information on the forces that may shape signals of all modalities into their final forms. Again, thinking about priors and how they are updated over individual life histories offers a natural focus for such efforts. Furthermore, previous work has tended to focus repeatedly on the same group of study organisms, leading us to know a fair amount of detail about certain species and taxa, but comparatively little about others; as a result, it is also difficult to draw some broader phylogenetic conclusions about animal communication. In order to address these issues, it will be necessary to study non-traditional organisms in non-traditional habitats, including the deep sea. We may benefit from insights gained from studies of animal–plant, animal–bacteria and bacteria–bacteria systems, which, when examined alongside animal–animal systems, may enable us to make general inferences about communication among all life forms. Wherever such effort is directed, it is clear that statistical decision theory offers a very natural framework within which to investigate the outstanding issues in animal communication.

References

Arnold, K., Pohlner, Y. & Zuberbuhler, K. (2008). A forest monkey's alarm call series to predator models. *Behavioral Ecology and Sociobiology*, **62**, 549–559.

Ayasse, M., Paxton, R. J. & Tengö, J. (2001). Mating behavior and chemical communication in the order Hymenoptera. *Annual Review of Entomology*, **46**, 31–78.

Bailey, N. W. & Zuk, M. (2008). Acoustic experience shapes female mate choice in field crickets. *Proceedings of the Royal Society of London Series B: Biological Sciences*, **275**, 2645–2650.

Beckers, O. M. & Schul, J. (2008). Developmental plasticity of mating calls enables acoustic communication in diverse environments. *Proceedings of the Royal Society of London SeriesB: Biological Sciences*, **275**, 1243–1248.

Belanger, R. M. & Corkum, L. D. (2009). Review of aquatic sex pheromones and chemical communication in anurans. *Journal of Herpetology*, **43**, 184–191.

Blumstein, D. T. (1995). Golden-marmot alarm calls. I. The production of situationally specific vocalizations. *Ethology*, **100**, 113–125.

Borgia, G. (1985). Bower quality, number of decorations and mating success of male satin bowerbirds (*Ptilonorhynchus violaceus*): an experimental analysis. *Animal Behaviour*, **33**, 266–271.

Bradbury, J. W. & Vehrencamp, S. L. (2011). *Principles of Animal Communication, 2nd edn.* Sunderland, MA: Sinauer Associates.

Brenowitz, E. A. & Beecher, M. D. (2005). Song learning in birds: diversity and plasticity, opportunities and challenges. *Trends in Neurosciences*, **28**, 127–132.

Bro-Jorgensen, J. & Pangle, W. M. (2010). Male topi antelopes alarm snort deceptively to retain females for mating. *American Naturalist*, **17**, E33–E39.

Bruschini, C., Cervo, R. & Turillazzi, S. (2010). Pheromones in social wasps. *Vitamins and Hormones*, **83**, 521–549.

Bshary, R. & Würth, M. (2001). Cleaner fish *Labroides dimidiatus* manipulate client reef fish by providing tactile stimulation. *Proceedings of the Royal Society of London Series B: Biological Sciences*, **268**, 1495–1501.

Bush, S. L., Robison, B. H. & Caldwell, R. L. (2009). Behaving in the dark: locomotor, chromatic, postural, and bioluminescent behaviors of the deep-sea squid *Octopoteuthis deletron* Young 1972. *Biological Bulletin*, **216**, 7–22.

Bywater, C. L., Angilletta, M. J. & Wilson, R. S. (2008). Weapon size is a reliable indicator of strength and social dominance in female slender crayfish (*Cherax dispar*). *Functional Ecology*, **22**, 311–316.

Candolin, U. (2003). The use of multiple cues in mate choice. *Biological Reviews*, **78**, 575–595.

Caro, T. (2009). Contrasting coloration in terrestrial mammals. *Philosophical Transactions of the Royal Society B: Biological Sciences*, **364**, 537–548.

Christy, J. H., Backwell, P. R. Y., Goshima, S. & Kreuter, T. (2002). Sexual selection for structure building by courting male fiddler crabs: an experimental study of behavioral mechanisms. *Behavioral Ecology*, **13**, 366–374.

Coleman, S. W., Patricelli, G. L. & Borgia, G. (2004). Variable female preferences drive complex male displays. *Nature*, **428**, 742–745.

Collis, K. & Borgia, G. (1993). The costs of male display and delayed plumage maturation in the satin bowerbird (*Ptilonorhynchus violaceus*). *Ethology*, **94**, 59–71.

Costa-Leonardo, A. M. & Haifig, I. (2010). Pheromones and exocrine glands in Isoptera. *Vitamins and Hormones*, **83**, 521–549.

Dall, S. R. X. (2010). Managing risk, the perils of uncertainty. In D.F. Westneat & C.W. Fox, eds., *Evolutionary Behavioral Ecology*. Oxford: Oxford University Press, pp. 194–206.

Dall, S. R. X., Giraldeau, L.-A., Olsson, O., McNamara, J. M. & Stephens, D. W. (2005). Information and its use by animals in evolutionary ecology. *Trends in Ecology and Evolution*, **20**, 187–193.

Danchin, E., Giraldeau, L. A., Valone, T. J. & Wagner, R. H. (2004). Public information: from nosy neighbors to cultural evolution. *Science*, **305**, 487–491.

Delaney, K. J., Roberts, J. A. & Uetz, G. W. (2007). Male signalling behaviour and sexual selection in a wolf spider (Araneae: Lycosidae): a test for dual functions. *Behavioral Ecology and Sociobiology*, **62**, 67–75.

Dyakonova, V. & Krushinsky, A. (2008). Previous motor experience enhances courtship behavior in male cricket *Gryllus bimaculatus*. *Journal of Insect Behavior*, **21**, 172–180.

Eliassen, S., Jorgensen, C., Mangel, M. & Giske, J. (2007). Exploration or exploitation: life expectancy changes the value of learning in foraging strategies. *Oikos*, **116**, 513–523.

Ferveur, J.-F. (2005). Cuticular hydrocarbons: their evolution and roles in *Drosophila* pheromonal communication. *Behavior Genetics*, **35**, 279–295.

Fitch, W. T. & Hauser, M. D. (2002). Unpacking 'honesty': vertebrate vocal production and the evolution of acoustic signals. In A.M. Simmons, A.N. Popper & R.R. Fay, eds., *Acoustic Communication*. New York: Springer, pp. 65–137.

Fugere, V., Ortega, H. & Krahe, R. (2011). Electrical signalling of dominance in a wild population of electric fish. *Biology Letters*, **7**, 197–200.

Gera, C. & Srivastava, S. (2006). Quorum-sensing: the phenomenon of microbial communication. *Current Science*, **90**, 666–677.

Gordon, S. D. & Uetz, G. W. (2011). Multimodal communication of wolf spiders on different substrates: evidence for behavioural plasticity. *Animal Behaviour*, **81**, 367–375.

Gowaty, P. A. & Plissner, J. H. (1998). Eastern Bluebird (*Sialia Sialis*). In A. Poole & F. Gill, eds. *The Birds of North America*. Philadelphia, PA: Philadelphia Natural Academy of Sciences.

Grill, C. P. & Rush, V. N. (2000). Analysing spectral data: comparison and application of two techniques. *Biological Journal of the Linnean Society*, **69**, 121–138.

Groot, A. T., Classen, A., Staudacher, H., Schal, C. & Heckel, D. G. (2010). Phenotypic plasticity in sexual communication signal of a noctuid moth. *Journal of Evolutionary Biology*, **23**, 2731–2738.

Haddock, S. H. D., Moline, M. A. & Case, J. F. (2010). Bioluminescence in the sea. *Annual Review of Marine Science*, **2**, 443–493.

Hamblin, S. & Hurd, P. L. (2009). When will evolution lead to deceptive signaling in the Sir Philip Sidney game? *Theoretical Population Biology*, **75**, 176–182.

Harder, J. D. & Jackson, L. M. (2010). Chemical communication and reproduction in the gray short-tailed opossum (*Monodelphis domestica*). *Vitamins and Hormones*, **83**, 373–399.

Hebets, E. & Papaj, D. R. (2005). Complex signal function: developing a framework of testable hypotheses. *Behavioral Ecology and Sociobiology*, **57**, 197–214.

Heinze, J. & d'Ettorre, P. (2009). Honest and dishonest communication in social Hymenoptera. *Journal of Experimental Biology*, **212**, 1775–1779.

Holzer, B., Jacot, A. & Brinkhof, M. W. G. (2003). Condition-dependent signaling affects male sexual attractiveness in field crickets, *Gryllus campestris*. *Behavioral Ecology*, **14**, 353–359.

Houck, L. D. (2009). Pheromone communication in amphibians and reptiles. *Annual Review of Physiology*, **71**, 161–176.

Houston, A. I. & McNamara, J. M. (1999). *Models of Adaptive Behaviour, an Approach Based on State*. Cambridge: Cambridge University Press.

Hubbard, J. K. (2008). Female plumage coloration in eastern bluebirds, *Sialia sialis:* is it a sexually selected trait? Unpublished Master's thesis, College of William and Mary, Williamsburg, Virginia, USA.

Hubbard, J. K., Uy, J. A. C., Hauber, M. E., Hoekstra, H. E. & Safran, R. J. (2010). Vertebrate pigmentation: from underlying genes to adaptive function. *Trends in Genetics*, **26**, 231–239.

Huntsman, B. O. & Ritchison, G. (2002). Use and possible functions of large song repertoires by male eastern bluebirds. *Journal of Field Ornithology*, **73**, 372–378.

Hurd, P. L. & Enquist, M. (2005). A strategic taxonomy of biological communication. *Animal Behaviour*, **70**, 1155–1170.

Janik, V. M. (2000). The different roles of social learning in vocal communication. *Animal Behaviour*, **60**, 1–11.

Johnstone, R. A. (2001). Eavesdropping and animal conflict. *Proceedings of the National Academy of Sciences USA*, **98**, 9177–9180.

Johnstone, R. A. & Grafen, A. (1993). Dishonesty and the handicap principle. *Animal Behaviour*, **46**, 759–764.

Kight, C. R. (2010). Acoustics of anthropogenic habitats: the impact of noise pollution on eastern bluebirds. Unpublished PhD dissertation, College of William and Mary, Williamsburg, Virginia, USA.

Kuhl, P. K. (2004). Early language acquisition: cracking the speech code. *Nature Reviews Neuroscience*, **5**, 831–843.

Kulahci, I. G., Dornhaus, A. & Papaj, D. R. (2008). Multimodal signals enhance decision making in foraging bumble-bees. *Proceedings of the Royal Society of London Series B: Biological Sciences*, **275**, 797–802.

Laidre, M. E. (2009). How often do animals lie about their intentions? An experimental test. *American Naturalist*, **173**, 337–346.

Lea, A. J., Barrera, J. P., Tom, L. M. & Blumstein, D. T. (2008). Heterospecific eavesdropping in a nonsocial species. *Behavioral Ecology*, **19**, 1041–1046.

Leimar, O., Hammerstein, P. & Van Dooren, T. J. M. (2006). A new perspective on developmental plasticity and the principles of adaptive morph determination. *American Naturalist*, **167**, 367–376.

Lishak, R. S. (1984). Alarm vocalizations of adult gray squirrels. *Journal of Mammalogy*, **65**, 681–684.

Lugli, M., Yan, H. Y. & Fine, M. L. (2003). Acoustic communication in two freshwater gobies: the relationship between ambient noise, hearing thresholds and sound spectrum. *Journal of Comparative Physiology A*, **189**, 309–320.

Magrath, R. D., Pitcher, B. J. & Gardner, J. L. (2007). A mutual understanding? Interspecific responses by birds to each other's aerial alarm calls. *Behavioral Ecology*, **18**, 944–951.

Marler, P. & Slabbekoorn, H. (2004). *Nature's Music*. Amsterdam: Elsevier Academic Press.

Marler, P. & Tamura, M. (1962). Song 'dialects' in three populations of white-crowned sparrows. *Condor*, **64**, 368–377.

Mäthger, L. M., Denton, E. J., Marshall, N. J. & Hanlon, R. T. (2009). Mechanisms and behavioural functions of structural coloration in cephalopods. *Journal of the Royal Society Interface*, **6**, S149–S163.

Maynard Smith, J. & Harper, D. (2003). *Animal Signals*. Oxford: Oxford University Press.

McCowan, B., Doyle, L. R. & Hanser, S. F. (2002). Using information theory to assess the diversity, complexity, and development of communicative repertoires. *Journal of Comparative Psychology*, **116**, 166–172.

McNamara, J. M. & Dall, S. R. X. (2010). Information is a fitness enhancing resource. *Oikos*, **119**, 231–236.

McNamara, J. M. & Dall, S. R. X. (2011). The evolution of unconditional strategies via the 'multiplier effect'. *Ecology Letters*, **14**, 237–243.

McNamara, J. M. & Houston, A. I. (1980). The application of statistical decision-theory to animal behavior. *Journal of Theoretical Biology*, **85**, 673–690.

McNamara, J. M., Green, R. F. & Olsson, O. (2006). Bayes' theorem and its applications in animal behaviour. *Oikos*, **112**, 243–251.

Norman, M. D., Finn, J. & Tregenza, T. (1999). Female impersonation as an alternative reproductive strategy in giant cuttlefish. *Proceedings of the Royal Society of London Series B: Biological Sciences*, **266**, 1347–1349.

Nowicki, S., Peters, S. & Podos, J. (1998). Song learning, early nutrition and sexual selection in songbirds. *American Zoologist*, **38**, 179–190.

Patricelli, G. L., Uy, J. A. C. & Borgia, G. (2003). Multiple male traits interact: attractive bower decorations facilitate attractive behavioural displays in satin bowerbirds. *Proceedings of the Royal Society of London Series B: Biological Sciences*, **270**, 2389–2395.

Podos, J. (2001). Correlated evolution of morphology and vocal signal structure in Darwin's finches. *Nature*, **409**, 185–188.

Pope, D. S. & Haney, B. R. (2008). Interspecific signalling competition between two hood-building fiddler crab species, *Uca latimanus* and *U. musica musica*. *Animal Behaviour*, **76**, 2037–2048.

Pratt, S. C. (2005). Quorum sensing by encounter rates in the ant *Temnothorax albipennis*. *Behavioral Ecology*, **16**, 488–496.

Rabin, L. A., McCowan, B., Hooper, S. L. & Owings, D. H. (2003). Anthropogenic noise and its effect on animal communication: an interface between comparative psychology and conservation biology. *International Journal of Comparative Psychology*, **16**, 172–192.

Raguso, R. A. (2008). Wake up and smell the roses: the ecology and evolution of floral scent. *Annual Review of Ecology, Evolution, and Systematics*, **39**, 549–569.

Rendall, D., Owren, M. J. & Ryan, M. J. (2009). What do animal signals mean? *Animal Behaviour*, **78**, 233–240.

Rose, T. A., Munn, A. J., Ramp, D. & Banks, P. B. (2006). Foot-thumping as an alarm signal in macropodoid marsupials: prevalence and hypotheses of function. *Mammal Review*, **36**, 281–298.

Rosenthal, G. G. (2007). Spatiotemporal dimensions of visual signals in animal communication. *Annual Review of Ecology, Evolution, and Systematics*, **38**, 155–178.

Rowell, J. T., Ellner, S. P. & Reeve, H. K. (2006). Why animals lie: how dishonesty and belief can coexist in a signalling system. *American Naturalist*, **168**, E180–E204.

Schaedelin, F. C. & Taborsky, M. (2009). Extended phenotypes as signals. *Biological Reviews*, **84**, 293–313.

Schaefer, H. M., Schaefer, V. & Levey, D. J. (2004). How plant–animal interactions signal new insights in communication. *Trends in Ecology and Evolution*, **19**, 577–584.

Schmidt, K. A., Dall, S. R. X. & Gils, J. A. v. (2010). The ecology of information: an overview on the ecological significance of making informed decisions. *Oikos*, **119**, 304–316.

Scott-Phillips, T. C. (2008). Defining biological communication. *Journal of Evolutionary Biology*, **21**, 387–395.

Seyfarth, R. M. & Cheney, D. L., (2003). Signalers and receivers in animal communication. *Annual Review of Psychology*, **54**, 145–173.

Shabani, S., Kamio, M. & Derby, C. D. (2009). Spiny lobsters use urine-borne olfactory signaling and physical aggressive behaviors to influence social status of conspecifics. *Journal of Experimental Biology*, **212**, 2464–2474.

Shaw, K. L. (1996). Polygenic inheritance of a behavioral phenotype: interspecific genetics of song in the Hawaiian cricket genus *Laupala*. *Evolution*, **50**, 256–266.

Smith, W. J. (1965). Message, meaning, and context in ethology. *American Naturalist*, **99**, 405–409.

Stephens, D. W. (1989). Variance and the value of information. *American Naturalist*, **134**, 128–140.

Stephens, D. W. (1991). Change, regularity, and value in the evolution of animal learning. *Behavioral Ecology*, **2**, 77–89.

Stephens, D. W. & Krebs, J. R. (1986). *Foraging Theory*. Princeton, NJ: Princeton University Press.

Szalai, F. & Szamado, S. (2009). Honest and cheating strategies in a simple model of aggressive communication. *Animal Behaviour*, **78**, 949–959.

Terman, C. R. (1980). Factors influencing delayed reproductive maturation in prairie deermice (*Peromyscus maniculatus bairdii*) in laboratory populations. *Journal of Mammalogy*, **61**, 219–223.

Thiel, M. & Breithaupt, T. (2011). Chemical communication in crustaceans: research challenges for the twenty-first century. In T. Breithaupt & M. Thiel, eds., *Chemical Communication in Crustaceans*. New York: Springer, pp. 3–22.

Touhara, K. (2008). Sexual communication via peptide and protein pheromones. *Current Opinion in Pharmacology*, **8**, 759–764.

Wiley, R. H. (1994). Errors, exaggeration, and deception in animal communication. In L.A. Real, ed., *Behavioral Mechanisms in Evolutionary Ecology*. Chicago, IL: University of Chicago Press, pp. 157–189.

Wiley, R. H. (2006). Signal detection and animal communication. *Advances in the Study of Behavior*, **36**, 217–247.

Wiley, R. H. & Richards, D. G. (1982). Adaptations for acoustic communication in birds: sound propagation and signal detection. In D.E. Kroodsma & E.H. Miller, eds., *Acoustic Communication in Birds*, Vol. 1. New York: Academic Press, pp. 131–181.

Wilkins, H. D. & Ritchison, G. (1999). Drumming and tapping by red-bellied woodpeckers: description and possible causation. *Journal of Field Ornithology*, **70**, 578–586.

Wilkinson, G. S. & Dodson, G. N. (1997). Function and evolution of antlers and eye stalks in flies. In J.C. Choe & B.J. Crespi, eds., *The Evolution of Mating Systems in Insects and Arachnids*. Cambridge: Cambridge University Press, pp. 310–327.

Wyatt, T. D. (2010). Pheromones and signature mixtures: defining species-wide signals and variable cues for identity in both invertebrates and vertebrates. *Journal of Comparative Physiology A*, **196**, 685–700.

Zhang, D., Terschak, J. A., Harley, M. A., Lin, J. & Hardege, J. D. (2011). Simultaneously hermaphroditic shrimp use lipophilic cuticular hydrocarbons as contact sex pheromones. *PLoS ONE* **6**, e17720.

Commentary

The application of decision theory to communication seems entirely correct to me and completely in accordance with the proposals in my chapter (Ch. 4) for the transfer of information in communication. Bayesian decision theory in which the context of a signal influences the optimal response is also in accordance with John Smith's early emphasis on the importance of the contexts of signals (Smith, 1965).

In other places, I have proposed combining decision theory and signal detection theory to understand animal communication (Wiley & Richards, 1982; Wiley, 1994, 2000, 2006). To avoid confusion, I have used the terms decision theory (DT) and signal detection theory (SDT), whereas this chapter uses SDT for statistical decision theory. A combination of decision theory and signal detection theory is particularly useful in explaining the evolution of deception in communication, as explained in the references above. The trade-off a receiver faces in adjusting its threshold for response in a noisy context can force it to accept some deception.

It is also worthwhile emphasising that decision theory can illuminate the behaviour of signallers as well as receivers. They too face decisions, in this case when, where and what to signal. As a result of trade-offs arising in part from responses by inappropriate receivers (eavesdroppers), a signaller must adjust the optimal situations and level of signalling. These trade-offs can force it to accept some exploitation (eavesdropping) by inappropriate receivers, just as a receiver's trade-offs can force it to accept some exploitation (deception) by inappropriate signallers.

Smith, W. J. (1965). Message, meaning, and context in ethology. *American Naturalist*, **99**, 405–409.

Wiley, R. H. (1994). Errors, exaggeration, and deception in animal communication. In L. Real, ed., *Behavioral Mechanisms in Evolutionary Ecology*. Chicago, IL: University of Chicago Press, pp. 157–189.

Wiley, R. H. (2000). Sexual selection and mate choice: trade-offs for males and females. In M. Apollonio, M. Festa-Bianchet & D. Mainardi, eds., *Vertebrate Mating Systems*. Singapore: World Scientific Publishing Co., pp. 8–46.

Wiley, R. H. (2006). Signal detection and animal communication. *Advances in the Study of Behavior*, **36**, 217–247.

Wiley, R. H. & Richards, D. G. (1982). Adaptations for acoustic communication in birds: sound propagation and signal detection. In D. E. Kroodsma & E. H. Miller, eds., *Acoustic Communication in Birds*, Vol. 1. New York: Academic Press, pp. 131–181.

R. Haven Wiley

4

Communication as a transfer of information: measurement, mechanism and meaning

R. HAVEN WILEY

4.1 Introduction

No one seems ever to have doubted that animals can communicate with each other. The evidence for communication has always seemed obvious – responses by one individual to the actions of another. In his extended discussions of animal behaviour, Darwin for instance took communication by animals for granted. Although he cited many reports of animals' responses to each other, he never made them the subject of his studies. Instead, he focused on evidence for continuity between humans and non-human animals in the evolution of mental processes. In *The Descent of Man, and Selection in Relation to Sex* (1871), he made an extended case that animals express many of the same emotions that humans do, even such mental activities as deceit, revenge, humour, deliberation and reason. In *The Expression of the Emotions in Man and Animals* (1873), he elaborated on phylogenetic continuity in the expression of many emotions – although not all of those he had mentioned previously. Furthermore, his principle of antithesis, that contrasting emotions tended to be associated with contrasting actions, suggested that animals' actions evolved by natural selection to promote communication.

The basic components of communication are now widely recognised – signaller, signal and receiver. To confirm that communication has occurred, it is thus necessary to show that one individual has produced a signal – a pattern of stimulation – to which another individual has responded. Experimental investigation of this process began with the use of simple models by early ethologists such as Niko Tinbergen (1951). In recent decades, presentations of audio and

Animal Communication Theory: Information and Influence, ed. Ulrich Stegmann. Published by Cambridge University Press.

video recordings and even robotic models have resulted in extensive experimental analysis of communication by animals.

Yet Darwin's principal claim remains controversial. Is there continuity between mental processes of humans and those of other animals? Even if the differences prove to be qualitative, can we measure the magnitude of the differences? As Darwin recognised, one of the central issues in these controversies is communication. What do animals communicate? And how much do they communicate? These questions are often phrased in terms of information. What information is communicated by animals? And how much?

This chapter addresses these questions in four steps. First, it reviews the concept of information in communication and thereby concludes that all communication must involve a transmission of information. Second, it considers, but rejects, the argument that information and manipulation are incompatible. Third, it argues that the transfer of information depends on mental processes of categorisation and association. Fourth, it addresses the issue of information about mental states of other individuals and ourselves. It concludes with an element of necessary ignorance.

4.2 Communication as a transfer of information

It is probably not a coincidence that the three components of communication – signaller, receiver and signal – were first identified in the decades following the invention and deployment of the telegraph. De Saussure's (1916 [1959]) diagram takes the telegraph as a metaphor for human language, and Ogden and Richards (1923) elaborate the model by emphasising the mental processes of the signaller and receiver. Linguists and philosophers now use these models routinely in their discussions of communication.

Further advances in engineering and the widespread adoption of telephones and electromagnetic radiation for human communication eventually led to competition for communication. How many radio stations could simultaneously operate in one area? How many conversations could simultaneously use one telephone line? Investigation of these practical issues revealed that communication had limits. To understand these limits, it was apparent that communication had to be measured. Shannon's (1948, 1963) pioneering contribution was to propose a measure of information and then to use it to demonstrate mathematically that the properties of the connection between signaller and receiver – the channel – imposed a limit on the amount of information that could be transmitted in any period of time.

Shannon's measure of information in a set of i signals (H_o) equals $-\sum p_i \log_2 p_i$, with p_i being the probability of the ith signal. As Shannon explains, this particular expression is the only one that can satisfy our intuitive requirements for a measure of the amount of communication. This measure (H_O) is the number of binary decisions required to specify which signal in a message is next, or in other words to specify the occurrence of any one signal. It is thus the uncertainty in predicting the occurrence of any one signal. An informative message would have high uncertainty about the occurrence of any one signal (it would require many binary decisions to specify each signal's occurrence). Frequent use of just a few signals conveys less information than would many less frequent signals. An infrequent signal increases the amount of information in a message more than does a frequent signal.

A set of signals could consist of a sequence of signals in time or an arrangement of signals in space. Shannon's measure applies to both cases. In either case, identifying a set of signals often requires some method for segmenting the temporal or spatial continuity of an animal's actions into components. As Shannon shows, this segmentation is not necessary, because his conclusions still apply in the limit of continuously varying signals and responses. Nevertheless most attempts to measure information require segmentation of animals' actions into sets of signals and responses.

The concept of information as a measure of the degree of uncertainty in a pattern of signals contrasts with the usual concept of information as the degree of certainty a receiver acquires from signals. Shannon's definition of information thus seems contrary to any definition that others might accept as intuitively appropriate. The issue is whether information is a property of the structure of signals or of the state of the receiver.

The problems arising from the segmentation of actions and the nature of information have both resulted in distortions in how biologists think about information. Both have resulted in premature rejections of information in animal communication. The remainder of this section discusses the first of these issues, the segmentation of signals and responses. Subsequent sections take up the second issue, the receiver's state of mind.

The problem of segmentation arose during attempts to measure the amount of information in animals' displays. At the time it seemed that such measures would allow comparisons of communication by different species or different modalities. Attempts to measure the information in the displays of rhesus macaques and hermit crabs (Altmann, 1965; Hazlett & Bossert, 1965) consisted of identifying a set of distinct actions and then estimating the probability of each in particular contexts. Ethologists had become accustomed to describing ethograms, discrete categories of actions for each species. Measuring the information in displays was just one of a number of ways that ethograms could be used to quantify behaviour. It became apparent, however, that any measure of information depended on how the observer chose to segment the animals' actions. In some cases, such as the songs and stereotyped displays of some birds, actions seem relatively invariant and discrete, although only in a few cases has variation actually been measured (Wiley, 1973). As a rule, however, animals' displays, including those of monkeys and crabs, consist of variable and intergrading actions. When an observer segments these variable displays into discrete categories, the number of categories and their boundaries have unknown relevance for the animals involved. As a result, measuring the amount of information in animal displays seems arbitrary, and comparisons of different species seem fruitless. Only a few studies have followed these precedents (Dingle, 1969; Steinberg & Conant, 1974).

The problem of segmentation is not insurmountable, however. The problem lies not with segmentation of animals' actions in itself but with identifying a segmentation relevant to the species under investigation, rather than one imposed by a human observer. Behavioural and neurophysiological experiments can determine how individuals classify stimulation. Yet we often do not know as much as we should.

Consider recognition of conspecific individuals. Many experiments have shown that animals respond to signals from their own species but not from others. In addition, they respond to signals from particular individuals but not others (Wiley & Wiley, 1977; Falls, 1982; Godard & Wiley, 1995). Recognition of young by parental birds provides a good example. Beecher and his students, for instance, have shown that adult cliff swallows recognise their own young while they are still in the nest, whereas adult barn swallows do not (Beecher *et al.*, 1986). When nestling barn swallows were experimentally exchanged between nests, parents responded to nestlings from another nest just as much as to those of their own. In contrast, parent cliff swallows did not feed others' young under any conditions. Playbacks of nestlings' calls confirmed this difference between the two species in parental recognition of young. Furthermore, the calls of nestling cliff swallows vary more among individuals than those of barn swallows, as expected if they encode more information about individual identity. Because the nests of cliff swallows are clustered in dense colonies, while those of barn swallows are dispersed, only among cliff swallows might parents or young occasionally enter the wrong nest. Since cliff swallows build flask-shaped nests of mud, so the young inside are in nearly complete darkness, it makes sense that the nestlings' vocalisations have evolved to promote parental recognition.

Although parent cliff swallows recognise their own young at least collectively, it is not known whether or not they can go a step farther to recognise each of their young individually. Individual recognition of this sort would require that parents respond to each offspring in a distinctive way. Current experiments indicate only that parents distinguish familiar nestlings' calls from unfamiliar ones.

These classic experiments demonstrate two important points. First, animal communication does convey information, in this case the identity of offspring, and, moreover, the analogous signals of two different species can differ in the amount of information conveyed. Second, even in species for which transmission of information has been demonstrated, it is a more difficult task to determine how much information this is. In particular, we do not know whether parents recognise their young collectively or each one individually. The difference is between a binary discrimination (between categories of their own young and all others) and a more complex discrimination (between as many as six individual young). In this case the units of classification (individual organisms) are clear, and we understand something about how swallows of different species classify these units, but there remain open questions about the complexity of this classification (Wiley, 2013).

Even when units of classification are apparent, actual signals and responses themselves are likely to vary continuously or at least in complex ways. This complexity makes it difficult to measure the amount of information in signals. Beecher and colleagues (Beecher, 1989; Medvin, Stoddard & Beecher, 1993) have estimated the potential amount of information in the vocalisations of nestling barn and cliff swallows by measuring variation in many different features of frequency and timing and then reducing this variation to a set of independent principal components. They could then use the standard deviations of these principal components to estimate the potential amount of information, in binary units, that these vocalisations contain. This estimate is an upper limit for the amount of information transmitted from signaller to receiver. To determine the actual amount of information transferred would require experiments to document the association between variation in signals and variation in responses.

Haldane and Spurway (1954) had earlier used similar procedures to determine the amount of information transmitted by the waggle dances of honeybees. Variation in the directions of honeybees' foraging flights provided an estimate of the amount of directional information that foraging bees obtained from waggle dances. Error in the mean direction of foraging flights provided an estimate of the amount of information in the dances themselves. Haldane and Spurway concluded that the dances appeared to contain two to three bits of information more than the accompanying foragers received. Recent measurements have shown that variation in the directions of the dances themselves depends on the distance or nature (food or nest site) of the target (Towne & Gould, 1988; Weidenmüller & Seeley, 1999; Tanner & Visscher, 2010). Similar procedures have been used to estimate the amount of information in the odour trails of ants (Wilson, 1962).

These cases show that determining the amount of information in animal signals must clear some technical hurdles (Pfeifer, 2006), but they also indicate that this process is important if we wish to understand the complexity of animal communication. As discussed below, understanding the categorisation of stimulation by animals is critical for any understanding of the evolution of communication.

4.3 Manipulation versus information

Prior to the development of rigorous thinking about the evolution of cooperation, it had always seemed that communication was an example of cooperation. Signallers provided information that receivers used. In *The Behavior of Communicating* (1980), Smith took this point for granted. He identified the 'message' of a signal as the association between a signaller's action and its current state (its neural and physiological state, including its disposition to act in particular ways and its perception of its environment). Thus the message of a signal might be that the signaller is likely to fight if attacked, that it has just seen a predator approaching, that it is in excellent physical condition or that it is a particular species or individual. Marler (1961) had earlier discussed the ways in which signals are associated with states of signallers. Smith then identified the 'meaning' of a signal as the association between the signal and the receiver's responses. He made the important point that signals with the same message could have different meanings for receivers, as a result of differences in a receiver's context and state. Much of Smith's own work focused on determining the associations between the signals produced by birds and their contexts and states.

Although these early analyses assumed that communication had mutual advantages for signaller and receiver, they nevertheless emphasised two undeniable features of communication. Signals include information only by virtue of their associations with the states (including contexts) of signallers. They transmit information only by virtue of their associations with the responses of receivers.

Rejecting the assumptions that communication is necessarily mutually beneficial to the participants, Dawkins and Krebs (1978; Krebs & Dawkins, 1984) argued that signals instead evolve by natural selection to manipulate receivers to respond in ways that provide advantages for the signaller, regardless of any advantages for the receiver. This position, however, raised the question of why receivers should respond to signals in ways that were disadvantageous for them. A possible answer is that signallers exploit sensory biases of receivers, in other words constraints on the way receivers respond to signals (Guilford & Dawkins, 1991; Arak & Enquist, 1993; Endler & Basolo, 1998; Ryan, 1998). Such constraints might occur when receivers have evolved to respond to particular signals in another context. For instance, if females respond to particular signals in finding food or shelter, a signal mimicking these signals might stimulate a female to respond to a male when she otherwise would not. Alternatively receivers might respond to exaggerated signals not normally produced by signallers, examples of supernormal stimuli, as a result of the retention of ancestral constraints on their nervous systems or as a result of peak shift in learning (Hogan, Kruijt & Frijlink, 1975; Lynn, Cnaani & Papaj, 2005; ten Cate & Rowe, 2007). Both of these proposals assume that receivers have not yet evolved more discriminating responses to sensory input.

A revision of this position came when Grafen (1990) emphasised that receivers must on average receive benefits from their responses, otherwise natural selection would tend to eliminate those responses. As a rule receivers should respond only to signals that convey information about (are associated with some feature of) the signaller that is useful to the receiver. Grafen attempted to confirm Zahavi's (1977) proposal that the cost of a signal guarantees its honesty, because for one reason or another the cost is too great for a deceptive signaller to bear (see also Zahavi, 1997). Searcy and Nowicki (2005), in their review of the evolution of communication, confirmed the three relevant points in this theory of honest signalling: (1) to qualify as signals, actions must at least occasionally evoke responses from receivers; (2) receivers must on average benefit from their responses; and (3) signals must convey information about signallers in ways related to their costs. For instance, females respond to signals associated with high-quality mates, and these signals have higher costs than those associated with low-quality mates. Searcy and Nowicki identify many examples of animal communication that meet these criteria.

These conditions for honest communication are close to the position that Smith advocated earlier, with the addition of a stipulation that signals are honest on average. The message of a signal is its association with the state of the signaller. Receivers on average benefit from their responses. Communication is on average honest and thus normally advantageous for both signaller and receiver. This revised position leaves open the possibility for manipulation, which occurs when signallers can take advantage of receivers by mimicking a signal that would in other contexts evoke a response beneficial to the receiver or when receivers can take advantage of signallers by eavesdropping on signals that would in other contexts evoke responses beneficial to the signaller. In all such cases receivers and signallers benefit on average from communication, although on infrequent occasions they are manipulated to their disadvantage.

Numerous such cases of manipulation are now known. For instance, birds occasionally give false alarms for predators in order to gain access to food that is otherwise monopolised by more dominant individuals (Møller, 1988), and some primates practise deception routinely (Whiten & Byrne, 1988; Cheney & Seyfarth, 1991; Mitchell & Anderson, 1997). It is now apparent that signals must, as a result of natural selection, evoke responses that have advantages for both signaller and receiver, at least on average. Manipulation is thus the exception that proves the rule (Wiley, 1994).

Recent discussions of the role of information in animal communication emphasise one aspect of these conclusions or another but are not actually in conflict (Owings & Morton, 1998; Rendall, Owren & Ryan, 2009; Seyfarth *et al.*, 2010). Signals do convey information about the signaller, and yet sometimes signals are manipulative. Everybody can agree that communication has three basic components: signals include information (about the signaller or its situation), receivers respond (overtly or covertly, with high or low probability), and both signallers and receivers benefit on average.

These conclusions do not resolve all problems raised by information in signals. Most people feel that the information in signals is more than a correlation with the internal or external state of the signaller. Instead, most people feel that information is about something – about something the signaller perceives or thinks. De Saussure (1916 [1959]) emphasised the relationship between a signal and the signaller's mind, and Ogden and Richards (1923) added an external referent to make a triangular relationship – signal, mind and referent – necessary to understand the 'meaning of meaning'. In the following sections, I pursue an engineering approach to information in order to address the 'meaning of meaning'.

4.4 Communication as categorisation and association

So far I have used the term 'signal' loosely. Engineers in fact never seem much concerned with a definition of a signal, although ethologists have perennially wrestled with a definition. Maynard Smith and Harper (2003), like Grafen (1990) previously, emphasised that a signal must have evolved for the purpose of evoking a response. They maintain that the condition of evolution distinguishes signals from 'cues', which include inanimate sources of stimulation that influence animals' behaviour. They also distinguish two kinds of signals – indices and handicaps – based on whether or not a signal is reliable because it cannot be faked or has excessive costs. All signals have costs, but handicaps have "strategic costs", costs in excess of "efficacy costs" which are those "needed to transmit the information unambiguously" (Maynard Smith & Harper, 2003, p. 7).

Shannon and Weaver (1963) defined ambiguity as the uncertainty in responses to a given signal (as opposed to equivocation, uncertainty in signals for a given response). Ambiguity and equivocation are the two components of noise in any system of communication. Ambiguity is a relationship between a signal and responses, not a property of a signal. In the real world, as Shannon realised, there is no communication without noise – no communication without ambiguity. Communication can have more or less ambiguity (and equivocation), more or less efficacy, if you will, but there is no transition between efficacious and 'strategic' communication, as Maynard Smith and Harper maintain. All the costs of an evolved signal contribute to efficacy, to reducing ambiguity by evoking an appropriate response.

Instead I have proposed a definition of a signal that does not require an antecedent understanding of its evolution (Wiley, 1994). A signal is any pattern of energy or matter that evokes a response without providing all of the power for that response. For instance, if a tree falls, shoving someone out of the way is not communication (the shove is not a signal because it provides sufficient energy to effect the movement of the recipient). A shout, "Heads up!", on the other hand, is a signal, provided the receiver sometimes responds, for instance by jumping out of the way. By this definition, the sound of the cracking trunk is also a signal, so that, if the hearer jumps away, communication has also occurred.

Two points need clarification. First, a system of communication includes many such instances of signals, not just one. It is characterised by probabilities, not isolated instances. Communication occurs even if on some occasions the recipient does not move. Second, although this definition includes inanimate sources of signals (which Maynard Smith and Harper and others would term cues), there is no essential distinction between these and signals from animate sources. However, animate sources can evolve, which raises the possibility that the properties of signals become optimised for communication, as Darwin's principle of antithesis had suggested. Because a signal does not provide all of the power for a response, the receiver must provide some, often most, of the power for the response. The signal of course must provide enough power to affect the receiver's sensory organs.

A receiver thus must have a nervous system (or some other feature of its physiology), which perceives a signal and then associates it with a response, and a musculoskeletal system (or in some organisms just a muscular system), which produces the response. The engineering equivalents are transducers, gates (switches) and amplifiers. The definition of a signal thus also defines a receiver – a mechanism with transducer, gate and amplifier.

Second, this definition makes it clear that the receiver is in control of communication. A receiver is a decision-making mechanism. It categorises impinging stimulation into perceived signals and associates perceived signals with responses. Animate receivers can evolve and thus optimise responses to a signal. As I have discussed elsewhere (Wiley, 1994, 2006) and as Grafen (1990) had previously recognised, such receivers should in all cases benefit on average from their responses to signals. They should evolve to minimise responses to unreliable or deceptive signals. In communication there is always the possibility of some deception or error, but unless responses to signals provide some benefit on average to a receiver, responding should evolve to cease completely.

Instead of pursuing questions about the evolution of communication, I want to emphasise here the decision-making property of receivers. One of their essential properties is categorising the stream of incoming stimulation. This is the process often called segmentation, by which discrete objects or units are identified in the continuous flood of stimulation. It is the basis of perception – a relationship between the properties of stimulation and the properties of the sensory components of the receiver's nervous system (the sense organs and higher sensory centres of the nervous system). The examples of recognition of conspecifics above are clear cases of the categorisation of sensory input. In fact, all communication involves such categorisation.

Furthermore, a receiver must associate perceived categories of stimulation (signals) with responses. As Sherrington (1906) long ago emphasised, one important function of all nervous systems is to associate each perceived category of stimulation with a particular response or suite of responses. The motor components of the nervous system, which control the musculoskeletal system, become the 'final common pathway'. Categorisation of stimulation and association of the resulting categories with responses are the two fundamental properties of an animate receiver – and indeed of any nervous system.

The process of categorising stimulation raises a question about the perceptual demarcations of categories. In general terms the rules for demarcation could be learned or innate. By innate, I mean developing in the absence of sufficient external information to specify the resulting rule. For instance, the striate cortex of mammals includes cells that develop into stripe detectors that respond only to strips of light in particular orientations at particular locations in the animal's visual field. It is now well known that these cells develop before birth in the absence of any exposure to patterns of light such as stripes (Hubel & Wiesel, 1963). Their development requires only environmental conditions sufficient for normal development of the brain in general. After the eyes open, the further development of these cells depends on subsequent environmental conditions, both general (exposure to light regardless of pattern) and specific (exposure to particular patterns of light, such as predominantly horizontal or predominantly vertical stripes). Nevertheless, under normal conditions for brain development, these cells develop initially to detect specific features without exposure to patterns of light.

Songbirds learn features of their songs, but they begin the process of learning with innate predispositions to attend to certain patterns of sound (in some cases, components of conspecific songs) or to sounds in certain situations (Marler, 1984; Marler & Peters, 1988). Without these initial (innate) predispositions, it is hard to imagine how a naïve bird could identify in the flood of incoming stimulation what it is that it should learn.

The importance of predispositions for learning had previously been emphasised by Lorenz (1966). Chomsky (1959, 1986) made the same point about the development of language in human children. Much earlier, Kant (1793 [1961]) had elaborated his philosophy from similar arguments for innate categories in all rational thought. Association without predisposition leads to chaos. With predispositions, association can produce the extraordinary complexity of animal and human behaviour, much if not most of which is communication in one form or another.

The expanded brain of humans no doubt allows greater complexity in categorisation and association. Quantitative increase in components can, in some sense, lead to qualitative differences in performance. Of course, recognising a qualitative difference is itself a form of categorisation. Humans are perhaps predisposed to recognise categories of human and non-human animals. So caution should temper any conclusion that human and non-human brains differ categorically.

4.5 Communication of states of mind

If the nervous systems of organisms, their brains in particular, are mechanisms for categorising stimulation and for associating the resulting categories with responses, are they sufficient to produce minds? Whether brains are sufficient explanations of minds is, of course, an old question in philosophy – perhaps, in one form or another, the only question. If an organism's mind is sufficiently explained by its brain, then the minds of other organisms are revealed by their behaviour. This position, I suggest, is the essence of behaviourism (Morris, 1955; Bennett, 1976) (perhaps philosophical behaviourism is a better label, to distinguish it from psychological behaviourism). What a stimulus means to me, for instance, is entirely equivalent to how it changes my behaviour. The change might not be immediate or overt. In addition, because so much of behaviour is communication in one form or another, we should accept probabilistic changes in behaviour as meaning. Two signals would have different meanings if they evoked different probability distributions of responses, covert or overt, immediate or eventual.

With this point of view, a 'theory of mind' would consist of an ability to predict, at least probabilistically, other individuals' responses to stimulation (signals). Humans obviously can manage this feat. As was long ago pointed out to me, we would not dare to drive home if we could not predict other people's behaviour. It is also obvious that all animals can predict the behaviour of other individuals, at least probabilistically, and respond appropriately. This behavioural point of view thus implies that all animals have 'theories of mind'. Just as animals differ in complexity of associative learning, so their 'theories of mind' differ in complexity.

Mind, however, is not obviously equivalent to brain. This nagging reservation arises particularly when I consider my own mind. Sometime in the future neurophysiologists might be able to specify the precise state of every cell in my brain at a particular time. It might, for instance, become possible to specify exactly which neurons are activated when I see a particular tree or when I imagine the concept of treeness. Nevertheless, these neurons, it is easy to suppose, might not *be* my image of a tree nor my concept of a tree. The issue is whether observations of another organism's brain or behaviour are, or are not, enough to characterise its mind. Such thoughts raise many issues, but at the core of these issues are self-awareness and intention.

Evidence for self-awareness, it is often assumed, can come from reactions to mirrors. When an animal or human directs responses to its own body while viewing itself in a mirror, it seems that it must have an awareness of itself (Gallup, 1970, 2011; De Veer & Van den Bos, 1999). This ability, however, develops as a result of experience with mirrors. Humans without such experience are baffled by mirrors. Indeed, even photographs and recordings confuse people who lack experience of seeing or hearing themselves. Learning that visual images in a mirror can be associated with actions directed towards one's own body requires mastery of a chain of contingencies. It requires a complexity of learning that is evidently beyond the abilities of most animals. Yet it is not clear that the process differs qualitatively from other examples of associative learning. Furthermore, anyone who has tried using mirrors to view the back of the head, or, worse still, to direct actions there, becomes quickly disabused of any conclusion that self-awareness is equivalent to mastery of mirrors.

Normally our sense of self-awareness comes from introspection, just as does our sense of treeness or a particular tree. It is probable that association is important for this introspective self-awareness. We might associate all of our responses to sensory input with a common agent, in other words, our self. Once again, it might become possible, sometime in the future, to predict when a person is self-aware by determining the state of neurons in the brain, but making this connection would depend on the person's own report of self-awareness. Thus it is not clear that a description of neurons can ever be equivalent to self-awareness. Even one-to-one mapping of behaviour and brain might not guarantee existential equivalence of mind and brain.

I am trying to choose my words carefully here so as not to take a position that mind is, or is not, brain. The preceding arguments suggest that currently there is no indisputable evidence for or against either position. At least to my mind, if I may say so, it is not utterly obvious that mind is brain, nor that it is not. Nevertheless, a discussion of information in communication must include attention to the state of mind often thought to be crucial for human communication – intention.

Intentions (in the sense of preconceptions of actions) are often assumed to distinguish human communication from that of animals. When communicating, I intend to modify the recipient's mind, at least in some minimal way. When speaking of a tree, for instance, I intend for the listener to acquire an image of a tree somewhat like my own. As Wittgenstein (1968) has famously emphasised, this process requires that we have developed similar rules for using signals, or, as Shannon (1948) would say, for encoding and decoding signals. We must both associate the word 'tree' with a mental image such as 'generalised tree'. These rules are just as important when our intention is to deceive. Intentions are the basis for much human morality and justice. It has also been proposed that adopting an "intentional stance" (Dennett, 1987) facilitates communication or indeed all interactions with animate and perhaps even inanimate objects. What produces intentions? And how do we recognise them in others?

By introspection, my intentions seem connected to my awareness of my self as an agent. As described previously, this awareness might arise as a result of an association of my responses. It is thus a second-order association. Particular sensory inputs become associated with certain responses. Then these sensory–motor associations become associated with each other to produce a sense of agency. It is the patterns in my behaviour as a sentient and responsive organism that generate my sense of my self as an agent (so it appears to me on introspection). Can someone else study my intentions by studying my brain and behaviour? It is not clear that they can, because, just as with self-awareness, verification of my intentions requires my introspection.

If my intentions are a result of introspection, to pursue this argument, my willingness to attribute them to others must depend on empathy. I can of course, with enough study, predict the behaviour of others, in a probabilistic way, as discussed above. Yet, if mind is not behaviour, attributing mental states such as self-awareness and intentions can only occur by empathy. Empathy is attribution of mental states based on a sense of similarity between oneself and another. The more similar another person is to me, for instance in behaviour, the easier it is to empathise. Empathy can be extended to non-human animals, on the same basis, and even to plants and inanimate objects. To the extent that my automobile responds predictably to my input and my careful attention, I can empathise with it. It might well help me to communicate with my automobile to take an intentional stance and to empathise with it. The personification of many objects and features of the environment by peoples of many cultures could well have the same basis.

The two contrasting possibilities, that mind is brain or that it is not, thus lead to two contrasting views of information in communication. The first possibility leads to probabilistic predictions of behaviour, based on associations of contexts with responses. The second leads to introspection and empathy. If attributing states of mind to other organisms is equivalent to predicting their behaviour, then I regard all animals (as well as people) as having states of mind, and all as having theories of mind that allow them to respond to other individuals in appropriate ways. If attributing states of mind is not equivalent to predicting behaviour, then animals (and indeed other people or even machines) have states of mind depending on my ability to empathise with them.

I want to stress once again that I take no position on this polarity. It is not clear to me whether it will be possible, sometime in the future, to reduce my introspective sense of self-awareness, intention and meaning to the states of the neurons in my brain or to complexities in my behaviour. Thus it is also not clear to me that I can identify these states of mind in other individuals by studying their brains or behaviour. It is an uncertainty I can live with, however. I conditionally accept that mind is brain and proceed to analyse how animals communicate, how they categorise other individuals and their environment, how they associate sensory input with responses, how complicated these processes can be. Attributing states of mind, self-awareness and intentions to other humans is a necessary feature of our moral and legal systems. Attributing these states to other people, to non-human organisms and to inanimate objects is often an amusing diversion and might also help me to interact with them fruitfully. Insofar as I do anything more than predict or anticipate their behaviour, however, I engage in empathy.

To summarise, this discussion has led to three conclusions. (1) Communication consists of transmission of information from one individual to another. (2) If mind is behaviour, then all organisms communicate states of mind. (3) If it is not, then no communication transmits states of mind.

References

Altmann, S. A. (1965). Sociobiology of rhesus monkeys. II: Stochastics of social communication. *Journal of Theoretical Biology*, **8**, 490–522.

Arak, A. & Enquist, M. (1993). Hidden preferences and the evolution of signals. *Philosophical Transactions: Biological Sciences*, **340**, 207–213.

Beecher, M. D. (1989). Signalling systems for individual recognition: an information theory approach. *Animal Behaviour*, **38**, 248–261.

Beecher, M. D., Medvin, M. B., Stoddard, P. K. & Loeschke, P. (1986). Acoustic adaptations for parent–offspring recognition in swallows. *Experimental Biology*, **45**, 179–193.

Bennett, J. F. (1976). *Linguistic Behaviour*. London: Cambridge University Press.

Cheney, D. L. & Seyfarth, R. M. (1991). Truth and deception in animal communication. In C. E. Ristau, ed., *Cognitive Ethology: The Minds of Other Animals. Essays in Honor of Donald R. Griffin*. Hillsdale, NJ: Lawrence Erlbaum, pp. 127–151.

Chomsky, N. (1959). Review of B.F. Skinner, *Verbal Behavior*, New York, 1957. *Language*, **35**, 26–58.

Chomsky, N. (1986). *Knowledge of Language: Its Nature, Origin, and Use*. New York: Praeger.

Darwin, C. (1871). *The Descent of Man, and Selection in Relation to Sex*. New York: D. Appleton.

Darwin, C. (1873). *The Expression of the Emotions in Man and Animals*. New York: D. Appleton (1st edn. London: John Murray).

Dawkins, R. & Krebs, J. R. (1978). Animal signals: information or manipulation. In J. R. Krebs & N. B. Davies, eds., *Behavioural Ecology: An Evolutionary Approach*. Oxford: Blackwell, pp. 282–309.

Dennett, D. C. (1987). *The Intentional Stance*. Cambridge, MA: MIT Press.

De Veer, M. W. & Van Den Bos, R. (1999). A critical review of methodology and interpretation of mirror self-recognition research in nonhuman primates. *Animal Behaviour*, **58**, 459–468.

Dingle, H. (1969). A statistical and information analysis of aggressive communication in the mantis shrimp *Gonodactylus bredini* Manning. *Animal Behaviour*, **17**, 561–575.

Endler, J. A. & Basolo, A. L. (1998). Sensory ecology, receiver biases and sexual selection. *Trends in Ecology and Evolution*, **13**, 415–420.

Falls, J. B. (1982). Individual recognition by sounds in birds. In D. E. Kroodsma & E. H. Miller, eds., *Acoustic Communication in Birds*, Vol. 2. New York: Academic Press, pp. 237–278.

Gallup, G. G. (1970). Chimpanzees: self-recognition. *Science*, **167**, 86–87.

Gallup Jr, G. G., Anderson, J. R. & Platek, S. M. (2011). Self-recognition. In S. Gallagher, ed., *Oxford Handbook of the Self*. Oxford: Oxford University Press, pp. 80–110.

Godard, R. & Wiley, R. H. (1995). Individual recognition of song repertoires in two wood warblers. *Behavioral Ecology and Sociobiology*, **37**, 119–123.

Grafen, A. (1990). Biological signals as handicaps. *Journal of Theoretical Biology*, **144**, 517–546.

Guilford, T. & Dawkins, M. S. (1991). Receiver psychology and the evolution of animal signals. *Animal Behaviour*, **42**, 1–14.

Haldane, J. B. S. & Spurway, H. (1954). A statistical analysis of communication in '*Apis mellifera*' and a comparison with communication in other animals. *Insectes sociaux*, **1**, 247–283.

Hazlett, B. A. & Bossert, W. H. (1965). A statistical analysis of the aggressive communications systems of some hermit crabs. *Animal Behaviour*, **13**, 357–373.

Hogan, J. A., Kruijt, J.P. & Frijlink, J. H. (1975). 'Supernormality' in a learning situation. *Zeitschrift für Tierpsychologie*, **38**, 212–218.

Hubel, D. H. & Wiesel T. N. (1963). Receptive fields of cells in striate cortex of very young, visually inexperienced kittens. *Journal of Neurophysiology*, **26**, 994–1002.

Kant, I. (1961). *Prolegomena to Any Future Metaphysics* (translated by P. Carus), in particular Sections 23–24. Chicago, IL: Open Court Publishing. [1st edn in German 1783, 1st edn thus 1902].

Krebs, J. R. & Dawkins, R. (1984). Animal signals: mind-reading and manipulation. In J. R. Krebs & N. B. Davies, eds., *Behavioural Ecology: An Evolutionary Approach*, 2nd edn. Oxford: Blackwell Science, pp. 380–402.

Lorenz, K. (1966). *Evolution and Modification of Behavior*. London: Methuen.

Lynn, S. K., Cnaani, J. & Papaj, D. R. (2005). Peak shift discrimination learning as a mechanism of signal evolution. *Evolution*, **59**, 1300–1305.

Marler, P. (1961). The logical analysis of animal communication. *Journal of Theoretical Biology*, **1**, 295–317.

Marler, P. (1984). Song learning: innate species differences in the learning process. In P. Marler & H. S. Terrace, eds., *The Biology of Learning*. Berlin: Springer Verlag, pp. 289–309.

Marler, P. & Peters, S. (1988). The role of song phonology and syntax in vocal learning preferences in the song sparrow, *Melospiza melodia*. *Ethology*, **77**, 125–149.

Maynard Smith, J. & Harper, D. G. C. (2003). *Animal Signals*. Oxford: Oxford University Press.

Medvin, M. B., Stoddard, P. K. & Beecher, M. D. (1993). Signals for parent–offspring recognition: a comparative information analysis of the calls of cliff swallows and barn swallows. *Animal Behaviour*, **45**, 841–850.

Mitchell, R. W. & Anderson, J. R. (1997). Pointing, withholding information, and deception in capuchin monkeys (*Cebus apella*). *Journal of Comparative Psychology*, **111**, 351–361.

Møller, A. P. (1988). False alarm calls as a means of resource usurpation in the great tit *Parus major*. *Ethology*, **79**, 25–30.

Morris, C. W. (1955). *Signs, Language, and Behavior*. New York: G. Braziller.

Ogden, C. K. & Richards, I. A. (1923). *The Meaning of Meaning: A Study of the Influence of Language upon Thought and of the Science of Symbolism*. London: K. Paul, Trench, Trubner.

Owings, D. H. & Morton, E. S. (1998). *Animal Vocal Communication: A New Approach*. Cambridge: Cambridge University Press.

Pfeifer, J. (2006). The use of information theory in biology: lessons from social insects. *Biological Theory*, **1**, 317–330.

Rendall, D., Owren, M. J. & Ryan, M. J. (2009). What do animal signals mean? *Animal Behaviour*, **78**, 233–240.

Ryan, M. J. (1998). Sexual selection, receiver biases, and the evolution of sex differences. *Science*, **281**, 1999–2003.

Saussure, F. de (1959). *Course in General Linguistics*, C. Bally, A. Sechehave & A. Riedlinger, eds. (translated by W. Baskin). New York: Philosophical Library [1st edn in French 1916].

Searcy, W. A. & Nowicki, S. (2005). *The Evolution of Animal Communication: Reliability and Deception in Signaling Systems*. Princeton, NJ: Princeton University Press.

Seyfarth, R. M., Cheney, D. L., Bergman, T. *et al.* (2010). The central importance of information in studies of animal communication. *Animal Behaviour*, **80**, 3–8.

Shannon, C. E. (1948). The mathematical theory of communication, I and II. *Bell System Technical Journal*, **27**, 379–423, 623–656.

Shannon, C. E. & Weaver, W. (1963). *The Mathematical Theory of Communication*. Urbana, IL: University of Illinois Press.

Sherrington, C. S. (1906). *The Integrative Action of the Nervous System*. New York: Scribner.

Smith, W. J. (1980). *The Behavior of Communicating: An Ethological Approach*. Cambridge, MA: Harvard University Press.

Steinberg, J. B. & Conant, R. C. (1974). An informational analysis of the inter-male behaviour of the grasshopper *Chortophaga viridifasciata*. *Animal Behaviour*, **22**, 617–627.

Tanner, D. A. & Visscher, P. K. (2010). Adaptation or constraint? Reference-dependent scatter in honey bee dances. *Behavioral Ecology and Sociobiology*, **64**, 1081–1086.

ten Cate, C. & Rowe, C. (2007). Biases in signal evolution: learning makes a difference. *Trends in Ecology and Evolution*, **22**, 380–387.

Tinbergen, N. (1951). *The Study of Instinct*. Oxford: Clarendon Press.

Towne, W. F. & Gould, J. L. (1988). The spatial precision of the honey bees' dance communication. *Journal of Insect Behavior*, **1**, 129–155.

Weidenmüller, A. & Seeley, T. D. (1999). Imprecision in waggle dances of the honeybee (*Apis mellifera*) for nearby food sources: error or adaptation? *Behavioral Ecology and Sociobiology*, **46**, 190–199.

Whiten, A. & Byrne, R. W. (1988). Tactical deception in primates. *Behavioral and Brain Sciences*, **11**, 233–273.

Wiley, R. H. (1973). The strut display of male sage grouse: a 'fixed' action pattern. *Behaviour*, **47**, 129–152.

Wiley, R. H. (1994). Errors, exaggeration, and deception in animal communication. In L. Real, ed., *Behavioral Mechanisms in Evolutionary Ecology*. Chicago, IL: University of Chicago Press, pp. 157–189.

Wiley, R. H. (2006). Signal detection and animal communication. *Advances in the Study of Behavior*, **36**, 217–247.

Wiley, R. H. (2013). Specificity and Multiplicity in the recognition of individuals: implications for the evolution of social behaviour. *Biological Reviews*, **88**.

Wiley, R. H. & Wiley, M. S. (1977). Recognition of neighbors' duets by stripe-backed wrens *Campylorhynchus nuchalis*. *Behaviour*, **62**, 10–34.

Wilson, E. O. (1962). Chemical communication among workers of the fire ant *Solenopsis saevissima* (Fr. Smith). 2. An information analysis of the odour trail. *Animal Behaviour*, **10**, 148–158.

Wittgenstein, L. (1968). *Philosophical Investigations*, 3rd edn (translated by G. E. M. Anscombe). New York: Macmillan. [1st edn 1953].

Zahavi, A. (1977). The cost of honesty. *Journal of Theoretical Biology*, **67**, 603–605.

Zahavi, A. & Zahavi, A. (1997). *The Handicap Principle*. Oxford: Oxford University Press.

Commentaries

"These classic experiments demonstrate two important points. First, animal communication does convey information, in this case the identity of offspring, and, second, the analogous signals of two different species can differ in the amount of information conveyed." Do they? To us, this Procrustean linguistic interpretation has no explanatory value for the two swallow species' vocalisations and does not show that information has been conveyed. Rather, this description of signal and perceiver fits the concept of management/assessment: the natural history of cliff swallows provides the selective background, as described by Wiley, favouring parents who provide care when perceiving brood-specific calls in nestlings, but such is not the case in barn swallows. It is parents as perceivers of signals that control parental care which, in turn, selects for nestling signal structure, either favouring specificity or not. Management/assessment describes the interaction of signallers and perceivers, and highlights the importance of signal structure in the evolution of communication, not transmitted information with its supposed 'encoding and decoding'.

Eugene S. Morton and Richard G. Coss

Wiley makes 'signal' factive. X signals Y only if Y 'responds in some way'. As in, Tom informed Bob, only if Bob responds in some way. This is at least curious. Suppose Xs, as a type, constitute a repertoire of signals for Ys, as a type. Then a particular X does not signal Y if on this occasion something interferes and causes Y not to respond in any way (e.g. there is noise that drowns out what X sends, Y goes deaf, Y gets eaten). Curious to make it factive – doing so means signallers cannot fail when they signal.

Fred Adams and Steven M. Beighley

Response

Despite the comment by **Morton and Coss**, the fact remains that in one species of swallow individual nestlings have consistent differences in their calls and in the other species of swallow they do not. As 'information' is defined in my chapter (and by Shannon and Weaver), it is straightforward to conclude that analogous signals of the two species differ in the amount of information included. The degree to which parents respond differently to differences in nestlings' vocalisations determines the amount of information transmitted. Any benefits that nestlings gain from producing distinctive calls or parents gain from responding differently to them have important consequences for the evolution of this form of communication. In contrast, a full understanding of the evolution of communication does not require a concept of 'management/assessment'.

Contrary to the comment by **Adams and Beighley**, I am careful to state that communication is a probabilistic relationship. Receivers obviously do not respond to every occurrence of a signal. Even when they occur, responses are often covert or delayed. Nevertheless, to meet the basic criterion for communication, responses to signals must occur more often than by chance. Whatever the exact circumstances, the evidence for communication is a significant association (or correlation) between signals and responses. If noise masks a signal on some occasions, as it often does, communication can still occur. If noise masks a signal on all occasions, or if potential receivers all become permanently deaf (or otherwise unresponsive), then no communication can occur!

R. Haven Wiley

5

Natural information, intentional signs and animal communication

RUTH G. MILLIKAN

This is a volume about animal communication. One important question concerns whether animals communicate information, and to answer we first need to know what information is. Information is carried by signs. This chapter proposes a theory of signs and of information.

5.1 Root signs

Root signs include all signs that provide information (a notion to be examined). They are what constitute the basic materials in both nature and culture that can be used to support perception and cognition in animals including humans. That is what 'root sign' will mean in this chapter. If we want to understand how perception and cognition are possible, we first need to understand what root signs are and the various forms they can take. Many intentional signs, including both animal communication signs and the conventional signs of humans, are also (or 'contain' if you prefer) root signs that have the same meaning or content as do the intentional signs. Thus root signs are truly basic; all genuine information is provided by them, including the information contained in non-accidentally true intentional signs.

I call root signs that are not also intentional 'natural root signs'. Here are some examples. Despite first appearances, I will argue that they are all fundamentally alike.

(1) That the water is boiling is a sign that it has reached 212 degrees Fahrenheit.

Animal Communication Theory: Information and Influence, ed. Ulrich Stegmann. Published by Cambridge University Press.

(2) Black clouds are often a sign of imminent rain; fever is sometimes a sign of measles, other times of flu and so forth.

(3) Given a wooden frame made of four straight boards paired in length and properly nailed end to end in a closed figure, that the frame has equal diagonals is a sign, often used by carpenters, that the sides are parallel and the corners at right angles.

(4) That the head is like that of an elephant is a sign that the tail is like that of an elephant.

(5) 'O say can you see' sung to a certain tune is usually a sign that 'by the dawn's early light' is coming next.

(6) Bluster, who made the bomb I am to carry to Muggins, said that if I should suddenly hear it fizzing I should drop it dead and run, for that would be a sign that it was going off prematurely.

(7) The direction of the North Star is a sign of the direction of geographic north; the pull on the southern pole of the magnetosome in a northern hemisphere marine bacterium is a sign of the direction of lower oxygen concentration.

(8) That Jim has gone to the party is a good sign that that is where Jane is also.

(9) This certain quality of voice is a sign for me that it is Aino, my daughter, who is speaking.

(10) Travelling north from Route 89 on Wormwood Hill Road, the pond on the right is a sign that our house is coming up next.

(11) Suzy's mitten lying on the walk to the side door, given that it wasn't there earlier today, is a sign that Suzy is already home from school.

(12) That this man smells exactly as did the one who fed him yesterday is a sign, for Rover, that it is the same man.

5.2 Traditional descriptions of 'natural signs' do not capture natural root signs

The above examples are chosen in part to show why assumptions that seem frequently to be made about 'natural signs' and/or 'natural information' do not fit natural root signs. The notion 'natural information', for example, is sometimes used such that a fever would be said to carry disjunctive information or information about probabilities. The sense I am looking for is one in which what a given fever is a sign of depends on its actual cause. Analogously, tokens of 'it's raining' do not always carry the same information, for example the information that either it is raining or the speaker is lying. Whether a token of 'it's raining' carries the information that it is raining depends on whether it is raining.

One assumption often made is that 'natural signs' are always related by causal laws to what they signify. But in (3) the equal diagonals are not causes of the parallel sides and in (7) geographic north is not causally related to direction of the North Star nor is the direction of lower oxygen concentration causally related to the pull of the magnetosome. In (10) the pond on Wormwood Hill Road is not causally connected with my house – not a cause of it, not an effect of it, not an effect of a common cause. And in examples (8) to (11), the signs are signs of individuals, but there are no causal laws that concern individuals as such. (How there can be signs of individuals is interestingly neglected in the literature, although how knowledge of individuals is possible clearly turns on it.) In (12), the sign is of an identity relation, which is also an odd candidate for participation in causal laws. I would argue, as well, that having an elephant-like head and having an elephant-like tail (4) are not, as some think, each caused by being an elephant (see Millikan, 2012, on Matthen).

A second suggestion that has been made is that natural signs, signs carrying natural information, correspond to their signifieds with certainty, with 'a probability of 1' (Dretske, 1981). This is not just because there is no such thing as natural misinformation, no such thing as a natural sign token with a non-existent signified. The latter is a matter of definition for Dretske, not probability or natural necessity. The suggestion is that a natural sign is a sign of a certain physical type of which every token necessarily corresponds to a real signified of another type. If that this water is boiling is a natural sign that it is at 212 °F, then if any water boils (in this kind of situation) it must be at 212 °F. If you know how to read a certain kind of natural sign then, unlike knowing how to read a merely intentional sign, you cannot go wrong in taking every token just like it to signify something actual of the same kind as the other tokens do. What a wonderful support for knowledge that would be, as Dretske (1981) tried to show!

Dretske then qualified his claim, however, with a reference to "channel conditions", conditions that had to be assumed to be in place, mediating between sign and signified, to make the probability be 1. But unless presence of the right channel conditions is to be considered part of the natural sign itself, this undercuts the assumption of certainty. That the water is boiling will not be a sign that it has reached 212 °F if it is on top of Mount Everest or, indeed, almost anywhere not on the Earth. Knowing how to read a certain kind of sign by assuming that the channel conditions are right cannot yield certainty. Certainty about the channel conditions would have to be added.

Indeed, the kind of signs on which perception and cognition actually rest virtually never have forms, shapes or intrinsic properties that unfailingly correspond to the same sort of signified, nor are channel conditions that might produce unfailing correspondence (should they be known) univocally signed to senses like ours unless still further channel conditions which are not necessarily univocally signed are assumed. Actual animal cognition is not supported by infallible indicators. Tokens of signs that support actual perception/cognition do not carry their signifying types on their sleeves. Physical twins of root sign tokens (identical fevers, say) that are not of the same signifying types (or that do not signify at all) abound. Compare homonyms, which sound the same but are different words.

The capacities of humans and other animals to perceive and to know – systematically to acquire accurate perceptions and true beliefs – often appear to rest heavily on mere correlations in nature rather than necessities. In line with this, it has been suggested that we recognise a kind of natural information – Nicholas Shea (2007) calls it 'correlational information' – that is produced when there is a *non-accidentally continuing* correlation (typically assumed to be underwritten by a causal connection, but let us admit other kinds of non-accidental correlation as well) between one kind of thing and another, such that the probability of the one is raised given the other (Lloyd, 1989; Price, 2001; Shea, 2007). Lloyd, at least, is clear that where A types carry this kind of information about B types, an A token does not carry this information unless there actually exists a corresponding B token (Lloyd, 1989, p. 64). Considering correlational signs as candidates for a kind of root sign – signs that support perception and cognition – we need Lloyd's restriction. For example, no matter how high the non-accidental correlation between fever and measles is in the area, if Johnny's fever is caused by flu then his particular fever would not be, for our purposes, a correlational sign of measles.

An obvious difficulty for the view that correlational signs are root signs concerns the strength of correlation to be required. But more basic, I think, is that correlations and conditional probabilities are defined relative to reference classes. It could of course be that given all space-time as the reference class, the boiling of water does raise the probability that it is at 212 °F. But boiling is likely to raise the probability more that water is one or another of various other temperatures, there being no reason to think that one Earth-atmosphere is an especially common pressure. Similarly, we have no evidence that an elephant-like head at one end raises the probability of an elephant-like tail at the other throughout all space-time, and it is quite certain that the direction of the North Star does not raise the probability of that direction being geographic north universe-wide. If root signs were correlational signs, clearly the reference classes for these correlations would have to be restricted in some way. How then would we decide, for any candidate root sign token, what the boundaries should be for the restricted class by reference to which it would be required to be an instance of a correlation? How, for example, would we determine that, given this little bacterium right here now, the current direction of magnetic north is a root sign of lesser oxygen, given that the relevant correlation holds (probably) neither universe-wide nor (certainly) Earth-wide?

Whispering in our ear may be the reply that the relevant reference class is the Earth's northern oceans – because, well, 'that's where the correlation is'. But unfortunately, the correlation is lots of other areas the bacterium is in as well – myriad smaller areas (in some of which it may be higher) and also myriad larger areas, ones, for example, that overlap with or include the northern hemisphere. And the correlation fails to hold in various other areas the bacterium is equally in, perhaps in some smaller areas such as the very square yard right around the bacterium which could be affected by a bar magnet someone has dropped underneath or by bubbles coming up from a diver. And it certainly fails in various larger areas that include the southern seas. That there exists some correlation of some strength within some arbitrarily chosen reference class which includes this item surely cannot define for us what a root sign is given our purposes. It is not facts of this anaemic kind that underlie the possibility of perception and cognition. Besides, we should remember examples of signs such as the fizzing bomb in (6) and Suzy's mitten in (11). These are unique cases, the coincidence of sign with signified occurring only once.

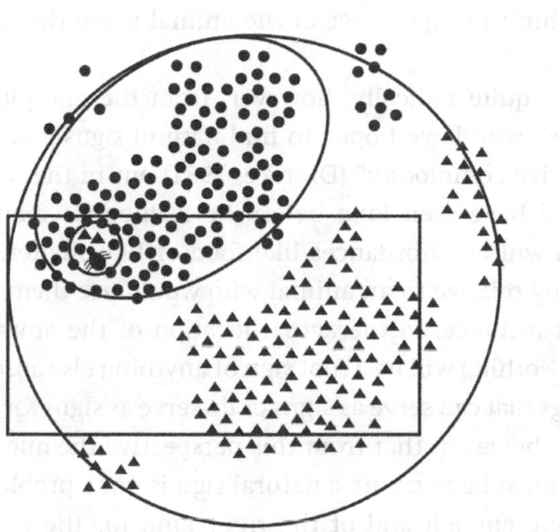

Figure 5.1 The reference class problem. The diagram represents a space-time continuum collapsed to two dimensions. The dots are centres of strong positive correlation of A with B, fading in strength outwards. The triangles are centres of strong negative correlation of A with B. Outside the dots and triangles there is little or no correlation of A with B. Assume that the bug is currently encountering some specific token A that is coupled with B. Which circumscribed area determines the reference class relative to which this specific token A is or is not, objectively, a correlational sign of B? Suggestion: the relevant area would be one that precisely encloses the past and ongoing path of the bug (or its species).

5.3 A reference class for determining root correlational signs

Clearly no cognising creature samples space and time randomly, or samples very much of it at all. If correlations or conditional probabilities are relevant to understanding what in nature supports cognition, I suggest that the only relevant or non-arbitrary reference class is the class of (candidate) signs that occur within the path of the animal that would read them, or if it is a species that learns to read them, within the various paths of the members of that species. The correlation must exist over the reference class that is this path, or over a portion or portions of this path that the animal must be able to distinguish, or over a long enough period of the animal's life for it to learn it. I am not suggesting that the reference class should merely *include* the animal's or animals' path(s) or relevant parts of it. That would raise exactly the same problem over again. The idea is that the relevant non-arbitrary reference class consists in the very samples sampled by the animal or species that uses a root sign, or of such samples as are further discriminable by it in some way as relevant. Useful correlations have to occur within the experience of the animals using them. Or they have to occur among things prior signs of which occur within the experience of the animal using them and so forth.

This changes the game quite radically, however, from the one played by theorists of 'natural signs', who have hoped to find natural signs and natural information as an "objective commodity" (Dretske, 1981) out in the world, as structures that God could have seen long before he fashioned creatures to harvest them. Root signs will be affordances like food or like shelter, things that are what they are only relative to an animal who would use them, in this case relative, in the first instance, to the actual location of the animal, not merely to its capabilities. Nothing will be a root sign of anything else absolutely. Rather, there will be things that can serve as signs or do serve as signs for a given animal or species. Notice, however, that from this perspective the question of how strong a correlation must be to create a natural sign is not a problem. The correlation must be strong enough and of the right kind for the particular animal to detect it, and for it to be possibly useful, given the animal's purposes, to bet on it. The underlying idea here is that *being able to serve as a natural sign* is what is basic rather than *being a natural sign.*

Strong correlations between things throughout all space and time are chiefly restricted to what follows from universal natural laws, these universal laws, as science knows, being hard to discern. But the space-time paths of individual animals and species often seem to be reference classes of very strong correlation between fairly numerous and fairly evident kinds of things. Suppose that we pause to wonder why this is so. Why are strong correlations in an animal's sampling past often good signs that these correlations will remain strong in its sampling future regardless of the strength of these correlations universe-wide? This, it seems to me, is really the fundamental question we should be trying to answer about root signs, about what makes cognition possible. Moreover, the answer generalises. It can foot an understanding of the nature also of root signs that are not correlational, as in examples (6), (11) and (12).

5.4 Answering the fundamental question

We need to superimpose two familiar facts. First, the path of an animal through space and time is continuous. It does not skip from one time and place to another. Similarly, a species spreads out over space and time on continuous individual paths that branch from one another, confined by natural selection within geographical areas with friendly properties. Second, the usual reason for the presence of local correlations is that things persist through time, staying in the same or connected locales, or that they self-maintain or cycle in the same or in connected locales or, in post-Archaeozoic times on Earth, that they reproduce or are reproduced (artifacts, animal signals, linguistic forms) in the same or in connected locales. Whether conditions, events or entities, much that is near the animal today will be near it tomorrow, or something much like it will be. Channel conditions remain in place, and events that manifest themselves through these channels recur. For these reasons, where there are good correlations in one portion of an animal's space-time path, frequently these correlations extend to other portions.

Mountains, valleys, rivers, oceans, the Earth's atmosphere, persist. Individual trees, rocks, houses, roads, paths, persist in definite places. Individual animals and plants and also species of these self-maintain, hence persist, remaining in roughly the same or connected areas. The Earth persists and rotates causing cyclical daily patterns, and it circles around the persisting Sun causing cyclical yearly patterns, cyclical weather patterns, and cyclical patterns in plant and animal behaviours. (It is not a natural law that black clouds tend to burst. Under more stable conditions they too would persist.) People cycle from home to work or school and back home again at fairly regular hours. Animal and plant species reproduce, stabilised by homeostasis in their gene pools and by natural selection in a continuing environment. Artifacts that work well or that please, songs and stories, red and green Christmas decorations, and steeples on churches are all numerously reproduced. Where local sampling shows correlations, typically the causes of the correlations are being actively preserved or cycled or reproduced and will continue to be so for some time through neighbouring times and places.[1] An animal's path typically persists among, crosses or overlaps the single or branching paths of many such persisting, cycling or reproducing items.

Travelling north up Wormwood Road, passing the pond on the right is repeatedly followed by passing our house because the relation between our house and the pond persists (10). In the circles I walk in, the peculiar quality of my daughter's voice is repeatedly reproduced by my daughter's larynx which persists in areas that frequently overlap mine (9). The correlation between the way south poles of magnetosomes point with lesser oxygen persists because the relation between magnetic north and the surface of the ocean persists as does the scarcity of other sources of magnetic fields on the Earth (7). The correlation between an elephant-like head at one end with an elephant-like tail at the other persists on Earth because elephants reproduce (4). The correlation between "O say can you see" and "by the dawn's early light" persists because the US national anthem is copied over and over by people who teach it to one another (5). The correlation of fever with measles persists because the measles virus reproduces in people and people reproduce thus reproducing the conditions that lead from the measles virus to the fever (2). The correlation between where Jim is to be found and where Jane is to be found persists because Jim and Jane and a certain bond between them each persists such as often to bring them together in the evenings (8).

Understanding why a correlation persists, what kind of endurings or cyclings or reproducings are accounting for it, can of course be a huge help in trying to project the more exact path or paths that a correlation will take, hence in reading signs. But it is not always necessary to know reasons. And many animals are born, live and die such that their life paths, taken entire, mark out reference classes in which many of the correlations they depend on actively persist. There is no need for them to recognise boundaries.

5.5 Generalising to non-correlational signs

A continuing correlation can be viewed simply as a very small recurring pattern, a repeated pattern of an A state of affairs being so-related to a B state of affairs. What repeats over and over is a black cloud moving overhead at a certain place and time with rain falling at that place shortly after that time, or an

[1] In Millikan (2004), where causes of correlations are being actively preserved or cycled or reproduced in this way I spoke of "locally recurrent natural signs". For reasons outlined above, I think I should not have, for there seems no way to define them as signs without reference to an animal that lives in or crosses the local areas within which they are found. Perhaps they should be called locally recurrent 'potential' signs, becoming root signs for an animal when they, or root signs of them, recur within its experience.

elephant-like head at one end of a thing that has an elephant-like tail at the other. What repeats in a sign-signed relation is a relation between a certain kind of sign and a certain kind of signed. Reading the sign is just completing the pattern.

Significant correlations between one thing and another require many repetitions of the one given the other. But in the case of extremely complex patterns, single recurrences may yield natural signs. When a very detailed complex pattern repeats even once in a nearby location, it is likely that the repetition is no accident, the chance of accident going down sharply with the detail and complexity of the pattern. Rather, the pattern has probably endured (it is the same individual again) or been repeated as a result of the persistence of conditions along with the cycling of events and/or some process involving reproduction or copying. Suppose that you encounter two detailed paintings that are exactly alike. Surely it is more than likely either that one has been reproduced from the other or both from some third – or perhaps the painting has just been moved. And if you find that one half of a detailed painting is exactly like one half of another, thus making it likely that the one has been reproduced from the other or from some third, or that it has been moved, then it is very likely that the other halves match as well. The pattern on one half can serve as a sign of the pattern on the other, but not, it seems, because of any background correlation in your experience.

Paintings are sometimes reproduced; elephants reproduce themselves. The shape, composition and structure of the whole elephant, all its parts and all their relations to one another – a concrete and very detailed pattern – keeps recurring. And this kind of pattern is large enough and complex enough that having observed enough of it on one occasion, parts of the pattern can serve you as signs of other parts on other occasions, even on a mere second occasion. Our world is chock-full of natural signs of this kind. The patterns that are whole alligators and whole daisies repeat, and also whole symphonies and whole Protestant wedding ceremonies and whole Toyota Camrys and whole Gothic churches and whole chairs and whole books (copies of them) and whole McDonalds restaurants.

The notion of a correlation has dropped far into the background here. A much broader notion of local pattern repetition and pattern completion emerges as the base principle explaining natural signs and the reading of natural information. It seems best to claim then that the *general* form that natural signs take is that of patterns that repeat within an animal's experience and that reading natural signs is just pattern completion. Natural sign reading may be based, at the one extreme, on observation of many repetitions of a very simple pattern, at the other extreme, on a single prior observation of a very complex pattern.

Having had it rain many times when black clouds form, I am prepared for rain the next time I see black clouds. Having seen only one whole elephant, I am prepared for the tail on the next.

It is often possible to recognise a complex repeated pattern from any of many different samplings of its features. An elephant may be recognised from the front or the back or the side, by the trunk, by the head, by the legs, by the tusks, by the tail, by the trumpet. Each of these may serve as a sign of an elephant and as a sign of each other elephant feature. Similarly, of course, a person or a building may be recognised from the front or the back or the side and so forth. A song may be recognised by hearing the beginning or the end or only a line in the middle. There are many ways to recognise a baseball game or a restaurant or a piano, also many ways to test for a chemical substance and so forth. Thus the completion of complex patterns is a doubly versatile way that nature affords of reading natural signs. Surely it is not just correlations of simple pairs of features but repeated clumpings of multiple features that supply the bulk of natural signs supporting cognition.

Natural signs result from endurances and repetitions of patterns along paths that criss-cross and interweave with the paths of the animals for whom these signs are affordances. Such patterns often criss-cross or interweave with one another as well. Repeated patterns may be superimposed on one another. If part of one pattern is recognised as such, then recognised as also being a part of a second superimposed pattern, pattern completion may reveal relations between various other parts of these patterns as well. Think of employing two maps that overlap to determine relations of places shown just on one to places shown just on the other. Compare recognising the repeated pattern that is small stray items lying outdoors where their owners have recently been, superimposed over the repeated pattern that is the owner of this mitten, Suzy, entering from school by the side door about this time of day (11). Bluster, who made the bomb I am to carry to Muggins, has mentally superimposed and chained together many small repeating patterns involving one simple kind of part that his bomb contains interacting with another simple part, which completed chain would determine it to go off as planned. But he knows of other sometimes repeated patterns that, superimposed, would include a hissing sound and immediate premature detonation, and it is this latter pattern that he is warning me about (6).

5.6 Animals' signs

Animals, by maintaining themselves hence persisting over time, by reproducing themselves and by exhibiting daily and seasonal behaviour cycles, introduce into nature innumerable kinds of root signs that may be read/interpreted by other animals. (Take 'interpreting' a sign here to be, simply, responding to it such as to guide behaviour or thought in a way that uses or takes account of what has been signified in accordance with an ability.[2]) Some of these root signs are of particular interest because purposively produced in order to be interpreted by conspecifics or, in some cases, by other species as well. The 'purposes' I have in mind here are natural purposes, as, for example, the purpose of the protective eye-blink reflex and of the eye itself. Especially important, I do not imply that when a root sign is produced purposively, its being read is a goal that is understood or represented in the psychology of the animal producing the sign, but only that the sign or sign-making activity was selected or tuned by natural selection, or by learning processes – or yes, possibly, by reasoning processes – for doing this job. (Elsewhere (Millikan, 1984, 2004 *inter alia*) I have argued that explicitly represented purposes are a sophisticated kind of natural purpose, so I do not mean altogether to exclude them here, but probably animals other than humans seldom produce signs with the explicit intention to do so.)

At least three kinds of correlational root signs produced by non-human animals are commonly believed to have derived from natural selection operating on both their producers and their interpreters with resulting benefit to both, hence to be purposively produced. First are signals indicating the current or immanent presence or the position of something of significance to species members or, sometimes, members of other species as well. Danger signals, signals indicating the presence of food, mating displays, growls and barks, and bee dances are such root signs whenever they actually correspond to the things they would signify for the usual reasons, that is, if they do not correspond accidentally. If there are signs that have evolved to indicate the health or strength of individual animals, such as prowess in fighting or the peacock's tail or the stotting of the gazelle, when these actually indicate as natural selection designed them to indicate, they too are root signs.

Second are signs designed to mark an individual as a member of its species so it may be recognised as such. The characteristic insignia marking many species of birds and also their species-specific songs are purposive root signs, as are the warning tail lashes and odour of the skunk and the rattling of a rattlesnake, which serve as warnings to many other animals by instinct.

Third are individual insignia – distinctive odours, distinctive calls – which serve many species that care about such things for re-identification of individuals. If individual signatures of this kind, easily discernable to conspecifics, have their origin in natural selection, then they too are purposive root signs. The

[2] 'Abilities' are described in Millikan (2000, Ch. 4).

principle underlying them is the simplest of all, the mere persistence over time of an individual with a distinctive stable property in a connected area. There may of course be other kinds of natural non-human animal signs that are purposive as well, perhaps having been selected for by learning mechanisms, or even by reasoning processes.

5.7 Intentional signs

Classically, natural signs were distinguished from conventional signs, which were considered to be used only by humans. Purposive human activities such as producing and interpreting conventional signs were not thought of as being part of nature, so the distinction between natural and conventional signs was assumed to be exclusive. Conventional signs could not also be natural signs, at least not natural signs having the same content. Animal signs, on the other hand, were not generally considered at all. From a perspective that takes all animals, humans and non-humans, along with their various purposive activities – whether these purposes are represented or not – to be part of nature, it is reasonable to draw, instead, two separate distinctions. We can draw a distinction, first, between signs that are root and those that are not; second, between signs that are 'intentional' and those that are not. That is, we recognise three basic kinds of signs: +root/+intentional, +root/–intentional and –root/+intenntional (–root/–intentional not being a sign at all).

I use 'intentional' in the traditional philosophical sense introduced by Brentano. Intentional signs are distinguished by the fact that they can be about non-existent things – non-existent objects or, more typically, non-existent states of affairs, that is, they can be false. Paradigmatically, they are signs produced by a system that has been designed to produce signs in a certain representational scheme for interpretation and use by a certain kind of cooperating 'consumer' system that has been designed, in turn, to interpret these signs (Millikan, 1984, 2004, 2005 *inter alia*), fruits of this design serving or having served both systems. The possibility of being false arises because these signs have as natural purposes to convey a definite kind of 'understanding' to an interpreter, that is, to alter an interpreter so as to take account of the thing or state of affairs that the sign signifies. This purpose cannot be served, of course, unless this thing or state of affairs is real. If it is not real, the sign is false. When intentional signs are true in accordance with their historically normal non-accidental ways of coming to be true, they will serve as root signs for any animal who can read them. If they are true by accident, however, they are not root signs of what they were designed to be of and do not carry their intentional content as information (compare a true belief that is not knowledge).

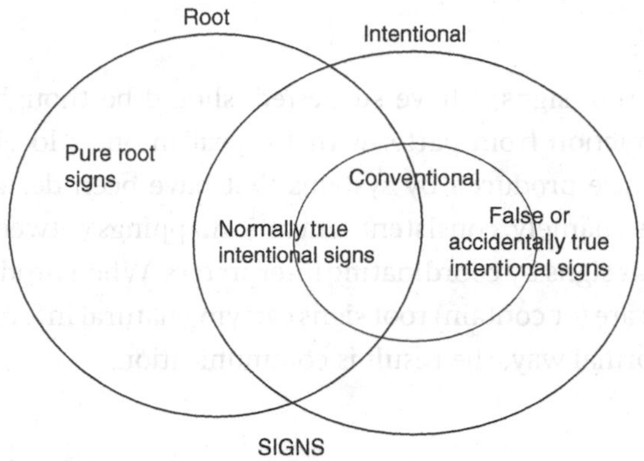

Figure 5.2 Examples of signs.

Natural +root: black clouds mean rain when actually followed by rain in the usual way.
Intentional +conventional +root: "It's raining" said upon seeing that it's raining.
Intentional +conventional –root: "It's raining" said when false, or when true but said lacking non-Gettiered evidence.
Intentional +conventional +root: a rabbit's danger thump upon seeing a dog.
Intentional –conventional –root: a rabbit's danger thump when there is no danger or when there is danger but what is dangerous is not what produced the thump.

Elsewhere I have argued that conventional signs are intentional signs that have evolved culturally in natural languages to serve cooperative purposes of speakers and hearers (Millikan, 1984, 2004, 2005 *inter alia*).[3] We thus derive the diagram in Figure 5.2.

5.8 Animal communication

Without caring to fight over words, it seems reasonable to consider that 'communication' takes place when an intentional sign is interpreted coincident with the purpose of its production by a cooperative interpreter in the normal way, a thing's purpose being – recall – something it was designed for doing. That is, it seems reasonable to set aside the Gricean analyses of 'meaning' and 'communication' (which I think seldom applies even to humans – Ch. 3 of Millikan, 1984), putting natural purposes in place of Gricean 'intentions'. Instinctively produced animal signals to conspecifics are then paradigm cases of intentional signs that often result in communication.

[3] Superimposed on these purposes may be other, sometimes conflicting, purposes derived from purposes of individual speakers (same references).

5.9 Conclusion

In sum, reading root signs, I have suggested, should be thought of as learning by pattern completion from patterns that repeat in one's locale for a reason. Intentional signs are produced by systems that have been designed to reproduce certain patterns, namely, consistent semantic mappings between signs and signifieds, to be read as signs by coordinating interpreters. When produced in a normal way, these signs are (or contain) root signs carrying natural information. When interpreted in a normal way, the result is communication.

References

Dretske, F. (1981). *Knowledge and the Flow of Information*. Cambridge, MA: MIT Press.

LLoyd, D. (1989). *Simple Minds*. Cambridge, MA: MIT Press.

Millikan, R. G. (1984). *Language, Thought and Other Biological Categories*. Cambridge, MA: MIT Press.

Millikan, R. G. (2000). *On Clear and Confused Ideas*. Cambridge: Cambridge University Press.

Millikan, R. G. (2004). *Varieties of Meaning*. Cambridge, MA: MIT Press.

Millikan, R. G. (2005). *Language: A Biological Model*. Oxford: Oxford University Press.

Millikan, R. G. (2012). Reply to Mohan Matthen. In D. Ryder, J. Kingsbury & K. Williford, eds., *Millikan and Her Critics*. Oxford: Basil Blackwell.

Price, C. (2001). *Functions in Mind; A Theory of Intentional Content*. Oxford: Oxford University Press.

Shea, N. (2007). Consumers need information: supplementing teleosemantics with an input condition. *Philosophy and Phenomenological Research*, **75**, 404–435.

Commentary

Millikan does what Rendall and Owren deem impossible: she cashes out the promissory note 'information'. She shows that 'informational' signalling is merely natural information, yet supports 'informationalist' approaches. She further shows how context powerfully modifies information's utility, even for something as starkly physical as boiling water – all the more so, we add, when information is in a relative feature (e.g. a higher rather than particular song rate), as in much signalling in networks.

Perhaps social exchange of natural information leads to articulated signalling systems. An alligator's head is underwritten by its consistent shape, but a mate's signal is underwritten by repeated interactions as a territory defender, provider etc. – sign upon sign. These 'channel conditions' include a history of signal exchanges and behavioural commitments – perhaps one route to language.

Andrew G. Horn and Peter McGregor

PART II INFLUENCE AND MANIPULATION

6

Communication without meaning or information: abandoning language-based and informational constructs in animal communication theory

DREW RENDALL AND MICHAEL J. OWREN

6.1 Introduction

Contemporary research in animal communication is heavily influenced by analogy to human language and language-related information constructs: it focuses on establishing the *meaning* of animal signals or how they *encode* and *transmit information*. This approach feels so natural that few stop to consider that linguistic and informational constructs are not givens (*a priorisms*) in animal communication, but represent a significant departure from the anchoring concepts of earlier research (Owren & Rendall, 2001; Owren , Rendall & Ryan, 2010). In fact, language-based and informational constructs became common in animal communication only with the rise of cognitivism in the middle twentieth century, and the result has been a double-edged sword. On the one hand, linguistic and informational constructs have had significant heuristic value and greatly raised the profile of the field. On the other hand, while the constructs are familiar and appear straightforward, they are not – at least as typically presented. We suggest they have proven fundamentally ambiguous and have put researchers out of step with core tenets of evolutionary biology. Hence, they are not strong conceptual pillars for a maturing science of animal communication.

To flesh out this argument, we first examine the origins of key ideas about information and cognitive representation in computer science,

Animal Communication Theory: Information and Influence, ed. Ulrich Stegmann. Published by Cambridge University Press.

linguistics and psychology, and their subsequent adoption by animal communication researchers. We then elaborate problems inherent to these ideas, not only in the field of animal communication, but also in the disciplines they were borrowed from. Finally, we outline a class of alternative frameworks for studying animal communication that are more consistent with core tenets of biological and evolutionary explanation, and are more in step with current research concerning the organisation of brains, bodies and behaviour.

6.2 Language, minds and computers: circular metaphors of the cognitive revolution

Linguistic and informational constructs now dominant in animal communication can be traced to two mutually reinforcing developments that sparked the 'cognitive revolution' (Miller, 1956; Chomsky, 1959; Neisser, 1967). One key development was technological – the advent of computer-based information-processing as a synthesis of formal logic (Turing, 1950) and physical symbol systems (*sensu* Newell & Simon, 1976). The other was the emergence of Chomskyan linguistics, based on the premise that language was an organic example of a physical symbol system (Chomsky, 1965).

Obvious parallels between computer systems and language systems made the computer an appealing metaphor for language. Quantitatively oriented linguists embraced the potential offered for formal logical and mathematical analysis of language structure. The key lay in the combinatorial power of syntax operating over arbitrary symbols. Such systems are computationally tractable so long as the forms of the symbols themselves are completely arbitrary and do not muddy the computations by having a logic of their own independent of the logic of the syntax that governs them. This emphasis helped to consolidate de Saussure's (1916) classic dictum of the *arbitrariness of the sign*. The view of language that emerged was of a system of arbitrarily structured symbol tokens stored and manipulated via rule-governed syntactical processes to create meaningful expressions that convey information. Language was seen as a natural system of information processing and transmission, and the computer metaphor for language was eponymously reified as *computational linguistics*.

The success of metaphorical, computer-based approaches to language also encouraged and reinforced tendencies to think about the brain (mind) in a similar way. This emerging cognitivist approach in psychology thus also relied on computer metaphors, again grounded in the supposition that mental processes can be modelled as a form of symbol manipulation via abstract rules. Later labelled the *computational theory of mind*, this approach moved beyond metaphor. Over time, the mind was not just *like* a computer, it effectively *was* a kind of computer. With computer metaphors forming a common ground, conceptions of language and brain became intertwined and mutually reinforcing. Indeed, mental processes were subsequently cast as a kind of *language of thought* (Fodor, 1975).

6.3 Cognitive ethology and the rethinking of animal communication

The promise of Chomskyan linguistics and digital computing for understanding the architecture of mental processing and complex behaviour was not lost on scientists of animal behaviour. Historically, issues concerning animal mental life had been central to comparative psychology, and after decades of the strictures of behaviourism, researchers were ready to embrace this prohibited topic once again. Just as language was seen to reveal the workings of human minds, communication systems in animals were seen as privileged windows on their minds (Griffin, 1974, 1995). Indeed, animals were proposed to demonstrate complex cognition in proportion to the degree to which their communication showed evidence of language-like properties. Language thus quickly emerged as a core metaphor for understanding animal communication, and was readily connected to the information-processing metaphors emerging in the study of cognition (Marler, 1961). The two emphases came together in the new field of *cognitive ethology*, a synthesis of animal behaviour and psychology.

The new approach took a large leap forward through seminal work on primate vocal communication by Seyfarth, Cheney and Marler. That work showed that vervet monkeys give acoustically distinct alarm calls to different predator types and that the calls alone elicit different escape responses (Seyfarth, Cheney & Marler, 1980a). Hence, the calls appeared to function as symbolic labels for the predators, much like human words. Because these sounds showed no iconic resemblance to the predators, they also seemed to exemplify the arbitrariness that de Saussure proposed for language. Here, then, was evidence of language-like communication in a monkey, with the promise of similarly human-like cognitive complexity. The implications for language evolution were tantalising, with equally rich prospects for the broader enterprise of language-oriented research in animals.

6.4 Animal signalling and language

It is difficult to overstate the influence of the vervet alarm-call research. It catalysed a generation of like-minded work on other primates, also searching for parallels to language and complex cognition. Soon, this approach spread to research on other species as well (Table 6.1), including animals with very

Table 6.1 *Examples of linguistic and informational constructs loosely used to support comparisons of animal signals to language. Examples trace the spread of such constructs from research on primates to research on other animal taxa.*

Author(s)	Explanations of signals, signalling or communication (*emphasis added*)
Seyfarth, Cheney & Marler (1980b)	"The qualitatively different responses elicited by experimental playbacks of leopard, eagle, and snake alarms demonstrate that alarm calls alone . . . *provided the monkeys with sufficient information* to make distinct and apparently adaptive responses . . . It is, of course, a difficult task to establish the precise *meaning* to the monkeys of each alarm type . . . There are limits to how far a *semantic* analysis of signals can be carried when it is based solely on the responses that those signals evoke. Nevertheless, it seems appropriate to conclude that the alarm calls of vervet monkeys *designate particular external referents*. Certainly the calls are *arbitrary* and *non-iconic* . . . one criterion for differentiating *symbols* from *icons* . . . This view of alarm calls as a form of *semantic* signalling, probably involving the formation of internal perceptual *concepts*, or *symbols*, contrasts with earlier interpretations . . . It therefore seems appropriate to interpret arousal-related properties of alarm calls as ancillary to more specific call features, supplementing and enriching the *meaning* of calls rather than serving as a primary basis for *meaning* . . . Having shown that alarm calls, whatever their motivational basis, can be used to *convey information* about external events, our next stop is to investigate whether calls used during social interactions function in a similar manner."
Cheney & Seyfarth (1988)	"Humans make judgments about the similarity or difference between words on the basis of an abstraction, their *meaning* . . . One method for determining how group-living animals assess the *meaning* of calls is through their ability to detect anomalous or unreliable signals. The results presented here suggest that the detection of unreliable signals is influenced by the ways in which animals assess and compare signals based upon their *meaning* . . . In the case of vervet monkeys, and perhaps other primates as well, selection may have favoured the ability to recognize 'spheres' of *meaning* and the *transfer of information* gained in one sphere to other, related ones. Individuals who have come to recognize that one type of call by a given signaller is unreliable appear to transfer their scepticism to other calls of broadly similar *meaning*, but not to calls whose *referents* are different."
Cheney & Seyfarth (1996)	"The alarm and contact calls of monkeys *provide information* about the signaller's current physical and mental states, but they are not deliberately given to inform or instruct others. Instead, listeners appear to *extract relevant information* about a call's function based on behavioral contingencies and their own experiences."

Table 6.1 (cont.)

Author(s)	Explanations of signals, signalling or communication (*emphasis added*)
Zuberbühler (2000)	"From the perspective of the call recipient, however, the difference between primate alarm calls and human linguistic utterances are less explicit. In this and other studies, it was the *meaning* of the stimuli, but not the acoustic features that explained the subjects' response patterns. These results extend this finding ... by showing that *semantic understanding can be based on arbitrary signals, as it is* [sic] *the case for word meaning.*"
Cheney & Seyfarth (2005)	"Here we review research on the vocal communication and cognition of non-human primates ... we conclude, first, that non-human primates' inability to represent the mental states of others makes their communication fundamentally different from human language. Second, while non-human primates' production of vocalizations is highly constrained, their ability to *extract complex information* from sounds is not. Upon hearing vocalizations, *listeners acquire information* about their social companions that is *referential, discretely coded, hierarchically structured, rule-governed, and propositional.*"
Slocombe & Zuberbühler (2007)	"Our first goal was to examine to what degree chimpanzee victim screams *conveyed information* about the nature of the conflict, thus *providing valuable information* for nearby receivers *deciding* whether or not to interfere. Previous research on macaques has revealed that callers produce acoustically distinct scream types that are *meaningful to listeners.*"
Evans & Evans (1999)	"Food-associated vocalizations have also been of interest for research addressing proximate questions, especially efforts to understand the *meaning* of animal signals. Some food calls may have properties like those of the highly specific alarm calls described in birds and monkeys and may *provide information* sufficient to evoke anticipatory feeding behaviour from conspecifics. If so, such food calls would be *'functionally referential'*."
Bugnyar, Kijne & Kotrschal (2001)	"*Signals may encode information* about attributes of the sender ... and about stimuli or events in the environment ... If such *signals provide receivers with sufficient information* to determine the context underlying signal production ... the signals are regarded as *functionally referential* ..."
Manser, Seyfarth & Cheney (2002)	"Recent work on suricates, an African mongoose, shows that animal alarm calls simultaneously *encode information* about both predator type and the signaler's perception of urgency."
Templeton, Greene & Davis (2005)	"If a species is preyed upon by different predators that use different hunting strategies or vary in the degree of danger they present, selection can favor variation in alarm signals that *encode this information*. Such variation in alarm signals can be used to *transfer information* about the type of predator, the degree of threat that a predator represents, or both."

different nervous systems, behaviours and evolutionary histories. More than 30 years on, however, vervet alarm calling remains not only the best-known and widely cited instance of language-like communication in animals – it *is* the best example. Despite intense interest, language-like, representational signalling has been reported in only some species, and then in just a fraction of those animals' signal repertoires. The majority of signals evince no language-like representations, and mediate routine activities such as social interaction, courtship and foraging. We have thus argued elsewhere against continued reliance on language-based metaphors in animal communication (Rendall, Owren & Ryan, 2009; Owren *et al.*, 2010), and here will highlight only some of the problems flagged in those critiques.

6.4.1 *Intentionality*

Among the most revealing conclusions to emerge from primate research is that these non-humans lack key social cognitive abilities that undergird human sociality and language. In language, words are imbued with meaning through the underlying communicative intentionality of both speakers and listeners. Speakers understand that words stand for, or represent, things in the world. Listeners also understand the representational relationship, and it is this shared understanding that allows productive communication. In short, word meaning hinges on implicit, reciprocal attributions about mental states, including what others do and do not know about the world, and how that knowledge can be modified through the use of words with shared representational value (Grice, 1957).

In contrast, such intentionality is largely absent in non-human primates. With the possible exception of some great apes, these animals do not attribute mental states to one another and, in their signalling, do not show sensitivity to the needs of perceivers (Cheney & Seyfarth, 1998, 2005). In fact, non-human primates appear to act largely in ignorance of the mental states and communicative needs of conspecifics in both signalling and wider patterns of social behaviour (Penn & Povinelli, 2007). Primate signallers even appear to be ignorant of the communicative value that their own signals can have (Cheney, Seyfarth & Palombit, 1996; Rendall, Cheney & Seyfarth, 2000).

6.4.2 *Development and neuroscience*

Such findings are buttressed by research showing that the mechanistic underpinnings of communication in human and non-human primates are also quite different. For example, speech production in humans is critically dependent on auditory experience and motor practice, is primarily governed by cortical circuits in the temporal and frontal lobes and is volitionally controlled

(Lieberman, 2002). In monkeys, however, vocalisations routinely emerge without any evident need to hear the sounds from others or to practise making them. Calling is furthermore governed primarily by subcortical structures of the limbic system, midbrain and brainstem, and is largely unaffected by cortical stimulation or damage (Jürgens, 2009). Overall, vocal production in primates is modulated primarily by emotion-related rather than volitional processes, appearing far more similar to spontaneous human emotional expressions, such as laughter and crying, than to language (Owren, Amoss & Rendall, 2011).

Thus, despite superficial resemblances between some primate vocalisations and human words, there is a growing realisation that the mechanisms involved are fundamentally different. Indeed, Cheney and Seyfarth (1996, 1998) reached this conclusion themselves more than a decade ago, recently reiterating that "non-human primates' inability to represent the mental states of others makes their communication fundamentally different from human language" (Cheney & Seyfarth, 2005, p. 135). Although others have also echoed this conclusion (Tomasello, 2008; Hauser, 2009), this insight has had little effect on the field. Many primate researchers remain committed to interpreting signals as representational events, although now with the qualification that the reference involved is only *functional* rather than truly language-like. In adopting this stance, researchers acknowledge that communication in primates is not like language, yet still put comparisons to language in a central role. The unfortunate effect is to continue to imply substantive connections to language even in the face of contrary evidence regarding intentionality, vocal development and associated neural mechanisms.

6.5 Problems with information

While communication research on non-primates has not been so heavily influenced by the aura of human language, reliance on information-processing constructs is virtually ubiquitous (Table 6.2). Such constructs dominate to such a degree that formal definitions of animal communication are typically grounded in terms of information (see Table 1 in Rendall *et al.*, 2009). Similarly, most research is guided by a general informational model of communication like that depicted in Figure 6.1. Here again, this focus feels natural and intuitive, and has also become so deeply entrenched that few reflect on its validity or historical origins. However, recalling points just made, the two emphases are importantly linked: the current centrality of informational constructs derives directly from the synergy between language, computer and mind that spurred the cognitive revolution. The outcome was wholesale adoption of the idea that minds are information-processing systems, with communication

Table 6.2 *Examples illustrating how ubiquitously and loosely informal informational constructs are used in current animal communication research. This sample was drawn from five issues of the flagship journal* Animal Behaviour *(January–May 2011), which were the most recent issues available when this chapter was being drafted. The examples cover a wide range of species and topics. Quoted material is drawn from Abstract, Introduction or Discussion material providing general characterisations of the communication problems being studied. The core informational constructs used were never further clarified or defined, and none of the studies used information in its formal quantitative sense. Authors invoking cognitive constructs such as 'decision' and 'evaluation' did so without definition or clarification.*

Author(s)	Topic and taxon	Explanations of signals, signalling or communication (*emphasis added*)
Jordan *et al.* (2011)	Scent marking in mongoose	"To understand fully the function(s) of scent marking we need to consider not only the broad spatial patterns of scent deposition, but also both the *information content* of olfactory signals ... In general, glandular secretions tend to contain stable *category-specific information* ... and are less likely to *convey information* on, and vary with, reproductive physiology ... Excretory products are more likely to *contain and convey information* on reproductive state."
Whattam & Bertram (2011)	Signals of condition in field crickets	"Content-based signals are thought to evolve because of the *information content* they *provide* to the receiver. Such signals may function as multiple messages, each *relaying different information or types of information.*"
Judge (2011)	Effect of age and quality on male courtship success in field crickets	"In the fall field cricket, *G. pennsylvanicus*, age *information* is conveyed through calling song ... a longitudinal analysis may detect relatively subtle age-related changes in calling song, but these changes may not *convey enough information* for females to predict male age ... To examine the *amount of information* about male age relative to male morphology that is conveyed in song, I conducted three sequential canonical correlation and redundancy analyses."

Table 6.2 (cont.)

Author(s)	Topic and taxon	Explanations of signals, signalling or communication (*emphasis added*)
Green & Field (2011)	Status signalling in wasps	"Visual status signals are small patches of colour that *convey information* about an individual's competitive ability, or resource-holding potential (RHP), to an opponent."
Berg *et al.* (2011)	Individual recognition in parrotlets	"Contact calls function to coordinate activities between two or more individuals in many social animals ... *Signature information* seems particularly important when individuals need to identify each other in crowded, noisy or dangerous reproductive contexts. Green-rumped parrotlets have large, albeit poorly known, vocal repertoires and could have individual *information encoded* in additional call types."
Gordon & Uetz (2011)	Multimodal communication in spiders	"... multimodal communication, in which communication is defined by signals that *convey information* in more than one sensory modality or communication channel ... Interest in multimodal signalling has resulted in numerous (nonexclusive) hypotheses concerning the origin, nature and content of multimodal signalling: (1) signals in different sensory modes *contain the same information* ... (2) signals in different sensory modes each *provide different information* ... (3) signals in different sensory modes *contain information intended* for different receivers, or are used in different contexts ..."
Chaine *et al.* (2011)	Multiple status signals in sparrows	"In birds, research on status signals has largely involved the colour and area of distinct feather patches ... Multiple signals are traits that show some phenotypic independence and *convey* either *independent information* to the same receiver or *different information* to different receivers."
Nunes *et al.* (2011)	Nestmate recognition in stingless bees	"The cuticle of stingless bees, as in other social insects, is a rich source of *information* that is important for the regulation of their society ... Each individual in a colony

Table 6.2 (cont.)

Author(s)	Topic and taxon	Explanations of signals, signalling or communication (*emphasis added*)
		presents a blend of compounds on its cuticle that may also *carry information* regarding its sex, age, caste, group task as well as colony."
Antunes *et al.* (2011)	Individual variation in acoustic signals of sperm whales	"Securing the benefits of group living often requires mechanisms for group cohesion. These require the *exchange of information* through some form of communication ... With this in mind, we hypothesized that variation in particular coda types could potentially *carry information* about individual identity and therefore codas could *contain both group- and individual-level information* ... The present study also suggests that codas are *hierarchically coded signals* in which individuality *information* is *encoded* in finer variations in timing around the stereotyped rhythm of a given coda type. We suggest that studies of animal communication will benefit from considering the possibility of subtle *information coding* at different hierarchical levels that may otherwise be overlooked."
Barrera *et al.* (2011)	Predator avoidance in doves	"Animals identify potential risk by assessing various cues such as alarm calls and predator vocalizations ... However, these different cues provide *different information* ... We first demonstrated that predator-elicited wing whistles in zenaida doves are alarm signals ... Then, we studied the *relative information content* of these signals compared to vocalizations from a common predator, the red-tailed hawk ... Given that our results showed a greater reaction to predator sounds, we infer that the nonvocal wing whistle was less reliable, suggesting that reliability influences the receiver's *evaluation* of the *relative information content*."
Karubian *et al.* (2011)	Sexual signalling in fairy-wrens	"In the red-backed fairy-wren, bill coloration (and perhaps behaviour) appears to *provide information* on current status during the

Table 6.2 (cont.)

Author(s)	Topic and taxon	Explanations of signals, signalling or communication (*emphasis added*)
		breeding season ... whereas plumage coloration *provides information* on condition, circulating levels of androgens and, potentially, status during moult prior to the breeding season. These findings are consistent with the 'multiple messages hypothesis', which proposes that different ornaments *provide information* about individual quality at different stages of life."
Gruter & Ratnieks (2011)	Forager recruitment in bees	"In many social insects, successful foragers guide nestmates to food sources by *providing* route or location *information* (in their waggle dances) ... However, recent studies suggest that many workers that follow waggle dances ignore the vector *information* on leaving the nest ... It seems that the floral odours on the dancing bee are important ... Hence, social odour *information* can cause *informational ambiguity* if it is similar to private odour *information* linked to route memories."
Balsby & Adams (2011)	Flockmate recruitment in conures	"Identifying which individuals will make good group mates requires the ability to communicate motivational state and/or identity prior to fission-fusion events ... Vocalizations can *carry* a variety of *information*, including group/flock association, relatedness or geographical origin, as well as *information* on physical characteristics such as sex, age and condition, all of which may aid the *decision* of whether or not to recruit other individuals ... In fission-fusion societies, the *information exchanged* within a single vocal interaction may be sufficient to *decide* whether or not to recruit an individual or group."

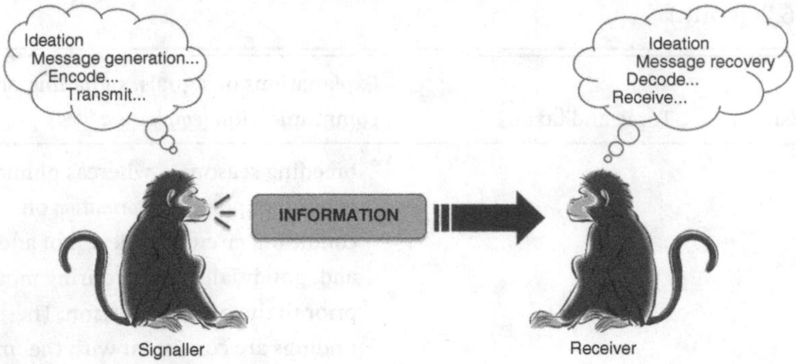

Figure 6.1 A schema illustrating core features common to language-based and informational models of communication. Communication involves the transmission of information, from signaller to receiver. Here, signaller ideation (thought, belief, motive) becomes a message encoded in the details of a physical signal transmitted to a receiver. The receiver receives the physical signal and decodes it to recover the intended message. This approach thus views signalling as a flow of packaged information from signaller to receiver. Additional implicit assumptions include that matching encoding and decoding mechanisms ensure transmission fidelity, and that the information transmitted is honest, because receivers are free to discount anything else. Figure redrawn from Rendall *et al.* (2009) with permission from Elsevier.

in all forms functioning to transmit that information. In other words, even when communication in a given species is not interpreted in language-based terms, closely associated notions of information-processing remain central (Rendall *et al.*, 2009; Owren *et al.*, 2010).

6.5.1 *'Information' is ambiguous*

One fundamental problem is that the information construct, as used by animal communication researchers, is inherently ambiguous. Although communication is frequently defined in informational terms, information itself is seldom defined or operationalised.[1] The most natural sense would be the one associated with formal information theory and the advent of digital computing, where information was defined quantitatively as uncertainty reduction

[1] In this sense, information has become the new phlogiston, something that cannot be seen, defined, measured or quantified but that is central to everything. The history of phlogiston theory should make us wary of such loose, sweeping constructs. We should be especially wary of the argument that information is a useful construct because it has supported a great deal of research in animal communication and can account for a great number of its findings (Seyfarth *et al.*, 2010). The same was once said of phlogiston, a flat Earth and geocentrism.

(Shannon & Weaver, 1949). Strangely, that is not the case. Information is instead almost always used in a looser, metaphorical sense that mirrors common discourse. Here, information becomes effectively equivalent to *meaning*: the information that a signal contains or transmits is what the signal *means*. However, the construct of meaning is notoriously slippery, and, as just reviewed, does not apply in its linguistic sense to animal communication. As a result, while being careful not to claim that animal signals convey meaning in a linguistic sense, researchers are then unable to explain what they do intend. Because terms such as information and meaning lie at the heart of current conceptions of animal communication, the field itself now rests on constructs that its practitioners are unable to define.[2]

6.5.2 *'Coding' is problematic*

Other core constructs of informational perspectives are similarly problematic. For example, informational characterisations of animal communication implicitly invoke some form of code. A signal's message is said to be *encoded* in the details of its physical form, information content that listeners recover through a *decoding* process. As with the term information, references to

[2] For example, Seyfarth *et al.* (2010) offer a recent defence of the information construct, yet similarly fail to define the term information. Instead, they appeal to a looser, informal conception wherein signals can be said to have information when they stand in predictive relation to some event or state of the world. Specifically, they argue that, just as a light predicts shock to a laboratory rat, so too does a vervet alarm call predict the presence of an eagle to other vervets. Just so, and if this is all they propose is entailed in vervet alarm calls, then there is nothing at all language-like about them and thus no basis for comparing them to language or inferring any implications for language evolution. We can, of course, agree that there is information *in the world* in the sense they propose, namely that predictive relationships abound and can be learned by animals (see Scott-Phillips, 2010 for more on this point). This hardly needs emphasising. However, what should be emphasised is that such information does not reside in the signals themselves but rather in the relationship between them and the events they co-occur with. This is, in fact, evinced in the very system Seyfarth and Cheney appeal to: naïve rats, in fact, do not avoid the light at first and, similarly, naïve infant vervets do not respond appropriately to eagle alarm calls at first (Seyfarth & Cheney, 1986). In both cases, the predictive relationship must be learned through a history of experience with the associations. The signals, by themselves, do not contain this information. To say that they do is to spirit into the signal itself the relationship it shares with events in the world and thus to fundamentally obscure the mechanisms by which signals actually function. Importantly, although vervet alarm calls do not actually contain information, we have argued elsewhere that their structure is nevertheless well designed to influence infant vervets directly but in ways that facilitate their learning of the predictive relationships between signals and predators, thereby acquiring appropriate escape responses that they specifically lack when young (Owren & Rendall, 2001; Rendall *et al.*, 2009; Owren *et al.*, 2010).

encoding and decoding are common (see Table 6.2), but remain tacit. There is, for instance, little attempt to explain what the unencoded or decoded versions of a message might be like.

In standard usage, the concept of encoding involves some process of signal translation or transduction: content in one domain is translated into a different, but corresponding form. Such content translations have been central to theories of human thought and communication. For example, the *language of thought* hypothesis (Fodor, 1975) proposes that mental processing occurs in a different form (an internal language) from the concrete form realised in spoken language. Similarly, Chomsky's original articulation of his theory of transformational or generative grammar (1965) proposed a fundamental distinction between the deep and surface structure of language. In our view, neither the deep structure nor the processes of transformation to surface structure could ever be substantively described, however, as is also the case for analogous notions of mental representation and encoding of animal signals.

6.5.3 *'Coding' is unnecessary*

More importantly, perhaps, there is often no need to appeal to an encoding process at all. Many animal signals mediate common social contexts such as aggressive competition for resources or attracting mates. Here, signals are proposed to *encode information* about relevant social or physical characteristics of signallers, such as their age, sex, body size, individual identity, emotional state or physical condition (see Table 6.2). However, in these and other common contexts, there is no need to invoke an encoding process – the dimensions are signalled directly. For instance, a large body naturally allows for a large vocal apparatus, which in turn tends to produce low frequency sounds (Fitch & Hauser, 1995). Hence, low frequency sounds are not somehow an *encoded translation* of large size. They are simply the direct acoustic manifestation of large size – what large size sounds like. Similarly, naturally occurring idiosyncracies in vocal anatomy yield subtle, corresponding differences in the sounds that different individuals produce (Rendall, Owren & Rodman, 1998). Those acoustic differences do not then somehow *encode information* about individual identity, they are just the acoustic manifestations of individual identity. In like fashion, particular emotional or motivational states can affect aspects of physiology (e.g. respiration) in ways that influence structural characteristics of vocal sounds produced; and variation in physical condition can influence the susceptibility of such sounds to perturbations induced by effortful performance displays. In all of these cases, structural differences in signals that are traditionally held to *encode* these different dimensions of size, identity, emotional state or physical condition are, in reality, just direct manifestations of the dimensions themselves. There is no need to posit an intervening translational process or code – instead, "the medium *is* the message" (McLuhan, 1964).

Similar points can be made about the other side of the information-transmission equation, where a separate, decoding process may rarely be required. Instead, signals can have relatively direct influence on perceiver sensory systems, physiology and behaviour.[3]

6.5.4 *Distinctive features and context*

By emphasising notions of encoding and decoding, informational approaches strongly encourage a view that the signal itself bears most of the load in communication. One consequence is that signals are seen as bundles of distinctive features, each one of which can be dissected out as a carrier of potentially unique information (see Table 6.2). The result is that there is relatively little emphasis on more holistic or integrated patterns of signal production and perception. A second, related effect is that researchers downplay or overlook many other factors influencing communication. These include a host of features of the social or environmental context that accompany signalling, as well as the variety of proximate motivations, predispositions and biases that signallers and perceivers bring to the interaction (Smith, 1977; Leger, 1993).

6.6 Language is not a fixed code

Returning to language, the view that emerged through Chomsky (1965) and others was both compatible with, and quickly became enmeshed in, contemporaneous computational and information-processing perspectives. It was

[3] Well-documented examples of such direct influence occur in a variety of fish, frogs, birds and insects (Cheng & Peng, 1997; Endler & Basolo, 1998; Wilczynski & Chu, 2001; Ryan & Rand, 2003; reviewed in Ryan, 1998), as well as in artificial neural networks (Enquist & Arak, 1993) and listener gene expression (Mello, Nootebohm & Clayton, 1995). In a classic example, spectral characteristics of the courtship signals of male túngara frogs, *Physalaemus pustulosus*, are proposed to have evolved to match pre-existing auditory sensitivity of conspecific females (Ryan, 1990). Female attraction to male calls is explained mechanistically by the way distinct components of the male call have evolved to maximally stimulate two complementary inner organs of females (reviewed in Ryan & Rand, 2003). Less dramatically, alarm vocalisations and common social calls produced by nonhuman primates (Owren & Rendall, 1997, 2001; Rendall & Owren, 2010) are not arbitrarily structured – as initially proposed – for instance most often being short, with abrupt onsets and broadband noisy spectra. These widely shared features are ideally suited for capturing and manipulating listener attention and arousal through direct links between the auditory periphery and brainstem regions regulating attention and arousal (also see Hartshorne, 1973; Searcy, 1992). Vocalisations can also have significant self-stimulation effects. For instance, Cheng (1992) found that the 'nest' coos of female ring doves stimulate hormone release in the caller herself, thereby helping to advance the courtship and mating process.

argued, for example, that language is too difficult for children to learn, and that the speech input that children receive is impoverished relative to the speech they eventually produce. To account for the surprising ease of language learning, Chomsky (1965) proposed an innate, and uniquely human, *language acquisition device* (LAD). The LAD was further argued to be an embodiment of *universal grammar* (UG), innate knowledge of the basic principles of grammar that underlie all languages. Early linguistic development is thus a process of setting language-specific parameters in the LAD rather than learning grammar from scratch. This perspective constitutes a *fixed-code* view of language (Harris, 1998), one in which grammar is rule-bound, words have fixed, universal meanings that encode abstract semantic constructs of thought, and the individual sounds of language form well-defined categories with specifiable acoustic and articulatory features. Yet, there are significant problems with the fixed-code approach at each of these levels.

6.6.1 *Grammar*

While Chomsky's proposals had immense influence, it proved impossible to specify the fixed, universal language features instantiated in UG. In later theory, therefore, Chomsky (1995) had to abandon the distinction between deep and surface structure, and dilute the principles and parameters proposed for UG. Even more damaging is the finding that language is, in fact, learnable from typical input.[4]

6.6.2 *Words*

Words have also been considered fixed, representing stable units with agreed-upon meanings. However, this view is strongly opposed by integrational linguists emphasising the role of individual experience and context. Harris (1981, 1998), for example, argues that word meanings are context-dependent and changeable based on each individual's language experience, the social circumstances in which words are used, and the semantic, grammatical and prosodic aspects of individual utterances (Cowley & Love, 2006). Hence, extra-linguistic factors such as context and pragmatics make word meaning inherently slippery and fluid rather than being stable and invariant.

[4] Here, neural networks can detect and 'learn' grammatical structure from statistical regularities in larger corpuses of language material, and relatively rich semantic knowledge can be developed through associative processes operating over very large corpuses of language material (Landauer & Dumai, 1997). In humans, even preverbal infants have been found to be sensitive to the statistical regularities of the speech stream (Saffran, Ashin & Newport, 1996) – which now appears to be much less impoverished than previously believed. Indeed, research has shown such structure to exist at multiple organisational levels, which can serve to bootstrap language learning (Kuhl, 2000).

6.6.3 *Speech sounds*

An early, serious challenge to the fixed-code view also arose in the search for invariance at the level of individual speech sounds. At an early stage, psycholinguists discovered that the acoustic signal does not provide the invariant cues to phones and phonemes they had believed to be present in the speech stream (Lisker & Abramson, 1967). In other words, although speech is psychologically experienced as a series of discrete phonemes, syllables and words, the physical input itself cannot be parsed into corresponding, individual units. Speech acoustics are actually far more variable and continuous over time, with phonetic segments overlapping forwards-and-backwards in the speech waveform.

This lack-of-invariance problem inspired a proposal that humans are innately endowed with a phonetic module – akin to Chomsky's LAD – that does the difficult perceptual work automatically. The early discovery of *categorical perception* (CP) appeared to confirm that proposal, showing that listeners parsed continuous acoustic variation into discrete psychological categories when listening to synthetic versions of stop consonants such as /b/ and /p/ (Liberman *et al.*, 1957). While this outcome was exactly the sort of specialisation expected of a native language endowment, the overall *speech is special* view that arose has also not fared very well. For example, both /b/ versus /p/ and other phonemic contrasts were later found to be processed categorically by rodents and monkeys as well (Kuhl & Miller, 1975; Kuhl & Padden, 1982), with the long-term lesson being that while written language may be relatively discrete and particulate, spoken language is not (Port, 2010).

6.6.4 *Speech and computers*

The real-world difficulties inherent to the fixed-code approach to language are illustrated by the decidedly meagre results of machine production and recognition of speech.[5] Nowhere has the effort been as great, or the returns as small, as in the continuing quest to develop computer speech recognition. Here again, lack of invariance creates formidable obstacles. As a result, while commercial speech-recognition software is now available, it functions by computing statistical best-guesses – which are often wrong. Even in the latest technology,

[5] While public agencies and private companies have long tried to develop machines capable of producing and comprehending fluent speech, the actual results have been modest with problems arising at each of the levels outlined above. Spoken language is, for example, rarely as well structured as written versions. Here, human listeners can take contextual factors into account to easily follow the broken and incomplete sentences that often characterise real-world speech. Machines cannot. The importance of semantic and other forms of context become quite obvious in machine translation of language. Performance can be reasonable for short, simple sentences that can be treated literally. However, even moderate complexity in the original material soon results in garbled output.

error rates are one to two orders of magnitude higher than they are for human listeners (reviewed in Furui, 2010). To achieve any level of success, programs have to be restricted to recognising either a very small number of words, or a larger number of words from only a few speakers. The most fruitful approach has been to limit the input to a single speaker who also first trains the software on pronunciations of known words. Functionally, the effect is to create a fixed code for that individual. However, the need to do so underscores that normative speech perception does not depend on such a code, instead being far more holistic, episodic and contextual in nature (e.g. Palmeri, Goldinger & Pisoni, 1993; Nygaard, Sommers & Pisoni, 1994; Johnson, 1997).

6.6.5 *Implications for fixed coding*

In spite of having deep, intuitive appeal, the fixed-code, particulate approach to language fails at multiple levels (Harris, 1981, 1998; Cowley & Love, 2006; Kravchenko, 2007; Port, 2010). The organisation and endowment of language no longer seems to plausibly lie in a set of narrowly circumscribed and innately specialised computational and perceptual modules. Instead, it seems to recruit a broad range of psychological processes, including simple but powerful associative and statistical learning abilities, and complex, context-based inference. Hence, while viewing the human language faculty as a discretely organised system is intuitive and compelling, this analogy to digital information-processing has little to say about how language production, perception and comprehension actually work in the brain.

6.7 How the mind ~~works~~ does not work

Recent developments in language theory are paralleled (naturally) by developments in theories of mind. The computer metaphor of mind, so intuitive in the early days of cognitivism, is now seen to have critical limitations and is gradually being eclipsed.[6] Foremost among its limitations is the emphasis on cognition as a disembodied, in-the-head phenomenon. In this view, perceptual input from the outside world is fundamentally transformed in creating an abstract mental code that is the basis of internal processing and representation. Behavioural responses then require a converse transformation from that code into motor commands. However, this *brain-as-computer* model appears adequate only for certain, representation-hungry tasks such as playing chess or doing

[6] "Interestingly, Claude Shannon, one of the developers of the mathematical theory of information, was skeptical that the brain was an information processor; he believed that processing information required a transmitter, a receiver, and an agreed-upon code, none of which is found in the brain" (Alva Noe, 2009, p. 156).

mental long-division (Clark, 1997). But these are relatively artificial and rarefied tasks. The bulk of quotidian behaviour and cognition is quite different, and is not well accommodated by the symbol-manipulation model of mind (Searle, 1980; Brooks, 1991; Clark, 1997; Dreyfus, 1999). Instead, ordinary behaviour and cognition is appreciated to be far more *embodied*, involving processes for behavioural control that entail relatively direct engagement with the environment via perception–action circuits that effectively bypass any need for internal representation, symbol transduction and processing. In addition, a great deal of what we have traditionally modelled as cognition is now acknowledged not to occur exclusively in one's head, but rather to be distributed to the world and our interaction with it (Hutchins, 1995; Clark & Chalmers, 1998; Clark, 2008; Wheeler & Clark, 2008). Indeed, a great deal of what we think of as uniquely human and complicated involves off-loading the demands of intensive internal processing to external supports in the environment.[7]

6.7.1 *Developments in artificial intelligence and robotics*

This conclusion is buttressed by research in artificial intelligence (AI) and robotics. These fields arose in conjunction with computer technology and were thus originally based on the same logic of symbol processing. They were widely anticipated to solve the problem of intelligence and to yield all manner of useful devices, but practical successes were slow to come (Dreyfus, 1999). This failing is argued to reflect a focus on symbol-crunching computational processes that, while generic and powerful, create insurmountable informational bottlenecks. Even simple tasks are hamstrung by the need, first, to re-represent internally many features of the external environment. An exhaustive, internal search must then combine this re-representation with stored knowledge to find and select among possible, situationally relevant response options. By the time a command for action has been issued, the situation is likely to have changed! Modern AI and robotics thus shows this

[7] For example, rather than commit to memory shopping lists, phone numbers and passwords, we commit them to pieces of paper or computer files, from which they can be retrieved whenever needed. We similarly store important personal items such as keys and glasses in locations that ensure we routinely encounter them on route to the habitual activities that will require them rather than in any number of other safer hiding places that are actually quite hard to remember! These are routine ways we off-load cognitive processing by marking the environment through our behaviour – sometimes deliberately, sometimes not – in ways that allow us simply to re-perceive, rather than remember (represent), important things. We also create a diversity of cognitive artifacts, like symbol manipulating calculators and computers, specifically to avoid cognitively demanding symbol manipulation tasks. In fact, perhaps our penchant for externalised symbol manipulating systems arises precisely to compensate for the weak symbol manipulation capacities of our brains.

emphasis on representation and symbol manipulation to be unproductive and unwarranted, and just to get in the way for many everyday tasks (Brooks, 1991; Dreyfus, 1999). Instead, functional behaviour can be achieved by peripheral perception–action loops that largely forgo representing the external world and instead capitalise on natural regularities and affordances inherent in the environment. In the words of Rodney Brooks (1991), "the world is its own best model". There is no need to re-represent it – just act on it.

The upshot is that models of mind based on the computer and on disembodied information processing and symbol manipulation increasingly appear to be substantively incomplete – if not largely wrong. They are appropriately giving way to alternatives that stress the active nature of cognition, and its more embodied and distributed nature. Such models of cognition are taking hold in research on human psychology but have yet to gain much purchase in the field of animal cognition (cf. Grasse, 1959; Gallese *et al.*, 1996; Barrett, 2011).

6.8 Metaphors, explanatory place-holders and true explanations

Metaphor is a powerful mode of human thought (Lakoff & Johnson, 1980), as well as an important reasoning tool that naturally also influences scientific thought. In science, metaphors often have heuristic value in the early stages of a discipline. Without a mature theoretical edifice in place, young disciplines frequently turn to other fields for constructs with which to provide initial characterisations of their own core phenomena.

6.8.1 *"The price of metaphor..."*

However, metaphors come at a cost. One is the risk that the metaphors become circular and self-sustaining, like those of the cognitive revolution. There is also the risk of unwarranted, often unwitting reification. Over time, a metaphor becomes so familiar that it slides gradually into a literal account of core phenomena. Hence, "the price of metaphor is eternal vigilance"[8] – regular re-evaluation of explanatory constructs is needed to avoid such pitfalls. In the normal course of things, as a discipline matures, its metaphors evolve and ultimately give way entirely to more concrete accounts of focal phenomena.

In animal communication, language-based metaphors had heuristic value during an important stage in the development of the field. The focus on language properties in the early vervet monkey research made good sense. Language was

[8] This quote is often attributed to Arturo Rosenbleuth and Norbert Weiner but typically either without citation details or with details that do not actually contain the quoted material (Rosenbleuth & Weiner, 1950). We have tried unsuccessfully to find the original quote. Given that, we simply continue the tradition of attributing the aphorism to them. It carries the same cautionary value no matter the source.

familiar and provided a ready benchmark for comparison in a field just finding its feet. It also made sense to seek evolutionary precursors to language among non-human primates. Given the expanding appeal of computer technology and information-processing models of human communication and cognition, applying similar constructs in animal communication research also seemed natural.

6.8.2 *Abandoning language and information metaphors*

Nonetheless, a variety of evidence now suggests that the language and information metaphors that have coloured research in animal communication have run their course and should be abandoned. Evidence of their limitations comes both from the field of animal communication where the metaphors have been applied, and from the domains of human language and cognition whence the metaphors originated.

In animal communication, the constructs have proven both too restrictive and too loose to cover the broad range of animal signalling phenomena. They are too restrictive because their common language-based and informational focus unduly narrows the focus of study and limits the range of questions asked, problems investigated and alternatives considered (Rendall *et al.*, 2009). The concepts are simultaneously too loose because their core linguistic and informational explanatory constructs – *information, meaning, encoding, decoding* – are vaguely defined and rarely operationalised. One outcome has been the emergence of theoretical hybrids that blur otherwise central distinctions in ethological and evolutionary enquiry. The idea of *functional reference*, for example, conflates mechanism and function in signalling, as well as the potentially disparate roles of signallers and perceivers.[9] Ultimately, notions such as

[9] The incoherence is most simply illustrated in a concurrent conceptual development, specifically the proposal that the meaning of animal signals can be conceived of as lying on a continuum between endpoints anchored by purely motivational signals and purely referential ones (Marler, Evans & Hanser, 1992). According to this proposal, the motivational end of the continuum involves signals that simply reflect and convey the internal emotional or motivational state of the signaller, while the referential end reflects the extent to which perceivers can draw inferences about external events upon hearing the signals. In other words, one end of the continuum concerns the mechanisms underlying signal production, and the other concerns the functional consequences for listeners of receiving and interpreting the signals. The notion that a given signal can be attributed meaning and placed at a single location on this continuum thus involves blending the mechanisms of signalling with its potential functions, and merges the distinct roles of signaller and perceiver in the process. As a result, either the distinction between the motivational and referential endpoints evaporates and with it the entire notion of a continuum between them, or any given signal must be said to exist simultaneously at multiple locations on the continuum depending on whose perspective is being considered and whether one is focused on either the mechanisms or the functions of signalling.

information and coding cannot be cashed out in terms of standard concepts used in biological and evolutionary theory. As a result, they operate in support of only 'as if' theories that focus on putative functional abilities, but masquerade as accounts of the underlying mechanisms involved.

At best, constructs such as information and coding provide functional, systems-level descriptions of "how it is WE CAN UNDERSTAND that", but not "how it IS that" (Craver, 2006). As such, they are only explanatory place-holders that have little or nothing to say about the actual mechanisms governing the system. The more detailed understanding needed – true explanation – goes beyond metaphorical description to account for the real underlying mechanisms themselves.

Outside the field of animal communication, traditional Chomskyan, computational and information-processing approaches are now regarded as quite incomplete – even as models for human language and human minds. At best, these conceptions are caricatures promoted by the disembodied information-processing logic of the computer. They are now slowly being abandoned in favour of alternative and more pluralistic approaches that are markedly different from those that originally spawned the cognitive revolution. It is ironic that research in animal communication continues to adhere to explanatory metaphors that have largely been abandoned in the fields they were borrowed from.

6.9 Summary of criticisms

Summarising the main points of our critique:

(1) Animal communication research has been guided by analogies to language and related information-processing constructs.

(2) That emphasis flowed from the cognitive revolution, which was founded on the computer as a metaphor for minds, languages and communication systems generally.

(3) Linguistic and computational constructs have not been clearly articulated and defined in animal communication research and ultimately have not fared well – even signals that at first seemed most language-like have proved very unlike language.

(4) At the same time, research in language and cognition has moved on, and these fields no longer adhere so strictly to computational and informational metaphors.

(5) One must therefore ask why animal communication researchers are bent on using loose and outmoded constructs borrowed from fields that themselves no longer adhere to them.

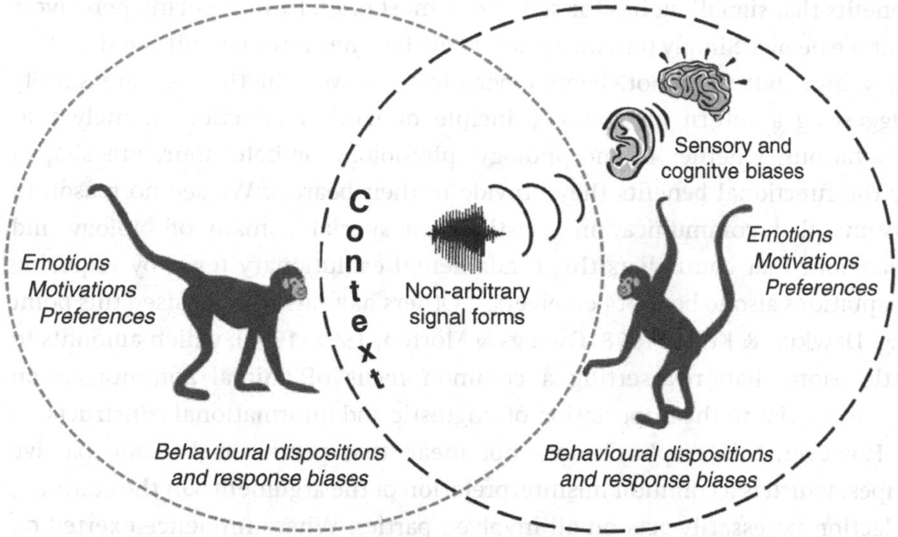

Figure 6.2 A schema illustrating some important features of non-informational alternatives to animal communication. Functionally, communication is dynamic, both in real time and in evolutionary time, and involves an iterated process of reciprocal influence and resistance by signallers and perceivers with overlapping spheres of influence. The details of the physical signals are important and are central to the functions they serve, including exerting relatively direct influence on perceiver's sensory, motivational and cognitive systems. Signals may be honest owing to selection pressure on perceivers to resist anything else. Honesty is not assumed, however, because historical, mechanistic constraints and the multi-functional nature of perceptual systems can leave perceivers susceptible to influence. Other factors affecting signalling dynamics include sensory, motivational, cognitive and behavioural biases, and associated predispositions in signallers and perceivers alike. Such predispositions are necessarily shaped by both species (phylogenetic) and individual histories, as well as being modulated in real time by specific features of the social and environmental context.

6.10 Alternative approaches to animal communication

To end on a more positive and productive note, we will briefly consider how future research in animal communication could be organised without recourse to linguistic and informational constructs (outlined schematically in Figure 6.2).

6.10.1 *Functional re-orientation around influence rather than information*

First, we suggest a fundamental re-orientation of research around the broad functional principle that signal evolution is ultimately organised by the benefits that signalling has for signallers, most often by influencing perceivers (but see below). Simply put, for signals to evolve, they must benefit the signaller. They may, but need not, benefit perceivers as well. In this, we are simply suggesting a return to a core principle of natural selection, namely that adaptations, whether of morphology, physiology or behaviour, are shaped by the functional benefits they provide to their bearers. We see no reason to assume that communication constitutes a special domain of biology and behaviour that contradicts this fundamental evolutionary tenet by requiring adaptations also to benefit perceivers.[10] Others have also emphasised this point (e.g. Dawkins & Krebs, 1978; Owings & Morton, 1997, 1998), which amounts to little more than re-asserting a common focus of animal communication research prior to the importation of linguistic and informational constructs.

However, this emphasis does not mean that perceivers become passive dupes, which is a common misinterpretation of the argument. On the contrary, selection necessarily acts on all involved parties. Where influence exerted on perceivers is not ultimately in their interests, they will be selected to resist signaller effects. Nonetheless, it cannot be assumed *a priori* that selection for perceiver resistance trumps selection on signaller influence. This assumption has become entrenched in some contemporary frameworks where signal honesty is offered as a putative axiom of communication (Zahavi & Zahavi, 1997; Maynard Smith & Harper, 2003; Searcy & Nowicki, 2005). But honesty is only one possible signalling outcome. Signalling systems can deviate from honest equilibria for a variety of reasons, including historical contingency, latent sensory biases, physiological and neurological constraints, and trade-offs created by the multi-functional nature of perceptual systems (Ryan, 1990, 1998; Guilford & Dawkins, 1991; Cummings, 2007). Hence, while the focus on honesty gives veto power to perceivers and yields a relatively one-sided view of the communication process, the focus on influence is broader and more widely applicable. It

[10] In a recent response to these arguments, Seyfarth *et al.* (2010) demur that our proposed focus on influence is inappropriate. In support, they cite an example we have often used, namely of the conflict that routinely occurs even between mothers and offspring over the timing and amount of investment provided by mothers, particularly at the stage when they are weaning offspring. In this context, offspring of many species produce long bouts of loud, harsh, chaotically structured calls that we have argued are not well designed to transmit information but are well designed to stimulate maternal attention and arousal, to preclude habituation to their noxious effects, and ultimately to wear down maternal resistance. Seyfarth *et al.* argue that it is wrong to characterise this interaction, and many others, as involving conflict and influence because all infants ultimately do get weaned. This argument patently conflates the outcome of a process with the process itself. If it were valid, then it would also be true that because the Great War ultimately ended there was in fact no conflict or influence ever involved.

acknowledges the dynamic nature of real-time signalling, with signallers and perceivers playing important and potentially distinct roles in an iterated, reciprocal process of influence and resistance (Owings & Morton, 1998). It acknowledges that signalling systems are dynamic in evolutionary time as well.

6.10.2 *Mechanistic re-orientation*

Second, we suggest an associated mechanistic re-orientation away from the representational and intentional processes that have preoccupied language-oriented research and that are, in fact, also an implicit focus of work grounded in informational constructs. Whether they know it or not, researchers relying on information and coding constructs to understand animal communication are implicitly positing that signals are inherently representational in nature (Owren *et al.*, 2010).

Instead, the field must update its views on perception and cognition. Following the points above, research should move away from the passive, disembodied and exclusively 'in-the-head' views of cognition inspired by computer metaphors and embrace alternative perceptual-cognitive frameworks that emphasise the dynamic, embodied and distributed nature of perception, cognition and action (e.g. Thelen & Smith, 1994; Hutchins, 1995; van Gelder, 1995; Dreyfus, 1999; Clark, 2001, 2008; Noe, 2009). The latter frameworks are grounded in the elemental and unassailable logic that organisms are characterised by a fundamental, ongoing engagement with themselves, with others and with the physical environment around them. Their basic challenge is therefore to monitor and manage this engagement in ways that maximise benefits while minimising costs. This focus entails a number of subsidiary emphases, including how affective and motivational systems complement cognitive processes in guiding behaviour so as to effectively influence as well as respond to others; how such systems are influenced and primed by contextual factors; how quotidian tasks may be organised by fairly direct links between perception and action that bypass the need for central, evaluative processes; and how proximate sensory and perceptual biases can facilitate some opportunities for action and constrain others. It might also include increased consideration of the extent to which behaviour, including communication, serves important self-regulatory or self-stimulatory functions (cf. Cheng, 1992; reviewed for bird song in Riters, 2011).

6.10.3 *Contextual factors*

Finally, we suggest looking beyond the physical signals themselves to consider the diversity of contextual factors involved in communication. Contextual factors have sometimes been studied to good effect, but have not been a continuing priority. Instead, as noted earlier, informational perspectives have assumed that the signals are doing the bulk of the work. The physical signals are, of course, central and must be a continuing focus. However, it is well established that social and environmental factors can influence physiological, perceptual and motivational systems that are instrumental in an organism's ongoing flow of behaviour (e.g. Siegel *et al.*, 2000; Galef & Laland, 2005).

We do not imagine this scenario is somehow complete, or even necessarily very novel. Indeed, much of what we propose is anticipated by previous work (von UexKull, 1910; Gibson, 1979; Jarvilehto, 2009). However, we do see the *kind* of approach we advocate as markedly different and both more pluralistic and more plausible than traditional language-based and informational perspectives that reduce this great variety of factors to unitary and enigmatic constructs such as *meaning* or *information*. The latter kind of explanatory reduction may seem a great simplification, in some sense, but ultimately it grossly underspecifies and obscures most of what needs explaining about animal communication and takes the study of it well outside the realm of normative ethological and evolutionary enquiry.

References

Antunes, R., Schulz, T., Gero, S. *et al.* (2011). Individually distinctive acoustic features in sperm whale codas. *Animal Behaviour*, **81**, 732–730.

Balsby, T. J. S. & Adams, D. M. (2011). Vocal similarity and familiarity determine response to potential flockmates in orange-fronted conures (Psittacidae). *Animal Behaviour*, **81**, 983–991.

Barrera, J. P., Chong, L., Judy, K. N. & Blumstein, D. T. (2011). Reliability of public information: predators provide more information about risk than conspecifics. *Animal Behaviour*, **81**, 779–787.

Barrett, L. (2011). *Beyond the Brain: How Body and Environment Shape Animal and Human Minds*. Princeton, NJ: Princeton University Press.

Berg, K. S., Delgado, S., Okawa, R., Beissinger, S. R. & Bradbury, J. W. (2011). Contact calls are used for individual mate recognition in free-ranging green-rumped parrotlets, *Forpus passerinus*. *Animal Behaviour*, **81**, 241–248.

Brooks, R. (1991). Intelligence without representation. *Artifical Intelligence Journal*, **47**, 139–159.

Bugnyar, T., Kijne, M. & Kotrschal, K. (2001). Food calling in ravens: are yells referential signals? *Animal Behaviour*, **61**, 949–958.

Chaine, A. S., Tjernell, K. A., Shizuka, D. & Lyon, B. E. (2011). Sparrows use multiple status signals in winter social flocks. *Animal Behaviour*, **81**, 447–453.

Cheney, D. L. & Seyfarth, R. M. (1988). Assessment of meaning and the detection of unreliable signals by vervet monkeys. *Animal Behaviour*, **36**, 477–486.

Cheney, D. L. & Seyfarth, R. M. (1996). Function and intention in the calls of non-human primates. *Proceedings of the British Academy*, **88**, 59–76.

Cheney, D. L. & Seyfarth, R. M. (1998). Why animals don't have language. In G. B. Pearson, ed., *The Tanner Lectures on Human Values*. Salt Lake City, UT: University of Utah Press, pp. 174–209.

Cheney, D. L. & Seyfarth, R. M. (2005). Constraints and preadaptations in the earliest stages of language evolution. *Linguistic Review*, **22**, 135–159.

Cheney, D. L., Seyfarth, R. M. & Palombit, R. (1996). The function and mechanisms underlying baboon 'contact' barks. *Animal Behaviour*, **52**, 507–518.

Cheng, M.-F. (1992). For whom does the female dove coo? A case for the role of self-stimulation. *Animal Behaviour*, **43**, 1035–1044.

Cheng, M.-F. & Peng, J. P. (1997). Reciprocal talk between the auditory thalamus and hypothalamus: an antidromic study. *NeuroReport*, **8**, 653–658.

Chomsky, N. (1959). Review of *Verbal Behavior*, by B. F. Skinner. *Language*, **35**, 26–57.

Chomsky, N. (1965). *Aspects of the Theory of Syntax*. Cambridge, MA: MIT Press.

Chomsky, N. (1995). *The Minimalist Program*. Cambridge, MA: MIT Press.

Clark, A. (1997). *Being There: Putting Brain, Body, and World Together Again*. Cambridge, MA: MIT Press.

Clark, A. (2001). *Mindware: An Introduction to the Philosophy of Cognitive Science*. Oxford: Oxford University Press.

Clark, A. (2008). *Supersizing the Mind: Embodiment, Action, and Cognitive Extension*. Oxford: Oxford University Press.

Clark, A. & Chalmers, D. (1998). The extended mind. *Analysis*, **58**, 7–19.

Cowley, S. & Love, N. (2006). Language and cognition, or, how to avoid the conduit metaphor. In A. Duszak & U. Okulska, eds., *Bridges and Walls in Metalinguistic Discourse*. Frankfurt/Main: Peter Lang, pp. 135–156.

Craver, C. F. (2006). When mechanistic models explain. *Synthese*, **153**, 355–376.

Cummings, M. E. (2007). Sensory trade-offs predict signal divergence in surfperch. *Evolution*, **61**, 530–545.

Dawkins, R. & Krebs, J. R. (1978). Animal signals: information or manipulation. In J. R. Krebs & N. B. Davies, eds., *Behavioural Ecology: An Evolutionary Approach*. Oxford: Blackwell Scientific, pp. 282–309.

Dreyfus, H. (1999). *What Computers Still Can't Do*. Cambridge, MA: MIT Press.

Endler, J. A. & Basolo, A. L. (1998). Sensory ecology, receiver biases and sexual selection. *Trends in Ecology and Evolution*, **13**, 415–420.

Enquist, M. & Arak, A. (1993). Selection of exaggerated male traits by female aesthetic senses. *Nature*, **361**, 446–448.

Evans, C. S. & Evans, L. (1999). Chicken food calls are functionally referential. *Animal Behaviour*, **58**, 307–319.

Fitch, W. T. & Hauser, M. D. (1995). Vocal production in non-human primates: acoustics, physiology and functional constraints on 'honest' adverstising. *American Journal of Primatology*, **37**, 191–219.

Fodor, J. (1975). *The Language of Thought*. Cambridge, MA: Harvard University Press.

Furui, S. (2010). History and development of speech recognition. In F. Chen & K. Jokinen, eds., *Speech Technology: Theory and Applications*. New York: Springer, pp. 1–16.

Galef, B. G. Jr & Laland, K. N. (2005). Social learning in animals: empirical studies and theoretical models. *Bioscience*, **55**, 489–499.

Gallese, V., Fadiga, L., Fogassi, L. & Rizzolatti, G. (1996). Action recognition in the premotor cortex. *Brain*, **119**, 593–609.

Gibson, J. J. (1979). *The Ecological Approach to Visual Perception*. Boston, MA: Houghton Mifflin.

Gordon, S. D. & Uetz, G. W. (2011). Multimodal communication of wolf spiders on different substrates: evidence for behavioural plasticity. *Animal Behaviour*, **81**, 367–375.

Grasse, P. P. (1959). La reconstruction du nid et les coordinations inter-individuelles chez Bellicosi-termes natalensis et Cubitermes sp. La theorie de la stigmergie: essai d'interpretation du comportement des termites constructeurs. *Insectes Sociaux*, **6**, 41–83.

Green, J. P. & Field, J. (2011). Interpopulation variation in status signalling in the paper wasp *Polistes dominulus*. *Animal Behaviour*, **81**, 205–209.

Grice, P. (1957). Meaning. *Philosophical Review*, **66**, 377–388.

Griffin, D. R. (1974). *The Question of Animal Awareness*. New York: Rockefeller University Press.

Griffin, D. R. (1995). Windows on animal minds. *Consciousness and Cognition*, **4**, 194–204.

Gruter, C. & Ratnieks, F. L. W. (2011). Honeybee foragers increase the use of waggle dance information when private information becomes unrewarding. *Animal Behaviour*, **81**, 949–954.

Guilford, T. & Dawkins, M. S. (1991). Receiver psychology and the evolution of animal signals. *Animal Behaviour*, **42**, 1–14.

Harris, R. (1981). *The Language Myth*. London: Duckworth Publishers.

Harris, R. (1998). *Introduction to Integrational Linguistics*. Oxford: Permagon Press.

Hartshorne, C. (1973). *Born to Sing*. Bloomington, IN: Indiana University Press.

Hauser, M. D. (2009). The possibility of impossible cultures. *Nature*, **460**, 190–196.

Hutchins, E. (1995). *Cognition in the Wild*. Cambridge, MA: MIT Press.

Jarvilehto, T. (2009). The theory of the organism-environment as basis for experimental work in psychology. *Ecological Psychology*, **21**, 112–120.

Johnson, K. (1997). Speech perception without speaker normalization: an exemplar model. In K. Johnson & J. Mullenix, eds., *Talker Variability in Speech Processing*. New York: Academic Press, pp. 145–166.

Jordan, N. R., Manser, M. B., Mwanguhya, F. *et al.* (2011). Scent marking in wild banded mongooses: 1. Sex-specific scents and overmarking. *Animal Behaviour*, **81**, 31–42.

Judge, K. A. (2011). Do male field crickets, *Gryllus pennsylvanicus*, signal their age? *Animal Behaviour*, **81**, 185–194.

Jürgens, U. (2009). The neural control of vocalization in mammals: a review. *Journal of Voice*, **23**, 1–10.

Karubian, J., Lindsay, W. R., Schwabl, H. & Webster, M. S. (2011). Bill coloration, a flexible signal in a tropical passerine bird, is regulated by social environment and androgens. *Animal Behaviour*, **81**, 795–800.

Kravchenko, A. V. (2007). Essential properties of language, or, why language is not a code. *Language Sciences*, **29**, 650–671.

Kuhl, P. K. (2000). A new view of language acquisition. *Proceedings of the National Academy of Sciences USA*, **97**, 11850–11857.

Kuhl, P. K. & Miller, J. D. (1975). Speech perception by the chinchilla: voiced-voiceless distinction in alveolar plosive consonants. *Science*, **190**, 69–72.

Kuhl, P. K. & Padden, D. M. (1982). Enhanced discriminability at the phonetic boundaries for the voicing feature in macaques. *Perception and Psychophysics*, **32**, 542–550.

Lakoff, G. & Johnson, M. (1980). *Metaphors We Live By*. Chicago, IL: University of Chicago Press.

Landauer, T. K. & Dumais, S. T. (1997). A solution to Plato's problem: the latent semantic analysis theory of the acquisition, induction, and representation of knowledge. *Psychological Review*, **104**, 211–240.

Leger, D. W. (1993). Contextual sources of information and responses to animal communication signals. *Psychological Bulletin*, **113**, 295–304.

Liberman, A. M., Harris, K. S., Hoffman, H. S. & Griffith, B. C. (1957). The discrimination of speech sounds within and across phoneme boundaries. *Journal of Experimental Psychology*, **54**, 358–368.

Lieberman, P. (2002). On the nature and evolution of the neural bases of human language. *Yearbook of Physical Anthropology*, **45**, 36–62.

Lisker, L. & Abramson, A. S. (1967). Some effects of context on voice onset time in English stops. *Language and Speech*, **10**, 1–28.

Manser, M. B., Seyfarth, R. L. & Cheney, D. L. (2002). Suricate alarm calls signal predator class and urgency. *Trends in Cognitive Sciences*, **6**, 55–57.

Marler, P. (1961). Logical analysis of animal communication. *Journal of Theoretical Biology*, **1**, 295–317.

Marler, P., Evans, C. S. & Hauser, M. D. (1992). Animal signals: motivational, referential, or both? In H. Papousek, U. Jürgens & M. Papousek, eds., *Nonverbal Vocal Communication: Comparative and Developmental Approaches*. Cambridge: Cambridge University Press, pp. 66–86.

Maynard Smith, J. & Harper, D. (2003). *Animal Signals*. Oxford: Oxford University Press.

McLuhan, M. (1964). *Understanding Media: The Extensions of Man*. New York: McGraw Hill.

Mello, C., Nootebohm, F. & Clayton, D. (1995). Repeated exposure to one song leads to a rapid and persistent decline in immediate early gene's response to that song in zebra finch telencephalon. *Journal of Neuroscience*, **15**, 6919–6925.

Miller, G. A. (1956). The magical number seven, plus or minus two: some limits on our capacity for processing information. *Psychological Review*, **63**, 81–97.

Neisser, U. (1967). *Cognitive Psychology*. New York: Apple-Century-Crofts.

Newell, A. & Simon, H. (1976). Computer science as empirical enquiry: symbols and search. *Communications of the Association for Computing Machinery*, **19**, 113–126.

Noe, A. (2009). *Out of Our Heads*. New York: Hill and Wang.

Nunes, T. M., Mateus, S., Turatti, I. C., Morgan, E. D. & Zucchi, R. (2011). Nestmate recognition in the stingless bee *Frieseomelitta varia* (Hymenoptera, Apidae, Meliponini): sources of chemical signals. *Animal Behaviour*, **81**, 463–467.

Nygaard, L. C., Sommers, M. S. & Pisoni, D. B. (1994). Speech perception as a talker-contingent process. *Psychological Science*, **5**, 42–46.

Owings, D. H. & Morton, E. S. (1997). The role of information in communication: an assessment/management approach. In D. H. Owings, M. D. Beecher & N. S. Thompson, eds., *Communication. Perspectives in Ethology*, Vol. 12. New York: Plenum Press, pp. 359–390.

Owings, D. H. & Morton, E. S. (1998). *Animal Vocal Communication: A New Approach*. Cambridge: Cambridge University Press.

Owren, M. J. & Rendall, D. (1997). An affect-conditioning model of nonhuman primate vocalizations. In D. H. Owings, M. D. Beecher & N. S. Thompson, eds., *Communication. Perspectives in Ethology*, Vol. 12. New York: Plenum Press, pp. 299–346.

Owren, M. J. & Rendall, D. (2001). Sound on the rebound: returning form and function to the forefront in understanding non-human primate vocal signaling. *Evolutionary Anthropology*, **10**, 58–71.

Owren, M. J., Amoss, R. T. & Rendall, D. (2011). Two organizing principles of vocal production: implications for non-human and human primates. *American Journal of Primatology*, **73**, 530–544.

Owren, M. J., Rendall, D. & Ryan, M. J. (2010). Redefining animal signaling: influence versus information in communication. *Biology and Philosophy*, **25**, 755–780.

Palmeri, T. J., Goldinger, S. D. & Pisoni, D. B. (1993). Episodic encoding of voice attributes and recognition memory for spoken words. *Journal of Experimental Psychology: Learning, Memory and Cognition*, **19**, 309–328.

Penn, D. C. & Povinelli, D. J. (2007). On the lack of evidence that chimpanzees possess anything remotely resembling a 'theory of mind'. *Philosophical Transactions of the Royal Society of London, Series B: Biological Sciences*, **362**, 731–744.

Port, R. F. (2010). Language as a social institution: why phonemes and words do not live in the brain. *Ecological Psychology*, **22**, 304–326.

Rendall, D., Cheney, D. L. & Seyfarth, R. M. (2000). Proximate factors mediating 'contact' calls in adult female baboons and their infants. *Journal of Comparative Psychology*, **114**, 36–46.

Rendall, D., Owren, M. J. & Rodman, P. S. (1998). The role of vocal tract filtering in identity cueing in rhesus monkey (*Macaca mulatta*) vocalizations. *Journal of the Acoustical Society of America*, **103**, 602–614.

Rendall, D., Owren, M. J. & Ryan, M. J. (2009). What do animal signals mean? *Animal Behaviour*, **78**, 233–240.

Riters, L. V. (2011). Pleasure seeking and birdsong. *Neuroscience and Biobehavioral Reviews*, **35**, 1837–1845.

Rosenbleuth, A. & Weiner, N. (1950). Purposeful and non-purposeful behavior. *Philosophy of Science*, **17**, 318–326.

Ryan, M. J. (1990). Sensory systems, sexual selection, and sensory exploitation. *Oxford Surveys in Evolutionary Biology*, **7**, 157–195.

Ryan, M. J. (1998). Receiver biases, sexual selection and the evolution of sex differences. *Science*, **281**, 1999–2003.

Ryan, M. J. & Rand, A. S. (2003). Mate recognition in tungara frogs: a review of some studies of brain, behavior, and evolution. *Acta Zoologica Sinica*, **49**, 713–726.

Saffran, J. R., Aslin, R. N. & Newport, E. L. (1996). Statistical learning by 8-month-old infants. *Science*, **274**, 1926–1928.

de Saussure, F. (1916/1986). *Course in General Linguistics*, C. Bally & A. Sechehaye, eds. (translated by R. Harris). La Salle, IL: Open Court Publishing.

Scott-Phillips, T. (2010). Animal communication: insights from lingustic pragmatics. *Animal Behaviour*, **79**, e1–e4.

Searcy, W. A (1992). Song repertoire and mate choice in birds. *American Zoologist*, **32**, 71–80.

Searcy, W. A. & Nowicki, S. (2005). *The Evolution of Communication: Reliability and Deception in Animal Signaling Systems*. Princeton, NJ: Princeton University Press.

Searle, J. (1980). Minds, brains and programs. *Behavioral and Brain Sciences*, **3**, 417–457.

Seyfarth, R. M. & Cheney, D. L. (1986). Vocal development in vervet monkeys. *Animal Behaviour*, **34**, 1640–1658.

Seyfarth, R. M., Cheney, D. L., Bergman, T. *et al.* (2010). The central importance of information in studies of animal communication. *Animal Behaviour*, **80**, 3–8.

Seyfarth, R. M., Cheney, D. L. & Marler, P. (1980a). Monkey responses to three different alarm calls: evidence for predator classification and semantic communication. *Science*, **210**, 801–803.

Seyfarth, R. M., Cheney, D. L. & Marler, P. (1980b). Vervet monkey alarm calls: semantic communication in a free-ranging primate. *Animal Behaviour*, **28**, 1070–1094.

Shannon, C. E. & Weaver, W. (1949). *The Mathematical Theory of Communication*. Urbana-Champaign, IL: University of Illinois Press.

Siegel, S., Baptista, M. A. S., Kim, J. A., McDonald, R. V. & Weise-Kelly, L. (2000). Pavlovian psychopharmacology: the associative basis of tolerance. *Experimental and Clinical Psychopharmacology*, **8**, 276–293.

Slocombe, K. E. & Zuberbühler, K. (2007). Chimpanzees modify recruitment screams as a function of audience composition. *Proceedings of the National Academy of Sciences USA*, **104**, 17228–17233.

Smith, W. J. (1977). *The Behavior of Communicating*. Cambridge, MA: Harvard University Press.

Templeton, C. N., Greene, E. & Davis, K. (2005). Allometry of alarm calls: black-capped chickadees encode information about predator size. *Science*, **308**, 1934–1937.

Thelen, E. & Smith, L. (1994). *A Dynamic Systems Approach to the Development of Cognition and Action*. Cambridge, MA: MIT Press.

Tomasello, M. (2008). *Origins of Human Communication*. Cambridge, MA: MIT Press.

Turing, A. M. (1950). Computing machinery and intelligence. *Mind*, **59**, 433–460.

Van Gelder, T. (1995). What might cognition be, if not computation? *Journal of Philosophy*, **92**, 345–381.

Uexküll, J. von (1910). Die Umwelt. *Die neue Rundschau*, **21**, 638–649.

Whattam, E. M. & Bertram, S. M. (2011). Effects of juvenile and adult condition on long-distance call components in the Jamaican field cricket, *Gryllus assimilis*. *Animal Behaviour*, **81**, 135–144.

Wheeler, M. & Clark, A. (2008). Culture, embodiment and genes: unravelling the triple helix. *Philosophical Transactions of the Royal Society Series B*, **363**, 3563–3575.

Wilczynski, W. & Chu, J. (2001). Acoustic communication, endocrine control, and the neurochemical systems of the brain. In M. J. Ryan, ed., *Anuran Communication*. Washington, DC: Smithsonian Institution, pp. 23–35.

Zahavi, A. & Zahavi, A. (1997). *The Handicap Principle: A Missing Piece of Darwin's Puzzle*. Oxford: Oxford University Press.

Zuberbühler, K. (2000). Interspecies semantic communication in two forest primates. *Proceedings of the Royal Society of London Series B*, **267**, 713–718.

Commentaries

I welcome Rendall and Owren's (RO) criticism of the encoding–decoding model (EDM) of animal communication, but I reject their inference that if information is not encoded in a signal, it is not carried by such a signal.

According to EDM, a signaller encodes information by transforming it into an arbitrarily selected equivalent suitable for transmission, and a recipient decodes the signal transmitted by applying the code in reverse to recover the original piece of information.

But senders and receivers of animal signals do not have access to any shared system of rules for transforming pieces of information back and forth into arbitrarily selected equivalents. As RO have argued elsewhere, in competitive contexts a cooperative convergence on a shared code cannot be posited, and the ability to communicate by means of a shared code requires a network of coordinated intentions beyond the cognitive reach of non-human animals.

RO suggest that some endorse a weaker understanding of encoding and decoding, according to which signals can be said to encode information anytime "they stand in predictive relation to some event or state of the world".

This is the notion of information I discussed in my chapter, where I argued that signal X carries *predictive information* about state of affairs Y just in case $P(Y \text{ given } X) \neq P(Y)$. When this is the case, X and Y are said to be statistically correlated.[1] A 'predictable relationship' between X and Y is instantiated when their correlation is strong enough to allow X to reliably predict Y (or not-Y).

The encoding and decoding metaphors are positively misleading with respect to predictive information. Saying that alarm calls encode information about predators is like saying that smoke encodes information about fire. This phrasing suggests that some process of rule-based transformation takes place between fire and smoke. We know instead that a straightforward causal relation underwrites the correlation between them.

The same holds for the correlation between predators and alarm calls, except that fire causes smoke directly, whereas predators cause alarm calls by means of signallers. I conclude with RO that the encoding and decoding metaphors are detrimental. But it does not follow that animal signals do not contain or carry information.

RO argue that information "does not reside in the signals themselves but rather in the relationship between them and the events they co-occur with". These remarks are motivated by an important realisation, but they go too far.

[1] They are positively correlated when $P(Y \text{ given } X) > P(Y)$, and negatively correlated when $P(Y \text{ given } X) < P(Y)$.

The realisation is that what information a signal carries is contingent upon what a recipient can predict from it, which is in turn contingent upon what the recipient already knows. RO correctly point out that a light predicts shock for a fear-conditioned rat, but not for a rat just introduced into the conditioning box. Similarly, a snake alarm call predicts snakes for adult vervet monkeys, but not for infants.

Since different recipients make different predictions (or no predictions) from the same signal, RO conclude that the information is not in the signals themselves. My view is instead that information resides neither in the recipient independently of the signal nor in the signal independently of the recipient. It is in the signal itself by virtue of what a potential recipient can predict upon receiving it. This makes the capacity to carry predictive information fundamentally *relational*: it is a capacity that a signal expresses when paired with the right recipient.

The predictive information relation should then be interpreted as a three-place relation: signal X carries information about Y relative to background knowledge *k* by virtue of a capacity of X to allow a potential recipient in background knowledge *k* to predict Y or not-Y from the signal.[2]

Encodable information (non-natural meaning) and predictive information (natural meaning) differ in several respects (Grice, 1957; Scarantino & Piccinini, 2010). The one I wish to emphasise in conclusion is that whereas it is up to senders what encoded information recipients receive, and all recipients decode the same information from the same signal, recipients can pick up predictive information that senders never intended to provide, and the same signal carries different predictive information to different recipients.

Scarantino, A. & Piccinini, G. (2010). Information without truth. *Metaphilosophy*, **41**, 313–330.

Andrea Scarantino

There is much to agree with in Rendall and Owren's (RO) chapter. Their emphasis on influence clearly accords with my view that communication is, by definition, a matter of effects rather than information (Scott-Phillips, 2008; Scott-Phillips & Kirby, Ch. 18 of this volume). Moreover, I agree with their demands that animal signalling theory should be oriented around functional benefits. However, I do not see why the reorganisation they call for is based only around the benefits that

[2] This entails that the probability functions *P*(*Y* given *X*) and *P*(*Y*) determining whether or not *X* carries information about *Y* must reflect *all* the background knowledge relevant to the context of inquiry (e.g. inquiry into the behaviour of a fear-conditioned rat, or of an adult vervet monkey).

signalling has for signallers. (RO do acknowledge that signals can benefit receivers, but they do not see it as a requirement.)

In the conclusion, RO appeal to a return to the basic principle of natural selection that adaptations are shaped by the benefits they provide to their bearers. Yet communication is the emergent consequence of the interaction of two adaptations, one for signalling and one for receiving (Scott-Phillips *et al.*, 2012). So while RO are correct that we should not assume that "selection on receiver resistance trumps selection on signaller influence", neither should we do the opposite. As a result, any reorganisation of animal signalling theory should be based around the benefits of influence to both signallers (the influencers) and receivers (the influenced).

I note that RO pick up on the same issue in their commentary on my co-authored chapter in this volume. I expand on these issues in my response.

Scott-Phillips, T. C. (2008). Defining biological communication. *Journal of Evolutionary Biology*, **21**(2), 387–395.

Scott-Phillips, T. C., Blythe, R. A., Gardner, A. & West, S. A. (2012). How do communication systems emerge? *Proceedings of the Royal Society of London Series B: Biological Sciences*, **279**, 1943–1949.

Thomas C. Scott-Phillips

There is little to disagree with in this chapter, except the vehemence with which Rendall and Owren deride informational accounts. Perhaps we are mellower because the excesses of the cognitive revolution did not railroad work on birds. True, it is "difficult to overstate the influence of the vervet alarm-call research", but it seems that Rendall and Owren have done just that.

Rendall and Owren seem to be advocating the very approach we advocate, yet we find informational constructs interesting and useful, while they find them unrealistic and misleading. Given that we are so in tune with their main message, we suggest that on the latter points we agree to disagree. After all, wasn't it Smith (1977), the whipping boy of anti-information approaches, whose career stressed the importance of context?

Andrew G. Horn and Peter McGregor

Response

Informational constructs in animal communication theory. Are we ready to cut the apron-strings? We appreciate commentaries by **Horn and McGregor**, **Scarantino** and **Scott-Phillips**. We are delighted they express general agreement with the thrust of our critique, namely that many language-based metaphors and related constructs arising from the cognitive revolution (e.g. signal encoding and decoding), are generally not apt characterisations of animal signalling phenomena, and that other common constructs, such as the concept of information, deserve additional scrutiny. That consensus is encouraging and suggests progress can be made on updating and clarifying the core theoretical constructs that undergird and motivate future research in the field. Of course, complete consensus may take time and be difficult to achieve. Commentators expressed general agreement with us, but they did not endorse everything in our critique and highlighted some specific points of divergence. We wholly respect these differences and have no desire to discount or dismiss them with further arguments. However, in the interests of continuing the discussion and motivating additional opportunities for it, we attempt some response.

Signallers versus receivers. **Scott-Phillips** agrees that animal communication is not about *information* but about *influence*. However, he is concerned that our characterisation places too much emphasis on signallers and not enough on receivers. He emphasises that animal signalling theory "should be based around the benefits of influence to both signallers (the influencers) and receivers (the influenced)". We wholly agree that receivers (perceivers) are as important as signallers. Indeed, we (like others, e.g. Owings & Morton, 1998) have emphasised the inherent bidirectionality of communication, "...signallers and perceivers play important and potentially distinct roles in an iterated, reciprocal process of influence and resistance". However, we do certainly acknowledge that our arguments involve foregrounding the role of signallers in as much as it is evolutionarily axiomatic that signals must ultimately be beneficial to them, or else they would not signal. We feel obliged to reiterate this basic point because it is sometimes overlooked in theorising that champions the principle of signal honesty. We agree receivers should be (and are) inherently skeptical, but we do not accept that they can simply ignore anything but honest signals, thereby forcing signallers to be honest. That would be a very one-sided view of signalling indeed, and one that is, as argued elsewhere, committed to an informational and cooperative view of communication we feel is inappropriate. It is also contradicted by diverse evidence that perceivers are not free to discount signals but instead, owing to a variety of mechanistic and functional factors, can be quite susceptible to signal influence. At bottom, signalling must benefit signallers but need not benefit receivers, and being clear about that is the basis for any special emphasis we place on signallers. Otherwise, we are in full agreement with Scott-Phillips that signallers and perceivers are equally important foci in animal communication theory. It is a further question whether or not signalling necessarily involves perceiver adaptation, which is taken up in commentary accompanying Scott-Phillips' chapter.

What does information add? **Scarantino** agrees that signals do not encode information and that talk of signal encoding and decoding is misleading. However, he feels we go too far in rejecting informational constructs entirely. He maintains that signals that do not *encode information* can nevertheless be said to *carry information* insofar as they bear a predictive relationship to events or actions. Thus, the vervet monkey's leopard alarm can be said to carry information about that predator because it reliably occurs in the presence of a leopard. This basic association defines an indexical relationship in C. S. Pierce's classic typology of signs, wherein an index (distinct from either icon or symbol) is a sign that denotes by virtue of its spatio-temporal association with the thing denoted. Using Scarantino's example, smoke can be a signal: it can index (or point to) fire because it is predictably associated with fire. We agree. Smoke indicates the presence of a fire, and vervet alarm calls indicate the presence of a predator. Of course, an important corollary then is that vervet alarms, like smoke, are not at all like language. In language, signs (words) denote specifically *not* by spatio-temporal associations with their designate, but via symbolic relationships to them that are established by convention. As Scarantino, we, and others in the volume emphasise, the latter requires a shared code and "coordinated intentions beyond the cognitive reach of non-human animals". So, we agree entirely that vervet alarm calls, and many other animal signals, qualify as indexes that point to, or indicate, things in the world but do not symbolise them. They are, therefore, quite unlike language.

What we do not fully understand is what is added by re-describing well-defined indexical relationships as 'carrying information'. Specifically, what is gained by parsing the relationship between vervet alarms and leopards as "vervet alarms *carry information* about leopards"? We understand the sense of information Scarantino intends, but do not see the benefit provided by an informational characterisation of the straightforward indexical relationship. Although harmless enough on its own, this kind of informational re-description can also actually be detrimental in encouraging further linguistic and informational characterisations (e.g. signal encoding and decoding, intentionality, representation). In fact, Scarantino seems to agree that such characterisations are unfounded, misleading and draw attention away from more fundamental ethological and evolutionary questions.

To wit, it is more than 30 years since the original description of language-like, symbolic signalling in vervet alarm calls. What we now know is that, lacking the fundamental intentional and representational properties of words, these alarm signals are, in fact, not language-like or symbolic. Revealingly, we do not yet know much about how the alarm call system does work. For example, we do not know what the selected, adaptive function of the calls is. Is it to warn kin? Is it to signal to predators that they have been detected? Similarly, we do not know what the proximate mechanisms are that motivate production of alarm calls, nor what the mechanisms are that determine listener responses. These are common and basic features of animal communication systems that should be central in ethological research but that seem to have been cast aside.

We suggest that these details are missing for the alarm call system of vervets (and for many other cases) because investigators have been preoccupied with trying to characterise signalling systems in linguistic or informational terms. As argued, these characterisations are fundamentally out-of-step with basic tenets of ethology and evolutionary biology, and, in the end, have proven misleading. But there is an even greater potential risk associated with informational characterisations: namely that, because of the natural familiarity and intuitive appeal of linguistic and informational constructs, applying them to animal signalling can create an unjustified impression of having explained the core phenomena involved. In reality, and as just noted, the resulting explanations are not substantial. They leave fundamental holes in our understanding of animal signalling, as illustrated by the much-studied and celebrated phenomenon of vervet alarm calling.

Is the case against linguistic and informational constructs overstated? **Horn and McGregor** see general agreement between our respective approaches, but also wonder if the excesses of the cognitive revolution are being overstated. Specifically, while the now familiar constructs on linguistics and information encoding may have infected research on primate communication, they have not had such an influence on bird research. Thus, while acknowledging our concerns, Horn and McGregor are reluctant to abandon informational constructs and still find them "interesting and useful". We accept their suggestion that, on this, we might simply "agree to disagree". But, prompted to respond, we have to wonder whether their reluctance to abandon informational constructs is not, in fact, evidence of exactly the kind of pervasive influence we propose them to have had?

Drew Rendall and Michael J. Owren

Owings, D.H. & Morton, E.S. (1998). *Animal Vocal Communication: A New Approach.* Cambridge: Cambridge University Press.

7

Information in animal communication: when and why does it matter?[1]

SAHOTRA SARKAR

7.1 Introduction

Organisms communicate. This claim is not as innocuous as it may initially seem. Consider the case of the Hawaiian field cricket, *Teleogryllus oceanicus*. The male remains stationary and sings in the evenings (Zuk, Simmons & Cupp, 1993; Zuk, Rotenberry & Tinghitella, 2006; Bretman & Tregenza, 2007). The song attracts the acoustically orienting fly, *Ormia ochracea*, which lays first-instar larvae on the male or in its immediate vicinity. The larvae emerge about a week later and burrow into the male, killing it. The effect is relatively strong: in the island of Kauai, the singing morph of *T. oceanicus* was largely replaced by a novel silent morph within 20 generations (Zuk *et al.*, 2006). It is clear that the individuals of the two species interact, and even that the behaviour of *T. oceanicus* individuals influences the behaviour of *O. ochracea* individuals. But do the former *communicate* with the latter? Is it even appropriate to say that there has been miscommunication? The evolutionary origins of male singing in *T. oceanicus* obviously cannot lie in attracting *O. ochracea*; rather, singing presumably evolved to attract roving females which use song characteristics to identify conspecifics and perhaps, if sexual selection is assumed, to assess the quality of potential mates (Zuk & Simmons, 1997; Bretman & Tregenza, 2007).

Next, consider, the honeybee (*Apis mellifera*). Worker bees indicate the distance and direction of foraging sources and potential nesting sites to nestmates

[1] For help with developing the arguments of this chapter, thanks are due to Colin Allen, Steve Downes, Justin Garson and Ulrich Stegmann.

Animal Communication Theory: Information and Influence, ed. Ulrich Stegmann. Published by Cambridge University Press.

using a 'waggle dance'; the distance to the targeted location is specified by the duration of the waggle component of the dance, the direction by the angle of the dance to the sun (Cadena, 2011). A recent experiment analysed the waggle dance of bees deprived of sleep for a night (Klein *et al.*, 2010). Sleep deprivation did not detectably affect the duration of the waggle component; however, there was a significant increase of variance in directionality compared with bees used as controls. Many sleep-deprived bees specified an incorrect direction to the foraging location. In this case, communication is clearly occurring; what is at hand may be an exemplary case of miscommunication. But, should this communication be viewed as a transfer of *information*, as the authors of the study interpret their results (Klein *et al.*, 2010, pp. 22707–22708)? This is the question that is at stake in this chapter, which expresses some skepticism about the utility of 'information' in animal behaviour studies in general and not only with respect to communication. However, before proceeding any further, some clarification of the use of 'communication' may prove helpful.

The analysis below will assume that not all interactions constitute communication – in particular, cases such as the *T. oceanicus–O. ochracea* interaction discussed earlier do not. At the very least, communication will be assumed to require – and this is not an uncontroversial assumption (see Pfeifer, 2006) – that an action typically "evoke[s] in partners behavior harmonious with the future behavior of the actor",[2] and that it evolved for that reason. These are supposed to be necessary but not sufficient conditions; in particular it captures the situation in which an interaction leads to enhanced fitnesses of both interacting agents, which is often presumed in models of communication (see, e.g., Hurd and Enquist, 2005). But harmony with future behaviour may be interpreted more broadly to permit measures other than enhanced fitness. These conditions exclude the possibility that there was communication between *T. oceanicus* and *O. ochracea*; we will return to the case of the sleep-deprived honeybees in Section 7.5. The distinction being made here is similar but not identical to the traditional distinction between cues and signals, with only the latter being an evolved feature for the purpose of coordinating behaviour. Usually this point is made by stating that signals, but not cues, evolved to convey information, but the critical point is that the relevant distinction can be made without invoking the concept of information. Moreover, until that concept is adequately clarified, the question whether cues can provide information without constituting communication will also remain open. The conceptual point – or claim – is that, if

[2] This is Haldane and Spurway's (1954) characterisation of "social releasers". Following Owren, Rendall & Ryan (2010, p.756 note) and as is standard practice in the relevant literature, no distinction will be made between animal communication and signalling.

'information' is unnecessary even for communication, the question whether cues are construed in informational terms is not of much interest.

7.2 Information and biology

Any discussion of the use of 'information' in biology should bear in mind two potentially relevant historical points and four critically relevant logical ones. The two historical points are:[3]

- Although 'information' as an item of instruction or training goes back to Chaucer in 1386 and, as a description of communicated knowledge, at least to 1450, the idea that it can be used *technically* (and, in fact, quantitatively) only derives from Fisher in 1925. Soon after, in 1928, it was used informally in the neurosciences by Adrian (1928) while, simultaneously, Hartley (1928) used the term formally in developing a theory of communication through signal transmission. Neither usage followed Fisher's (1925) sense: it was never obvious what 'information' was uniformly trying to capture in all these contexts, which raises the question of whether there is any unique entity that the term does capture. However, systematic use of 'information' in biology only follows Shannon's (1948) seminal development of mathematical communication theory (MCT), including a measure of information which is often also referred to as 'entropy' because of its formal identity with entropy as defined in statistical mechanics. (The Shannon measure will be discussed in some detail later in this section.) In genetics, the use of 'information' began only in 1953. In the study of animal communication, informal use dates back at least to von Frisch in 1950 and Benveniste in 1953;[4] the explicit invocation of MCT began with Haldane and Spurway's (1954) use of the Shannon measure to analyse von Frisch's data on bee (*Apis mellifera carnica*) dances. The point to emphasise is that the use of 'information' in biology – including genetics and behavioural biology – is of remarkably recent vintage. Generations of modern (that is, post-Darwinian) biologists got by with no recourse to 'information'.
- The late 1940s and 1950s also saw the emergence of large-scale digital computation, which transformed society both materially and intellectually. Associated with these developments were what have

[3] Relevant historical details are from Heims (1991), Sarkar (1996a, 2004), Kay (2000) and Garson (2003).

[4] See von Frisch (1950) and Benveniste (1953); Griffin also uses the term informally in his introduction to von Frisch's book.

come to be called the information sciences, including Norbert Wiener's 'cybernetics'. As many historians of science have documented, this period was characterised by widespread anticipation that these sciences would transform all traditional disciplines and, perhaps, human society itself. Eigen (1971, p. 467) even attributed to Wiener the view that "information be regarded as a new variable of physics". Cybernetic metaphors (including information) were rampant in the social sciences of the period,[5] and it is possible (as Sarkar, 1996a, 1996b argued for the case of genetics) that 'information' may have entered the biological lexicon as no more than a metaphor masquerading as a theoretical concept.

These historical points raise the *prima facie* possibility that there was no scientific (experimental or theoretical) need that 'information' fulfilled; rather, scientific discourse followed the fashion of the times in embracing a new metaphor.

The logical points that follow accentuate that worry. There are four relevant logical points:

- MCT, which is what is typically meant by 'information theory', envisions a situation in which communication consists of signal transmission over a channel. In Shannon's (1948) model,[6] a source produces a message to be communicated. An encoder associates with the message some 'object' which is suitable for transmission over the channel. The decoder operates on the output of the channel, and a decision is made as to the identity of the message. There is no certainty that the output is the same as the input – or even very close to it – because of 'noise' introduced in the channel. The goal of Shannon's analysis was to make both the class of permissible inputs and the probability of identifying the correct input as large as possible while constrained by the physical properties of the channel. 'Information' was supposed to capture the uncertainty associated with the transmitted 'object' and Shannon proposed a measure for it, $-\Sigma_i p_i \log_2 p_i$, where p_i is the prior probability (interpreted as expected frequency) of the ith unit. Two aspects of this measure are important: (i) it does not consider the process of encoding and decoding; and (ii) although, in principle, the transmitted 'object' can have any

[5] As Bar-Hillel (1952, p. 11) put it: "The words 'cybernetics' (and its derivatives) and 'information' were surely the two most used, and misused, members of the scientific vocabulary of the fifties."

[6] The contrast, here, is with Wiener (1948). Wiener's model did not include encoding/decoding processes – see Ash (1965, p. v) and references therein for relevant detail.

structure, Shannon assumed it to have a natural linear (that is, sequential) organisation. Independent of any particular measure (and Shannon explicitly noted that there were many related possibilities) is the crucial point that any MCT-information measure has its value specified by the frequencies of events – transmission of signals, in the case of animal communication. As Shannon explicitly pointed out, MCT-information had nothing to do with the content of a message, what it means or says.

- The Shannon measure ($-\Sigma_i p_i \log_2 p_i$) was used to quantify diversity in ecology starting in 1953, with p_i interpreted as the relative proportion (frequency) of the ith species in an ecological community.[7] The motivation was that this measure (that is, the formula, $-\Sigma_i p_i \log_2 p_i$) provided a natural quantification of the evenness (or equitability) of an ecological community while also partly incorporating the richness of the community (that is, the number of species in it). In what follows, this interpretation of the measure will be called DT-information (with 'DT' for 'diversity theory'). There is a logical connection between this interpretation, that is, DT-information, and MCT-information. If we generalise to collections of different types of entities (rather than only species), and *if* information is *generated* at the source before transmission, the diversity at the source measured by DT-information is numerically equal to the MCT-information entering the transmission process before potential reduction through noise introduced in the channel. However, DT-information, though thus related to MCT-information, is not identical to the latter: it makes sense to use DT-information even when there is no communication, for instance, as noted earlier, to measure the diversity of ecological communities. It does not make sense to use MCT-information in this way. Thus, so far, there are two different interpretations of the same measure ($-\Sigma_i p_i \log_2 p_i$), one as diversity, DT-information, and one as information transmitted through a channel, MCT-information, sometimes also appropriately called 'transinformation' (for 'transmitted information'). The amount of the latter available at the onset of a signal transmission process may well be the 'diversity' at the source; nevertheless the two entities are conceptually distinct. One source of confusion in many discussions has been the conflation of these two interpretations.[8] It deserves emphasis that 'MCT-

[7] See Good (1953); this use was systematically advocated by Margalef (1958) while MacArthur (1957) used it as a measure of ecological stability. For a discussion of this history, see Sarkar (2007).

[8] See Halliday and Slater (1983).

information' will only be used here when there is transmission of information and not when all that is at stake is diversity, for instance the diversity of a signal repertoire.[9]

- In contrast to these construals, content is the focus of what, following standard logical terminology since the 1930s (Sarkar, 1992), has been called *semantic* information. The canonical work is that of Carnap and Bar-Hillel (1952) who took the pre-systematic (that is, customary) information content of a claim to be the class of those possible states (of the universe) that it excludes. The explication (roughly, formalisation) of this concept of information led to two distinct concepts, one corresponding to surprisal (the inverse of the probability) and the other, substantive value (Bar-Hillel, 1952). For purely formal reasons, the latter was quantified again using the Shannon measure ($-\Sigma_i p_i \log_2 p_i$) but, now, p_i is the (logical) probability of the ith claim.
- In other words, the Shannon measure has at least three different interpretations, each of which corresponds to a different construal of 'information'. Which of these interpretations, if any, are relevant to animal communication? As we shall see, each interpretation has its advocates but none is unproblematic. Part of the confusion – or, at least, the controversy – about the topic lies in the fact that proponents of the use of 'information' often glide from one use to another without notice. Moreover, those who seem to use semantic information never use the Shannon measure explicitly, in spite of the Carnap–Bar-Hillel theory, and often use the term colloquially without specifying what is being *theoretically* assumed about the concept. As many critics have pointed out, explicit explication of 'information' has been lacking not only in animal communication studies but throughout biology (Allen & Hauser, 1993; Sarkar, 1996a; Owren *et al.*, 2010; Maclaurin, 2011).

In what follows we will briefly examine all three construals of information to assess what each contributes – or may contribute – to animal communication studies.

7.3 MCT-information

Even those who are generally skeptical of the value of 'information' (especially semantic information) in animal communication studies often assume that the use of MCT-information is straightforward (see, e.g., Owren

[9] Indeed, 'transinformation', when used appropriately, should also be restricted to contexts which include transmission. However, that term will not be used in this chapter again in order to avoid even a semblance of conflation.

et al., 2010). But, as we shall see, there is ample ground for caution (Pfeifer, 2006). In Section 7.2 we mentioned Haldane and Spurway's (1954) pioneering analysis of the quantity of information transmitted through the waggle dance of bees. This was followed by Wilson's (1962) quantification of the MCT-information transmitted by the odour trail of the fire ant, *Solenopsis saevissima*. These ants indicate the location of food sources by extruding their stings and dragging them over the surface, thus releasing a pheromone at frequent intervals along a trail. The pheromone creates a vapour tunnel that other ants can sense with their antennae. The ants that are recruited follow the tunnel before the pheromone signature dissipates. If several ants discover the food source, they all release pheromones making the vapour tunnel more intense and longer lasting.

To justify the quantification of the information using the Shannon measure, Haldane and Spurway (1954) argued that natural selection would favour reasonably accurate but not perfect MCT-information transmission.[10] Wilson (1962) implicitly endorsed this claim but also provided an independent argument for the optimisation through natural selection of MCT-information that depended on its quantification through the Shannon measure. He argued that the MCT-information transmitted by the honeybee dance was roughly equal to that transmitted through the fire ant odour trail. The former transmitted 3.6–7.3 bits per dance (2.5–4.0 bits about direction and 1.1–3.3 bits about distance). The latter transmits 2.4–8.4 bits per trail (~3–5 bits about direction and ~2 bits about distance). Wilson (1962) envisioned no other explanation of this apparently remarkable numerical concordance between the relevant pairs of numbers other than optimisation through natural selection. Obviously, without the quantification through the Shannon measure, we would not have noticed this numerical concordance. (We will address problems with Wilson's claim later.)

Both these studies continue to inspire the use of MCT-information in animal communication studies (see, e.g., McCowan, Hanser & Doyle, 1999; Gherardi & Pieraccini, 2004). The idea is to use the Shannon measure for inter-specific comparisons which may lead to insights of evolutionary significance. But there are potentially insurmountable problems (Pfeifer, 2006). In the discussion below, following Maynard Smith and Harper (2003), we will assume that we can operationally identify which behaviours or structures constitute signals that are part of animal communication systems.[11] Roughly, these are behaviours or

[10] Perfect transmission would not be preferable because a dance could have been inaccurate, conditions might have changed, there might be other nearby food sources etc.

[11] See Pfeifer (2006) for skepticism on this count. Stegmann (2005) critically discusses Maynard Smith and Harper's (2003) account.

structures that change another individual's behaviour, increase the fitness of the source (sender) and have evolved for that reason.

Problems arise when we begin individuating signals. Recall that, to deploy the Shannon measure, we must estimate the frequency of each signal that is part of a message. This means we must identify each unit signal so that they can be counted and their frequencies estimated.[12] Both Haldane and Spurway (1954) and Wilson (1962) individuated directional signals at a resolution of 1 degree, leading to 360 possible signals, presumably because the circle is conventionally resolved into 360 degrees.[13] But this is entirely arbitrary with no biological (or mathematical) basis. We have no reason to believe that 360 is the correct size for the potential directional signal repertoire for either bees or fire ants; we have no reason to presume that the size of the repertoire is the same for both species. A different resolution of directionality would change the numerical value of the Shannon measure, and the concordance on which Wilson (1962) relied is an artifact of this choice.

Using MCT-information credibly to make claims about its evolution or optimisation will require canonical individuation of signals of all taxa of interest. For directional specification in bee dances or fire ant odour trails, this has never been accomplished. However, this is not to suggest that canonical individuation will never be possible. One possibility would be to analyse the perceptual discriminatory capabilities of receivers of signals.[14] At present, we do not have any such general account for most species.[15] But, even after that, much empirical work would remain to be done, for instance, to ascertain which of the distinguished putative signals constitute part of the message and which are only noise (at the source).

Recent attempts in this direction have not been more convincing. For instance, Gherardi and Pieraccini (2004) have analysed the agonistic interactions of the crayfish, *Procambarus acutus acutus*, during the formation of dominance hierarchies. Agonistic interactions were defined as sequences of behavioural patterns

[12] In probability theory this is part of the problem of defining the reference class. There are further subtleties which will be ignored here because they are not likely to be relevant. For instance, what matters is not only the members of the reference class but the order in which they are presented.

[13] Haldane and Spurway's (1954) analysis had an additional problem: von Frisch's data were not recorded at this high degree of resolution. This issue further underscores the claim that the apparent concordance of MCT-transmission through bee dances and fire ant odour trails is probably entirely spurious.

[14] On this point, see, especially, Hauser (1996).

[15] Allen (in his contribution to this volume, Ch. 13) recognises this problem while attempting a back-of-the-envelope calculation of MCT-information transmission between meerkats (*Suricata suricatta*).

(what are being called signals here) when an opponent approached the other (with the end of the sequence specified by a separation of the two individuals out of each other's reach). The signal set was specified as consisting of 20 behavioural patterns (antennule flicking, moving backward, casual approach, interlocked, chela strike, direct approach, freezing, grasping, hugging, moving forward, motionless, meral spread, no observable change, pushing, retreat, tail flipping, touching, walking below, walking over, and other). Though the individuation was based on biological experience (even though it may seem to be arbitrarily concocted), the study does not suggest that it was in any sense unique.[16] The point is not to criticise this particular study which was much more self-conscious than most studies about pitfalls in the use of MCT-information. Rather, it is hard to see how, in cases such as these, arbitrariness in signal individuation can be avoided so that we have non-arbitrary estimates of the frequencies required to compute the Shannon measure for MCT-information.

In some cases, such as songs of birds or cetaceans, individuation of signals appears to be relatively unproblematic.[17] However, we shall see in Section 7.4 that many, perhaps most, studies on these organisms have reported DT-information rather than MCT-information. The most important worry about all these studies is that, a half-century after Haldane and Spurway (1954) and Wilson (1962), it remains unclear whether any biological insight has emerged from the use of MCT-information in animal communication studies. Perhaps this is the reason, as Gherardi and Pieraccini (2004) noted, that after a flurry of studies using MCT-information in the 1960s and 1970s, its use in behavioural ecology has largely disappeared.

7.4 DT-information

Since the 1980s, once the initial excitement over MCT-information had waned, most studies that have claimed to use MCT-information appear to report nothing more than DT-information insofar as they are only concerned with the structure of the signal repertoire of animals and not at all with the process of communication between individuals.[18] For instance, McCowan *et al.* (1999) analysed the the whistle vocalisations of the bottlenose dolphin, *Tursiops truncatus*;

[16] It also notes that chemical signals may have been missed since they were not recorded as part of the experimental design.

[17] At least they can be individuated using statistical criteria, for instance through the use of *k*-means cluster analysis in the case of bottleneck dolphin whistles (McCowan *et al.*, 1999).

[18] Sometimes this is at least implicitly recognised – see, for instance, McCowan *et al.* (1999) and McCowan, Doyle and Hanser (2002).

McCowan *et al.* (2002) followed with an analysis of the vocalisation patterns of the squirrel monkey, *Saimiri sciureus*.[19] In both cases patterns changed during development. More recently, Grimsley, Monaghan & Wenstrup (2011) analysed the vocalisations of mice at different developmental stages to compare signal repertoires and found that they, too, change significantly during development. None of these studies was concerned with what happens to the signal sequence after emission at the source, that is, its transmission along a channel and reception at the receiver. But these are critical components of Shannon's model which specifies MCT-information. Ignoring them means that we have no interest in the transmission of information: we are only interested in the uncertainty/complexity/diversity at the source. In other words, we are measuring DT-information.

Many of these studies also used a Zipf plot, which is a log–log plot of the frequency of signal units against their rank order (McCowan *et al.*, 1999, 2002).[20] What is sometimes called Zipf's law is the claim that this plot is linear (with a slope of about −1 for words and letters of almost all human languages). By and large, the signal repertoire studies mentioned earlier reported linear Zipf plots. Given linearity, structural change of a signal repertoire is indicated by a change of slope of Zipf plots, and these studies duly recorded such changes. In part, these results are not unexpected: it would have been more surprising if signal repertoires did not undergo structural changes during development. However, the observation that the Zipf plots are linear, that is, Zipf's law holds, may be more interesting.[21] It *may* indicate some structural similarities between these species' vocalisations and human language but this is, at present, no more than speculation.

Two points are most pertinent here. First, these structural studies of signal repertoires are related to communication only because there is good reason to believe that they are used for this purpose. However, as emphasised earlier, they do not address the process of communication directly. The use of the Shannon measure should be viewed as the use of DT-information. It is logically related to MCT-information only in the sense indicated in Section 7.2. In this sense it is incorrect to claim that these studies use MCT-information as many of their authors at least implicitly seem to do.

[19] Besides the Shannon index both studies also computed higher-order entropies, but this complication is not relevant to the issues treated in this chapter.

[20] For criticism of the use of Zipf's law, see Suzuki, Buck & Tyack (2005); for a reply, see McCowan *et al.* (2005).

[21] Suzuki *et al.* (2005) have argued that it is artifactual and that even a random process may generate straight-line Zipf plots. However, this point is irrelevant to the claim that differences in slopes of linear Zipf plots (in fact, in the shape of the Zipf plots) are indicative of differences in the structure of signal repertoires.

Second, Zipf plots are a statistical tool conceptually unrelated to information in any of its interpretations. However, it is formally trivial to show that changes in the slopes of these plots (when linear) imply changes in the values of the Shannon measure (for DT-information). This means that changes in the Shannon measure can also be used to infer that the signal repertoire structure changes during development. But the slope of the linear Zipf plots presumably provides a more sensitive indicator of structural change in signal repertoires than the Shannon measure alone. In this sense, what is most interesting in these studies goes beyond the use of DT-information.

For both bottleneck dolphins and squirrel monkeys, the Shannon measure increases in value between the infant and the adult stage (McCowan *et al.*, 2002).[22] The increase is slight but may be interpreted as an increase of complexity/diversity in the signal repertoire of these species during the course of development. If this pattern is also found for other species, then it may lead to some insight about what happens to animal communication systems during development in the sense that we may have a useful quantitative measure of complexity/diversity increase during development. It is too early to tell where these analyses will take us. But prospects for the utility of DT-information in animal communication studies look much better than that of MCT-information. However, all the problems with the individuation of signals and distinguishing signal from noise affect the potential utility of DT-information in exactly the same way that they affect MCT-information.

7.5 Semantic information and colloquial correlates

We turn, finally, to semantic information. The use of semantic information concepts in animal communication studies, even when not quantified, has been comprehensively criticised lately (Owren *et al.*, 2010) and is being widely debated in this volume. The discussion here will therefore be very brief in order to avoid unnecessary repetition.

It does not appear that any animal communication study has used the Carnap –Bar-Hillel theory and its associated interpretation of the Shannon measure. This is not surprising given that the Carnap–Bar-Hillel theory has been rarely explored in any context, partly because of the difficulty of credibly assigning logical probabilities to the relevant statements. What is more troubling is that animal communication studies that have focused on the content of

[22] But higher-order entropies show a reverse trend; this confounds any interpretation of developmental changes using such complexity measures.

signal sequences have made no attempt to quantify information content except, as in rare cases, through the use of the Shannon measure interpreted as MCT-information (e.g., Martins, 1994). That assumes that content can be quantified using the frequency of signals, with lower frequency having higher content which, as Pfeifer (2006) has recently pointed out (perhaps too strongly), seems evolutionarily "ridiculous" (p. 329, n. 13). The point is that it is not credible that the rarest behaviours (signals) are always the ones that are the most evolutionarily useful (and, in that sense, the ones with the most content). Nevertheless, the issue of quantifying, or at least, ranking signal sequences on the basis of their presumed information content must be broached. If these sequences cannot be ranked at all, it will not even be possible to claim that one signal sequence has more information than another. If large sets of signal sequences must be ranked, the most plausible way of establishing an order is to introduce a quantitative measure. Moreover, such a quantitative measure would probably facilitate the exploration of mathematical or computational predictive models for the evolution of signalling systems.

Yet, most advocates of the use of semantic information in animal communication studies seem to eschew quantification altogether.[23] Rather, they use colloquial correlates which, when explicated, require that the content of signals be of a specified kind in order to be repositories of information. A variety of accounts have been offered as to what this specification of kind must be.[24] Almost all appeal to representation (in the sender – that is, the source of the signal – or in the receiver, or both) and evolutionary function. Now each of these questions is biologically interesting: when and in what form an animal has a representation of the state of the world (including the external environment), and how and why this form has evolved.

But the question that is most relevant here is what additional insight is provided by construing signals as bearers of semantic information.[25] Information-talk can be replaced by mechanistic accounts which use no

[23] An important exception is Dall *et al.* (2005) who invoke statistical decision theory but couch it in terms of information, which is entirely unnecessary. Rather, statistical decision theory is an alternative to semantic information-talk and not an explication of it. Discussing the merits of statistical decision theory – and there are many – is beyond the scope of this contribution (but see the Introduction of this book).

[24] For extended discussion of alternatives, see Allen and Hauser (1993) and Stegmann (2005, 2009).

[25] We could claim, of course, that all representation involves information. But we would then generate the problem of quantifying (or ranking) representation. Once again, an additional pertinent issue is why we would need both concepts, representation and information.

informational terms, as Dawkins and Krebs pointed out long ago.[26] Returning to the case of the honeybees and the waggle dance, which is typically interpreted in informational terms, the description of the system in Section 7.1 required no use of 'information'. No doubt, additional insight would be gained by elucidating the physiological mechanisms by which sleep deprivation affects behaviour, along with the neurological mechanisms associating direction and length of flights with the perceived physical features of the dances. The evolutionary origins of such mechanisms are obviously also of great interest. But it is far from clear what additional insight an informational interpretation of these mechanisms would provide.

Moreover, understanding the evolution of signalling systems also does not seem to require the use of the concept of information (Owren *et al.*, 2010). It is incumbent upon proponents of the use of informational concepts to produce evolutionary models that both use these concepts and cannot be recast without them, or, at the very least, that any such recasting would result in excessively unwieldy formulations. In particular, given some account of signal and benefit (for example enhanced fitness) it is possible to make sense of both communication and miscommunication. Communication was defined earlier to require the production of signals that typically invoke behaviour that benefits the sender and has evolved for that reason; *miscommunication* occurs when the sender receives no benefit in spite of transmitting a signal that typically invokes a behaviour that benefits the sender (and has evolved for that reason). Miscommunication is thus to be distinguished from sending 'dishonest' signals. However, miscommunication still remains a form of communication. Returning again to the case of the sleep-deprived honeybees (Section 7.1), some nestmates would waste energy and return after foraging unsuccessfully. This, in turn, would presumably negatively affect all members of the nest; at the very least, the misled bees would receive no benefit. There is thus a case of miscommunication, but we did not need to speak of information. Moreover, if we model such a system, we can quantify the loss of optimality (e.g. as a function of the departure from optimality of resources gathered relative to foraging effort) with no recourse to 'information'. If we interpret this measure as a component of fitness, there are interesting conceptual issues regarding whether these fitnesses must be frequency-dependent and whether selection is operating not only at the level of the individual.[27] But, once again, 'information' is irrelevant.

[26] See Dawkins and Krebs (1978), although they were later somewhat more sympathetic to both MCT-information and semantic information (Dawkins & Krebs, 1984).

[27] A similar story would have to be told for cases in which signals are accompanied by cost interpreted as a loss of individual fitnesses. See Sarkar (2008) on a presumed connection between frequency-dependent fitnesses and higher-level selection.

The situation might have been different if proponents of the use of semantic information had provided a quantitative measure of content which would permit the type of comparison that made MCT-information temporarily fashionable as discussed earlier and keeps DT-information relevant today. But no such account seems forthcoming. Meanwhile, conceptual parsimony would suggest eliminating talk of semantic information in animal communication studies.

7.6 Final remarks

Where does this leave us? There is as yet no knockdown argument establishing the irrelevance of the informational concepts in animal communication studies. Nonetheless, the case for usage is weak no matter which construal is at stake.

For MCT-information, much of the traditional mystique was generated by calculations that had as their basis arbitrary individuation of animal signals and, therefore, arbitrary assignment of frequencies. While canonical individuation of signals may be possible, for instance, using the perceptual discriminatory capacities of receivers, we are yet to find definitive studies that establish the utility of MCT-information in this way. Proponents of MCT-information are yet to make a convincing case for its relevance to animal communication studies. The situation is no better – and no worse – than the use of MCT-information for (human) natural language. Meanwhile, MCT-information appears to be best left to the context for which mathematical communication theory was developed: the transmission of digitised messages along well-defined channels.

For DT-information, assuming that signals are appropriately defined, there is no issue with measuring information as the complexity/diversity of the signal repertoire. Some interesting generalisations have been proposed, for instance changes in the slope of Zipf plots (which do not require explicit estimates of DT-information) during animal development. The same point could be made using the Shannon measure (that is, DT-information), although with less sensitivity. Most importantly, though, these developments are yet to provide palpable insights. Nevertheless, this may remain the most promising role for the use of information in animal communication studies.

For semantic information, the question is whether the concept is at all necessary. If communication occurs through signals, and we have an adequate notion of what benefits a sender, we can distinguish between communication and miscommunication without invoking any notion of information. Modelling communication systems does not require the use of any construal of information, and in the absence of a quantitative measure of semantic information, it is difficult to envision how the use of 'information' would even be helpful in modelling contexts. As noted at the end of Section 7.5, conceptual parsimony suggests abandoning a redundant concept from the theoretical repertoire of animal communication studies. The onus, in this case, is on the proponents of the use of informational concepts in animal communication studies to provide examples in which the use of these concepts are strictly necessary.

References

Adrian, E. D. (1928). *The Basis of Sensation: The Action of the Sense Organs.* New York: W. W. Norton.

Allen, C. & Hauser, M. (1993). Communication and cognition: is information the connection? In D. L. Hull, M. Forbes & K. Okrulik, eds., *PSA 1992: Proceedings of the Biennial Meeting of the Philosophy of Science Association*, Vol. 2. Chicago, IL: University of Chicago Press, pp. 81–91.

Ash, R. B. (1965). *Information Theory.* New York: Dover.

Bar-Hillel, Y. (1952). Semantic information and its measures. *Transactions of the Tenth Conference on Cybernetics.* New York: Josiah Macy Jr Foundation, pp. 22–48.

Benveniste, E. (1953). Animal communication and human language. *Diogenes*, **1**, 1–7.

Bretman, A. & Tregenza, T. (2007). Strong, silent types: the rapid, adaptive disappearance of a sexual signal. *Trends in Ecology and Evolution*, **22**, 226–228.

Cadena, V. (2011). Sleepless nights lead to miscommunication in honey bees. *Journal of Experimental Biology*, **214**, iv.

Carnap, R. & Bar-Hillel, Y. (1952). *An Outline of a Theory of Semantic Information.* Technical Report No. 247. Cambridge, MA: Research Laboratory of Electronics, Massachusetts Institute of Technology.

Dall, S. R. X., Giraldeau, L.-A., Olsson, O., McNamara, J. M. & Stephens, D. W. (2005). Information and its use by animals in evolutionary ecology. *Trends in Ecology and Evolution*, **20**, 187–193.

Dawkins, R. & Krebs, J. R. (1978). Animal signals: information or manipulation? In J. R. Krebs & N. B. Davies, eds., *Behavioural Ecology: An Evolutionary Approach.* Oxford: Blackwell, pp. 282–309.

Dawkins, R. & Krebs, J. R. (1984). Animal signals: mind-reading and manipulation. In J. R. Krebs & N. B. Davies, eds., *Behavioural Ecology: An Evolutionary Approach*, 2nd edn. Sunderland, MA: Sinauer, pp. 380–402.

Eigen, M. (1971). Self-organisation of matter and the evolution of macromolecules. *Naturwissenschaften*, **58**, 465–523.

Fisher, R. A. (1925). Theory of statistical estimation. *Proceedings of the Cambridge Philosophical Society*, **22**, 700–725.

Garson, J. (2003). The introduction of information into neurobiology. *Philosophy of Science*, **70**, 926–936.

Gherardi, F. & Pieraccini, R. (2004). Using information theory to assess dynamics, structure, and organization of crayfish agonistic repertoire. *Behavioural Processes*, **65**, 163–178.

Good, I. J. (1953). The population frequencies of species and the estimation of population parameters. *Biometrika*, **40**, 237–264.

Grimsley, J. M. S., Monaghan, J. J. M. & Wenstrup, J. J. (2011). Development of social vocalizations in mice. *PLoS ONE*, **6**(3), e17460.

Haldane, J. B. S. & Spurway, H. (1954). A statistical analysis of communication in '*Apis mellifera*' and a comparison with communication in other animals. *Insectes Sociaux*, **1**, 247–283.

Halliday, T. R. & Slater, P. J. B. (eds.) (1983). *Animal Behaviour: Communication*. Oxford: Blackwell Scientific.

Hartley, R. V. L. (1928). Transmission of information. *Bell System Technical Journal*, **7**, 535–563.

Hauser, M. D. (1996). *The Evolution of Communication*. Cambridge, MA: MIT Press.

Heims, S. J. (1991). *The Cybernetics Group*. Cambridge, MA: MIT Press.

Hurd, P. L. & Enquist, M. (2005). A strategic taxonomy of biological communication. *Animal Behaviour*, **70**, 1155–1170.

Kay, L. E. (2000). *Who Wrote the Book of Life? A History of the Genetic Code*. Stanford, CA: Stanford University Press.

Klein, B. A., Klein, A., Wray, M. K., Mueller, U. G. & Seeley, T. D. (2010). Sleep deprivation impairs precision of waggle dance signaling in honey bees. *Proceedings of the National Academy of Sciences USA*, **107**, 22705–22709.

MacArthur, R. H. (1957). On the relative abundance of bird species. *Proceedings of the National Academy of Sciences USA*, **43**, 293–295.

Maclaurin, J. (2011). Commentary on 'The Transmission Sense of Information' by Carl T. Bergstrom and Martin Rosvall. *Biology and Philosophy*, **26**, 191–194.

Margalef, R. (1958). Information theory in ecology. *General Systems Yearbook*, **3**, 36–71.

Martins, E. P. (1994). Structural complexity in the lizard communication system: the sceloporus gracious 'push-up' display. *Copeia*, **4**, 944–955.

Maynard Smith, J. & Harper, D. (2003). *Animal Signals*. Oxford: Oxford University Press.

McCowan, B., Doyle, L. R. & Hanser, S. F. (2002). Using information theory to assess the diversity, complexity, and development of communicative repertoires. *Journal of Comparative Psychology*, **116**, 166–172.

McCowan, B., Doyle, L. R., Jenkins, J. M. & Hanser, S. F. (2005). The appropriate use of Zipf's law in animal communication studies. *Animal Behaviour*, **69**, F1–F7.

McCowan, B., Hanser, S. F. & Doyle, L. R. (1999). Quantitative tools for comparing animal communication systems: information theory applied to bottlenose dolphin whistle repertoires. *Animal Behaviour*, **57**, 409–419.

Owren, M. J., Rendall, D. & Ryan, M. J. (2010). Redefining animal signaling: influence versus information in communication. *Biology and Philosophy*, **25**, 755–780.

Pfeifer, J. (2006). The use of information theory in biology: lessons from social insects. *Biological Theory*, **3**, 317–330.

Sarkar, S. (1992). 'The boundless ocean of infinite possibilities': logic in Carnap's logical syntax of language. *Synthese*, **93**, 191–237.

Sarkar, S. (1996a). Biological information: a skeptical look at some central dogmas of molecular biology. In S. Sarkar, ed., *The Philosophy and History of Molecular Biology: New Perspectives*. Dordrecht: Kluwer, pp. 187–231.

Sarkar, S. (1996b). Decoding 'coding': information and DNA. *BioScience*, **46**, 857–863.

Sarkar, S. (2004). Genes encode information for phenotypic traits. In C. Hitchcock, ed., *Contemporary Debates in Philosophy of Science*. Malden: Blackwell, pp. 259–274.

Sarkar, S. (2007). From ecological diversity to biodiversity. In D. L. Hull & M. Ruse, eds., *The Cambridge Companion to the Philosophy of Biology*. Cambridge: Cambridge University Press, pp. 388–409.

Sarkar, S. (2008). A note on frequency-dependence and the levels/units of selection. *Biology and Philosophy*, **23**, 217–228.

Shannon, C. E. (1948). A mathematical theory of communication. *Bell System Technical Journal*, **27**, 379–423, 623–656.

Stegmann, U. (2005). John Maynard Smith's notion of animal signals. *Biology and Philosophy*, **20**, 1011–1025.

Stegmann, U. (2009). A consumer-based teleosemantics for animal signals. *Philosophy of Science*, **76**, 864–875.

Suzuki, R., Buck, J. R. & Tyack, P. L. (2005). The use of Zipf's Law in animal communication analysis. *Animal Behaviour*, **69**, F9–F17.

von Frisch, K. (1950). *Bees: Their Vision, Chemical Senses, and Language*. Ithaca, NY: Cornell University Press.

Wiener, N. (1948). *Cybernetics: Or Control and Communication in the Animal and the Machine*. Cambridge, MA: MIT Press.

Wilson, E. O. (1962). Chemical communication among workers of the fire ant *Solenopsis saevissima* (Fr. Smith): 2. An information analysis of the odour trail. *Animal Behaviour*, **19**, 148–158.

Zuk, M. & Simmons, L. W. (1997). Reproductive strategies of the crickets (Orthoptera: Gryllidae). In J. C. Choe & B. J. Crespi, eds., *The Evolution of Mating Systems in Insects and Arachnids*. Cambridge: Cambridge University Press, pp. 89–109.

Zuk, M., Rotenberry, J. T. & Tinghitella, R. M. (2006). Silent night: adaptive disappearance of a sexual signal in a parasitized population of field crickets. *Biology Letters*, **2**, 521–524.

Zuk, M., Simmons, L. W. & Cupp, L. (1993). Calling characteristics of parasitized and unparasitized populations of the field cricket, *Teleogryllus oceanicus*. *Behavioral and Ecological Sociobiology*, **33**, 339–343.

8

Mitogenetic rays and the information metaphor: transmitted information has had its day

EUGENE S. MORTON AND RICHARD G. COSS

We dedicate this chapter to the late Professor Donald H. Owings (deceased 9 April 2011) who contributed the abstract that inspired the theoretical framework for this chapter. Don engaged in decades of ground-breaking research in the lab and field on how ground squirrels cope with their snake predators. We describe in our chapter Don's insights that emerged from this research that shaped the assessment/management construct.

About ten years ago a Russian investigator, Gurwitsch, reported that rapidly growing cells, such as the tip of an onion root, emit radiation of short wavelengths and are able to accelerate growth in neighboring cells ... Several hundred papers have followed in this field ... Some investigators find mitogenetic rays emitted by a variety of living tissues, and increased growth has been reported in yeast cells, young bacterial, and certain plants.

(Daniels, 1935)

The 'miracle of caryokinesis' was the starting point that stimulated Alexander G. Gurwitsch to carry out his famous 'mitogenetic' experiments in 1923 ... results confirmed his hypothesis of a weak radiation from cells, which is able to trigger the growth of other cells ... Both 'energetic' and 'informational' aspects have to be considered, namely radiation effective in activating molecules, and that involved in arranging them into larger units.

(Gurwitsch, 1988)

Animal Communication Theory: Information and Influence, ed. Ulrich Stegmann. Published by Cambridge University Press.

> **M-Rays' Existence Doubted**. 'Not proven' is the Scotch verdict returned by two critical biophysicists after a careful investigation of the disputed phenomenon of mitogenetic radiation, or M-rays ... they were unable to obtain any evidence ... of the existence of mitogenetic radiation. They therefore rest their case with a negative verdict, at the same time stating their willingness to reopen it again if supporters of the M-ray hypothesis come forward with positive evidence produced under really rigorous experimental conditions.
>
> (*Science Service*, 1938)

Scientific truth changes as we test, accept and discard hypotheses. The quotes above provide an example of the scientific process you may not remember. Mitogenetic rays were a trendy subject between 1924 and 1938. The originator pointed a growing onion root tip towards another and suggested that cell divisions in the second root increase owing to 'irradiation' from the first root tip. The irradiation was by 'mitogenetic rays' (M-rays). Hundreds of papers were published about them and many a PhD spawned. They never existed.

The concept of M-rays may sound silly now with our advanced thinking (but see VanWijk, 2001). But a current dilemma deserves the scrutiny afforded M-rays. We contend that 'information' as still applied, willy nilly, to the process, definition and function of animal communication is comparable to mitogenetic rays (Owings & Morton, 1998). They share certain elements. Messages are to information what mitogenetic rays were to changes in root growth. Both share the notion that something causes a change. M-rays increase cell growth rate; messages are decoded and cause changes in recipient behaviour. M-rays affect the rate of growth of cells that receive them. Information is carried and transmitted within a signal and causes changes in recipients. M-rays are a form of radiation whereas a message is an abstract property of entities and events (Smith, 1977). An informer informs another by conveying information so that the informed can interpret the meaning in the message and make choices. A major difference is that, if M-rays exist, they should be detectable.

Like phlogiston, the downfall of M-rays was that rays could not be found. The 'rays' turned out to be volatile substances, perhaps ethereal oils given off from crushed onion tissue (*Nature*, 1931). The downfall of 'transmitted information' might be that the alleged 'abstract properties' of messages are non-existent, like the rays (Font & Carazo, 2010). But showing that something does not exist is extremely difficult when there is nothing to shoot at. Instead, we use heuristic arguments for removing information, *as a causative agent*, from animal communication science.

We contend that the 'informational perspective' is not good science because it leads us astray from using form/function analysis (part of the evolutionary biology toolkit), substitutes for testing hypotheses (see Lakatos, 1970) and allows the powerful forces of anthropomorphism a long leash (Owings & Morton, 1998). We focus on transmitted information (TI) because of the convolution it represents. On the one hand, individuals produce signals; on the other, individuals that perceive these signals extract information from them. Therefore, there must be information in the signal that is extracted, which is TI. This assumption of TI initiates a series of biases, the most egregious being that it places the sender in control of the evolution of communication because its transmitted information causes things to occur. The alternate hypothesis, not previously considered, is that signals, like M-rays, do not contain TI. We question both the veracity and utility of TI, apart from our human predisposition favouring it. In its place we consider the assessment activities of perceivers, long considered important, but not fully embraced as the driving property of communication.

8.1 Anthropomorphism

'Information' is used in a metaphoric sense, a linguistic metaphor that encourages the search for speech-like coding in animal signals (Owings & Morton, 1998). We are coming to realise that metaphors are not rhetorical frills at the edge of how we think; they are the very heart of it (Geary, 2011). As a speech metaphor, information has such great intuitive appeal that it holds a central place for many who study animal communication (Box 1.2 in Owings & Morton, 1998). 'Information' used in a linguistic sense is bound to cause trouble in evolutionary and proximate analyses of animal communication. *A priori*, it adopts human traits as the basis for studying animal communication. This was not helped by the invention of writing, which elevates informative symbols as central to thinking itself (Donald, 1991; Gleick, 2011). Anthrozoology is the study of human–animal bonds and ties the roots of those bonds to culture and biology operating in collusion with the human capacity to infer the mental states of others. We find it easy to anthropomorphise about animals, since humans routinely attribute human characteristics to anything with a face, a voice, a trajectory (e.g. bears, bats, storms, the moon, ships). Deacon (1997, p. 52) pointed out that using human language as a basis to compare other species' communication "as exceptions to a rule based on the one most exceptional and divergent case" is a perverse analytical method. Why would a science adopt a concept like transmitted information when this undermines the goal of objectivity? It's like shooting yourself in the foot in the hope of winning a marathon.

We suggest that 'information' can be used as a shorthand to describe *to humans* what vocalisations can/could do. For example: "Vocalizations can provide information about a bird's behavioural state, quality or condition, and relationships with nearby animals" (Catchpole & Slater, 1995). But the term 'information' should not be used as if animals are providing something to each other. An example would be the statement: "When we ask why gaping is performed we are interested in the information borne by this display and how the interests of sender and receiver are affected." We would ask: "Affected by what, the information?" We would answer: "No, it's the signal itself, its physical form and how its form relates to its function. You are *not* interested in the information but in the accomplishment of the communication." Earlier, information content was not regarded as a commodity but a property or potential that only could be discussed in relation to responses (Marler, 1961). This is different from saying that information causes responses. In communication, *perceivers are independent of sender control but senders are not free from perceiver choice.*

This perceiver's perspective of information can be seen in the manner that humans evolved sophisticated skills to broadly assess various mental states. For example, the evolutionary advent of the modern human foot about 1.5 Myr ago fostered endurance running, allowing the capture of small and disabled prey (Carrier, 1984; Bramble & Lieberman, 2004). Assessment of prey vulnerability in relationship to their ease of capture was relatively simple. Complex assessment of prey behaviour by ancestral humans emerged more than 200 kyr ago during the prolonged 'arms race' in which a variety of game increased their wariness of humans or defensively attacked them (Thuppil & Coss, 2012), requiring humans to adopt stealthier hunting practices and projectiles (Larson, 2009). As with leopards deterred from hunting diana monkeys (*Cercopithecus diana*), the alarm calling of game as public announcements revealing hunter detection would mediate decisions over whether to continue hunting in the area (Zuberbühler, Jenny & Bshary, 1999).

The pursuit of TI, whether defined as knowledge, reduction of uncertainty, semiotics or displays, has dominated animal communication research from shortly after tape recorders suitable for fieldwork were invented. Over 55% of publications since 1955 use the informational perspective as the basis for generating hypotheses (Fig. 1.1 of Owings & Morton, 1998). As has been said, "... grounding the idea of communication in undefined informational constructs renders both those constructs and others that flow from them untenable" (Rendell, Owren & Ryan, 2009). For example, 'sharing information' implies that selection favours efficiency and the correct reception of signals (Wiley & Richards, 1982; Endler, 1993; Hauser, 1996; Bradbury & Vehrencamp, 2011). In birdsong studies, the primary sources of selection on singers are deemed to be correct signal reception to improve the performance of receivers, and honesty, enforced by females who discount all but honest signals of male quality via sexual selection (Gil & Gahr, 2002; Maynard Smith & Harper, 2003; Searcy & Nowicky, 2005). Signal-detection theory derived from acoustical engineering and information theory (Shannon & Weaver, 1949) is brought into play. This theoretical model considers human communication to involve channel-like information transmission in which the sender's meaning is encoded as a signal and the receiver decodes the signal to recreate the meaning (Arundale, 1999). Indeed, biologists use the information theory metaphor, as indicated by our use of *sender, receiver, transmit, channel, decoding* etc., even though most use the term 'information' in the dictionary sense of 'knowledge' (P. Marler, personal communication). Seyfarth and colleagues (2010) attempt to defend the informational perspective using information theory to define information (as a reduction of uncertainty in the recipient) even though this operates only at the syntactical level (focuses on the signal), so this construct tells us nothing about the significance of signals to the communicants (Cherry, 1957) (see also our reply to commentaries).

The information theory metaphor may underlie uncritical acceptance of information as a necessary 'content' of a signal much as do linguistic metaphors. Information, and efficiency in communicating it, makes evolutionary conflicts between participants amount to noise, something selection should eliminate. But, if we switch from a mechanistic engineering view of communication to a biological view, the perceivers must be deemed the driving force because their responses affect the value of communication for senders. Gordon Burghardt discussed this earlier (Burghardt, 1970). Perceivers determine the physical features of the signal and determine a signal's 'meaningful' content. Content refers to whatever a signal correlates with plus assessment by perceivers. Their responses most often reflect conflicts rather than cooperation or sharing and are important because they may form the basis for notable evolutionary events, such as song learning in songbirds (Morton, 1996).

The information perspective and its linguistic metaphorical roots promote human speech-based terms, such as honesty, costliness, retaliation and other attributes associated with game theoretic approaches to communication (e.g. Maynard Smith & Harper, 2003). Vehrencamp (2000) put it this way: "In signaling exchanges with conflicting sender–receiver interests, there will always be an incentive for senders to lie, exaggerate, or mislead in order to induce the receiver to choose the response preferred by the sender." We question that game theory predictions for communication are valid (Enquist *et al.*, 2002). Game theory's informational stance predicts that signals will rarely provide information about intentions (Dawkins & Krebs, 1978; Maynard Smith, 1979).

But cannot fighting/body size/energetic relationships provide the honest basis for communication to evolve to replace aggressive fighting? Does not ethological data show that displays are often derived from preexisting behaviours, emancipated from their former functions, and ritualised for a communicative function (e.g. Daanje, 1950; Tinbergen, 1952; Moynihan, 1955)? Where does 'honesty' come into that scenario? Is there a need to invoke 'external validity' to explain the veracity of communication?

We suggest that the purported need for checks on 'honesty' arises from the assumption that TI exists. However, built-in honesty comes in several forms that obviate the supposed value of TI. Energetic constraints relate to condition-dependent aspects of communication especially common in mate choice (e.g. Holzer, Jacat & Brinkoff, 2003) or resource-holding potential (e.g. López & Martín, 2011). Placing information as a go-between sender and receiver assures that the built-in honesty of communication will be overlooked and that TI will replace the stamina, strength and ability to survive risks that constitute fighting ability (Morton, 2000). Communication is based upon what it accomplishes for the sender or can be afforded by it, not supposed TI. And perceiver assessment of what signals correlate with, not signalling itself, is what determines the evolution and the substance of communication; active assessment produces 'honesty' in communication making the need to search for its roots in the sender a moot point.

The search for honesty in animal communication was based in part upon Maynard Smith and Harper's (2003) suggestion that only signals carrying 'true' semantic information could be evolutionarily stable owing to receiver retaliation. Hence, they too embraced the assessment process by perceivers as important to the semantic effects of signals, but they differ from our position because they fully embraced the informational perspective that signals carry semantic content about the sender (Stegmann, 2005). This is ironic because Dawkins and Krebs' (1978) game theoretic approach to communication downgraded TI. Our position is a logical extension for the assessor role, that a signal's semantic content is based solely upon the assessment process; the sender does not encode information in its signals.

If humans need to describe the 'information' in a signal, then it should be based upon the assessor's response. For example, in red deer (*Cervus elaphus*), roaring results in the buck with the highest roaring rate causing opponents to retreat (Clutton-Brock & Albon, 1979). "Then the winning male's higher-frequency roar would mean, to the opponent, the kind of behaviour this roar is evolutionarily designed to elicit in the opponent, i.e. the opponent's retreat. What one male signals to the other will therefore be 'Retreat!'"(Stegmann, 2005).

Because assessment is a proactive process, there is no need to imagine some transmitted information prods the perceiver into action; the signal does this.

There is no need to place TI as an intermediary between sender and receiver. Signals initiate a pragmatic process of self-interested regulation of perceiver behaviour (management) that works by exploiting connections established by their assessment activities. Indeed, the definition of a signal as *an act deployed to capitalise on assessment systems* captures the essence of communication (Owings & Morton, 1998).

Mimicry employs assessment in just this way. For example, some visual signals involving mimicry appear to be deceptive, such as the eyespot patterns displayed by a wide range of species. But 'deceptive information' is not being 'sent': eyespots simply capitalise on the perceiver's recognition that two facing eyes are characteristic of the interest of conspecifics or predators (Coss & Goldthwaite, 1995). Indeed, it should be kept in mind that Batesian kinds of mimicry are due to selection on the signallers by the assessment activities of perceivers, which in this case are the dupes as well. Batesian mimicry illustrates our proposition that assessment, generally, is the source of selection on signals, and there is no need to use TI to describe this selection.

Perhaps communication studies need a null hypothesis. In order to provide a null hypothesis, information must be replaced by aspects intrinsic to the individual. Prum (2010) suggests a null hypothesis for bird song: it may be *arbitrary*, simply communicating an individual's availability and motivation to mate, which has coevolved arbitrarily with a mating preference. It need not be influenced by additional sources of selection. However, birdsong is widely viewed as an *indicator* trait, carrying a wide range of 'information' about a singer's genetics, health, vigour etc., that makes singing 'honest' or 'dishonest'. As Prum (2010) points out, the potential arbitrary nature of birdsong is ignored; what we see, and what the birdsong literature for the past 50 years largely supports, is a case study in confirmationist research lacking simultaneous tests of the competing null hypothesis (see Platt, 1964).

8.2 Form and function

Human speech consists of words whose sounds are unrelated to their meaning (except for onomatopoeic words). Because of this, we learn what words mean and call this knowledge 'information'. Linguistic pragmatics, which deals with meaning in context, stresses functionality in communication (Scott-Phillips, 2010), as should communication in biological systems. But linguistic pragmatics assumes the arbitrariness of words and so excludes the properties of 'form' encompassing relationships between signal form and function. The speech metaphor allows us to assume *a priori* that the forms (i.e. physical structures) of animal signals, vocalisations in particular, are arbitrary. Speech consists primarily of arbitrary sounds (Fromkin, Rodman & Hyams, 2011). Arbitrariness may be an adaptation that ensures accurate learning of a parental language by children (Pinker & Bloom, 1990). However, for animal communication research, this deflects attention from relationships between signal structure and function. Forms are indubitably related to their functions in contexts where functions affect fitness. Recall the early work of Peter Marler (1955) on how the tonal structure of alarm calls in birds made them difficult to locate, whereas mobbing calls were easily located by their inter-aural arrival time differences; form is correlated with function.

This applies to communication in all modalities, but here we concentrate on the acoustic modality, that most affected by human speech; the general validity of the debated concepts should be extended to other forms of signalling as well. For example, Avilés and Soler (2009) found that chromatic components of nestling gapes (the signals) were associated with their parents' visual system (the perceivers), illustrating how nestling competition for perceiver care can affect the signal with no need to invoke 'information'.

While some signals (like indices) do not fit the arbitrary assumption, arbitrariness is the default stance of the information perspective. The physical structures of signals, measurable acoustic descriptions such as frequency and amplitude, as well as perceptual descriptions, such as harshness or tonality resulting from physical structures, are not usually considered part of the semantics of signals (Owings & Morton, 1997), even though harshness or noisiness can reveal the emotional state of the caller (Coss, McCowan & Ramakrishnan, 2007).

Bird song is a good example of form and function because it is well known that vagaries of the environment affect these long-distance signals (LDSs) as they propagate. LDSs have an 'active space' defined as the volume of air in which they are detectible. This 'active space' is maximised when components of the LDS avoid background noise and match frequencies for optimum sound propagation for the habitat (Brenowitz, 1982; Slabbekoorn & Smith, 2002). The 1970s saw a flurry of interest in sound propagation (Chappuis, 1971; Morton, 1975; Marten & Marler, 1977a, 1977b). Some frequencies were shown to propagate better than others depending upon habitat and height above ground. Bands of frequencies propagating best were sometimes called 'sound windows' (Waser & Brown, 1984; Ellinger & Hödl, 2003). Wiley and Richards (1978) and Michelsen (1978) highlighted reverberation and irregular amplitude fluctuations and predicted that LDSs should be tonal or modulated in different habitats based on these considerations. Structuring LDSs to attain maximum acoustic space is called the 'acoustic adaptation hypothesis' (reviewed in Boncoraglio & Saino, 2007; Tobias *et al.*, 2010). The acoustic adaptation hypothesis predicts that LDSs should be fine-tuned to habitat acoustics (e.g. Hunter & Krebs, 1979; Gish & Morton, 1981;

Nicholls & Goldizen, 2006; Tubaro & Lijtmaer, 2006). In many birds, learning may promote acquiring songs fine-tuned to an acoustic environment (Hansen, 1979; Morton, 1996) but even non-learning species show acoustic adaptation in their songs (Morton, 1975; Morton & Derrickson, 1996; Nemeth, Winkler & Dabelsteen, 2001; Seddon, 2005). Signal structure for these LDSs helps them propagate well. Less degraded signals make the sender appear close to perceivers, thereby grabbing their attention (Morton, 1986, 2012).

A more general way that structure relates to function in acoustic signals may reflect the origin of terrestrial vocal communication that began, at least by the Jurassic Period, in amphibians. Frogs and toads, unlike mammals and birds, continue to grow after sexual maturity and, with males, the best fighters are larger and older and generally preferred by females for mates. Big toads produce lower-pitched species-specific calls than smaller individuals. Anuran signals evolved to replace fighting owing to this pitch/size correlation. The source of selection was energy-based; it took less energy than evicting competitors by physically pushing them away. Experiments proved that the vocal signal alone is sufficiently intimidating to smaller toads that they move away from the calls of larger ones (Davies & Halliday, 1978). Form (lower pitch) is directly related to its function of repelling males and attracting females. Smaller males escape to live another day, and females are attracted by larger males because they have demonstrated their ability to survive.

There is no information 'sent'; instead a signal's content is whatever it correlates with plus assessment by perceivers. The direct communication of size we see in anurans, where competitors differ in size, cannot pertain to birds and mammals because these cease growing around the time of sexual maturation. Signals of size exist but reflect motivation, not absolute size. In this expressive sound symbolism (Morton, 1994; Owings & Morton, 1998, p. 104), signals by aggressive individuals are low-pitched while fearful or friendly individuals signal using higher pitch. Signals stand for size and can replace a sender's need to move around, replacing fighting and intimidation with less energy expenditure. Signal assessment produces this relationship. Communication is based on the immutable physical law that larger bodies have lower resonant frequencies (Morton, 1977; Scherer, 1985). Such signals can only be 'honest', but, again, this is a moot point.

Owren and Rendall (1997, 2001) added greatly to form/function analysis in their descriptions of primate communication by ascribing direct and indirect effects to vocalisations. They point out that acoustic startle, arousal and affective responses are directly mediated by the brainstem and other subcortical structures. Vocalisations such as primate squeaks, shrieks and screams may induce attention, arousal and affect by stimulating the primitive subcortical brain structures. For example in bonnet macaques (*Macaca radiata*), noisier vocalisations indicating higher states of physiological arousal can be the product of forceful diaphragm contractions, producing turbulence of the airflow through the open glottis and aperiodic vocalfold vibrations (Coss *et al.*, 2007).

Young animals and adult victims of aggression typically use these sorts of calls:

> Whether a steady stream of auditory pin-pricks or a full-fledged aural assault, these calling episodes by 'neglected' youngsters and victims of aggression are well designed to motivate receivers to relent, thereby 'turning off' the sounds. Abrupt onsets, click-like pulsing, dramatic modulations, or chaotic frequency spectra are also to be expected in alarm vocalisations, and provide another example of sounds that should be grounded in salient attention-and-arousal-inducing acoustic features. (Owren & Rendall, 2001)

This is a nice example of sensory exploitation, another idea that explains communication satisfactorily without recourse to TI (Ryan *et al.*, 1990).

Indirect effects include resonant sounds that are shaped by the vocal tract cavities of the caller. According to Owren and Rendall (2001) these reveal personal characteristics of the caller such as sex, body size and individual identity, and are often used at close range. Managers can use such vocalisations to influence assessor affect. When a dominant produces a threat call before or during an aggressive act the sound alone will produce desired effects through Pavlovian conditioning.

Owren and Rendall have opened up a rich new area for communication research, one that has barely been touched but may have far-reaching effects, particularly in species with obligatory sociality, like many primates and birds. The idea that managers might use signalling coercively via forms that function specifically to 'get into the head' of perceivers to control them seems full of potential. A male chicken (*Gallus gallus*), for example, gives a crooning low sound when he circles a hen while flicking one wing against the ground. Sometimes a cock will attract a hen to himself with the 'food call', designed to attract a hen to himself, even with no food evident, and when a hen gets near enough, he will start the crooning song and circling. Marler, Karakashian & Gyger, (1991) implied that the rooster was employing a signal with the intent to deceive. A more general explanation from natural history suggests that hens are safer near their rooster because he protects them against predators, so 'deceit' is unnecessary to attract them. Another possibility is that the cock's behaviour induces fear in the hen so that she will crouch in reaction and be easier for the cock to mate. In contrast, Satin Bowerbird bower construction and vocalisations may function to reduce female fear and induce her to stay in the bower and copulate (Patricelli, Coleman & Borgia, 2006). These 'psychological' aspects of signalling thus may affect social relations in many ways both indirectly, as in Pavlovian conditioning, or directly by capitalising on the sensory biases of perceivers (e.g. Ryan *et al.*, 1990).

8.3 Assessment and management

The assessment/management (A/M) concept was presented in Owings and Morton (1997, 1998). A/M defines the perceiver role (assessment) as a proactive process of determining what a signal is correlated with and the sender role (management) as a pragmatic process of self-interested regulation of the behaviour of others that works by exploiting the connections established by the assessment activities of surrounding individuals. The assessor does not need to be prodded into action by the receipt of information nor does the manager deal in information transfer.

There were three flashes of insight that inspired the A/M perspective by Donald Owings and his graduate student, David Hennessy (Owings & Hennessy, 1984). First was the discovery of the theoretical ideas of philosopher of science Steven Pepper (1942). Pepper described how in mechanistic thinking, stability is considered primary and change associated with events or forces needed to be explained. As the alternative, continuity could be considered as primary with the processes causing stability needed to be explained (see interpretation by Overton & Reese, 1981). Pepper used the term *contextualism* to label the process of studying temporal relationships of higher-order structure. As a variant of contextualism, control-systems theory (Powers, 1973) involves the study of multiple goal-directed reference signals and error-correcting feedback loops at higher levels of organisation that regulate behaviour over time.

The third and most dynamic insight influencing the assessment component of A/M was the proactive view of perception in the field of ecological psychology founded by James Gibson (Gibson, 1966). Gibson challenged the dogmatic position that perception is based upon inputs to the brain from sensory nerves; that impulses from these nerves comprise the messages of sense and are the only basis for perception:

> . . . the input of the sensory nerves is not the basis for perception . . . , but only the basis for passive sense impressions. These are not the data of perception, not the raw material out of which perception is fashioned by the brain. The active senses cannot be simply initiators of *signals* in nerve fibers or *messages* to the brain; instead they are analogous to tentacles and feelers. And the function of the brain when looped with

> its perceptual organs is not to decode signals, nor to interpret messages, nor to accept images. These old analogies no longer apply. The function of the brain is not even to *organise* the sensory input or to *process* the data . . . The perceptual systems, including the nerve centers at various levels up to the brain, are ways of seeking and extracting information about the environment from the flowing array of ambient energy. (Gibson, 1966, p. 5)

The formative structure of A/M was relatively complete when Owings and Hennessy argued that tail flagging by wild California ground squirrels (*Spermophilus beecheyi*) engaging tethered rattlesnakes had signalling properties that were "used to elicit a particular kind of performance from the target(s)" (Hennessy, 1980; Hennessy *et al.*, 1981). Greater formality of this idea was presented in the context that there are "multiple targets of signalling; multiple functions with respect to each target; the use of signals as probes; and the effect of self-regulation on signal structure" (Owings & Hennessy, 1984). Self-regulation has been an understated component of A/M in which, in addition to influencing others, the signaller itself is typically one target of its own behaviour.

Perceivers *assess* signals in context, and selection favours senders that respond to assessment by developing their signalling in light of assessment. A signal is an act deployed to get the most out of assessment systems. Signalling would be selected against if the process of assessment did not result in feedback. Indeed, communication might be defined by the process: communication is one individual signalling to manage the behaviour of others who, in their selfish interests, simultaneously assess these signals (Owings & Morton, 1998). This is in agreement with a definition focused on the signal rather than its supposed information:

> A signal is a packet of energy or matter generated by a display or action of one organism (the signaller) that is selected for its effects in influencing the probability pattern of behaviour of another organism (the receiver) via its sensory-nervous system in a fashion that is adaptive either to one or both parties. (Markl, 1983; see also Burghardt, 1970)

Information should be subsumed by the general statement that a signal's content is whatever it is correlated with plus assessment by perceivers and not used to signify something sent by the sender. The emphasis on information 'made available' by the signaller is an obstacle to determining the aspects of the signals that assessors respond to (Owings & Morton, 1998). Information is whatever assessors infer from the stimulus properties engendered by the signal (Figure 8.1). The signal itself has no information when viewed in isolation from receivers, so no TI is buried in the signal to be 'taken out'.

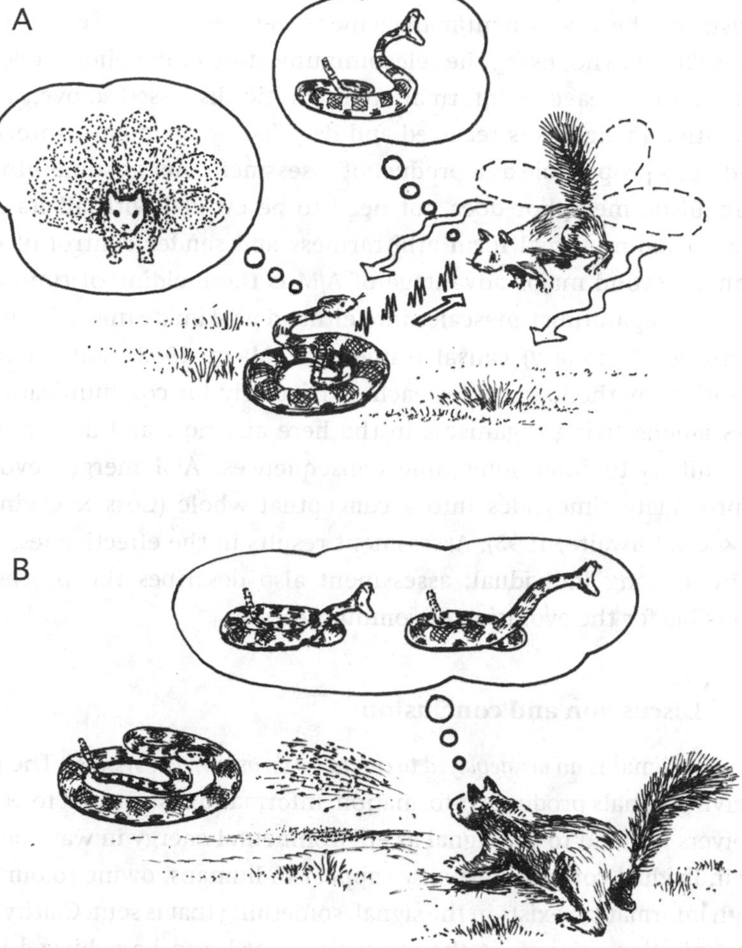

Figure 8.1 Comparison of two communication perspectives, one involving signalling to obtain information (see Rowe & Owings, 1990, 1996) (A), the other involving direct assessment without first receiving a signal (B), with both constructs employing behavioural assessment. In A, a California ground squirrel (*Spermophilus beecheyi*) confronts its northern Pacific rattlesnake (*Crotalis viridis*) predator by sending a deceptive signal that it is a much larger, more formidable adversary. This is accomplished by tail flagging with a heated tail that capitalises on the rattlesnake's infrared sensory ability (Rundus *et al.*, 2009). In turn, the rattlesnake rattles, signalling its intention to strike. The rattling click rate unintentionally reveals the snake's body size and temperature that constrains its striking distance. In B, the squirrel actively elicits this striking range information by throwing loose substrate at the snake to initiate its rattling.

Assessment/management has two things going for it, despite recent criticism of the assessment/management perspective by Seyfarth and colleagues (2010), who, using the telecommunications metaphor modelled after Shannon and Weaver's information theoretic discussed above, argue that information in signals is received and decoded by recipients. Information is placed in its proper role as a product of assessment, not as something sent, so the linguistic metaphor does not need to be evoked with all its attendant biases, including signal form arbitrariness and sender control of communication. A second major advantage of A/M is the melding of timescales. We are used to separating timescales into either a proximate (more immediate) or ultimate (evolutionary) causal framework (Mayr, 1988), and in describing appropriate methodologies for each. Particularly for communication, which occurs among living organisms in the here and now and does not fossilise to permit us to infer long time consequences, A/M merges evolutionary and proximate timescales into a conceptual whole (Coss & Owings, 1985; Coss & Goldthwaite, 1995). Assessment results in the effectiveness of signalling by a living individual; assessment also describes the process that is responsible for the evolution of communication.

8.4 Discussion and conclusion

A signal is *an act deployed to capitalise on assessment systems*. The process of perceiving signals produces information. Information is not sent to be received; perceivers respond to the signal as environmental energy in ways pertinent to their individual context. Responses appear to humans, owing to our biases, as though information exists in the signal, something that is sent. Clarity in animal communication science, at the conceptual level, can be achieved if the perceiver's role is given precedence in producing 'information'. We are not alone in this emphasis on assessment as the driver of communication. There has been a slow, but steady, flow of papers highlighting the perceiver role (e.g. Ryan & Rand, 1990; Guilford & Dawkins, 1991; Rendall *et al.*, 2009).

There is also more emphasis on function and form. Font and Carazo (2010; Carazo & Font, 2010) propose another meaning of information, *functional information*, which is "whatever information (in the semantic sense) can be extracted from the communication exchange that makes it adaptive for the receiver to respond to a given signal". We agree in part with their emphasis on the receiver-dependent (Stegmann, 2005) 'functional' notion of information, but their idea of information extraction still suggests that signals transmit 'informative content' rather than its emerging from perceiver assessment. We feel it is not necessary to include transmitted information in this paradigm.

The same transmitted information concept is used by Wagner and Danchin (2010) in their 'general taxonomy of biological information'. They define *intentional information* as "synonymous with Signal, which is a trait or behaviour produced by selection to intentionally transmit information, the adaptive function of which is to alter the behaviour of receivers to the benefit of the sender". Transmitted information is not necessary. Using Wagner and Danchin's definitions, but emphasising the receivers' importance, *intentional information* becomes: the result of assessment by perceivers based upon public information (information accessible to all) using their (the perceivers') private information (information possessed by an individual that is inaccessible to others) as a basis for making subsequent behavioural decisions. Their public information includes social and non-social information accessible to others. These decisions may or may not benefit the sender, depending on the average consequences of signalling. Signals and signalling evolve owing to these consequences/accomplishments (Burghardt, 1970), but information or content is just whatever the signal is correlated with and what perceivers infer or 'make' of the signal given their own private information, context, age, sex etc.; the signal itself does not have information if viewed in isolation from perceivers.

To expand further the idea of emergence from the perceiver's perspective, it is reasonable to argue that units of biological information are the cohesive regularities of relationships at different levels of organisation, with lower levels of organisation influencing higher levels of organisation (see Weber & Deacon, 2000). Analogous to the way that liquidity is not a property of individual water molecules, but results from their interactions, an individual fish does not have the property of a fish school. Within the school, individual fish perceive the relationships of neighbours and adjust their spacing accordingly, yielding cohesive regularities at the group level (Parrish, Viscido & Grünbaum, 2002). In this context, the emergent property of schooling organisation reflects the influence of the next lowest level of organisation, the multiple emergent properties of information engendered by the brain activities of fish perceivers. Similarly, one could view face-to-face interactions during communication as a changing flux of emergent properties with moment-to-moment regularities.

As for M-rays, Transmitted Information Existence Doubted. 'Not proven' is the Scotch verdict returned by three critical biologists after a careful investigation of the disputed phenomenon of transmitted information, or TI. They were unable to obtain any evidence of the existence of transmitted information. They therefore rest their case with a negative verdict, at the same time stating their willingness to reopen it again if supporters of the TI hypothesis come forward with positive evidence produced under really rigorous experimental conditions.

Acknowledgements

We sadly note the passing of Donald H. Owings before he was able to contribute directly to this chapter. We included his abstract in the manuscript so we count him as an author, in addition to much of the inspiration. We thank Giuseppe Boncoraglio, Gordon Burghardt and Ulrich Stegmann for many valuable suggestions for improving the manuscript.

References

Anonymous (1931). Mitogenetic rays. *Nature*, **127**, 214.

Avilés, J. M. & Soler, J. J. (2009). Sibling competition and conspicuousness of nestling gapes in altricial birds: a comparative study. *Journal of Evolutionary Biology*, **22**, 376–386.

Arundale, R. B. (1999). An alternative model and ideology of communication for an alternative to politeness theory. *Pragmatics*, **9**, 119–153.

Boncoraglio, G. & Saino, N. (2007). Habitat structure and the evolution of bird song: a meta-analysis of the evidence for the acoustic adaptation hypothesis. *Functional Ecology*, **21**, 134–142.

Bradbury, J. W. & Vehrencamp, S. L. (2011). *Principles of Animal Communication, 2nd edn.* Sunderland, MA: Sinauer Associates.

Bramble, D. M. & Lieberman, D. E. (2004). Endurance running and the evolution of Homo. *Nature*, **432**, 345–352.

Brenowitz, E. A. (1982). The active space of red-winged blackbird song. *Journal of Comparative Physiology*, **147**, 511–522.

Burghardt, G. M. (1970). Defining 'communication'. In J. W. Johnston, Jr, D. G. Moulton & A. Turk, eds., *Communication by Chemical Signals*. New York: Appleton Century-Crofts, pp. 5–18.

Carazo, P. & Font, E. (2010). Putting information back into biological communication. *Journal of Evolutionary Biology*, **23**, 661–669.

Carrier, D. R. (1984). The energetic paradox of human running and hominid evolution. *Current Anthropology*, **25**, 483–495.

Catchpole, C. K. & Slater, P. J. B. (1995). *Bird Song: Biological Themes and Variations*. Cambridge: Cambridge University Press.

Chappuis, C. (1971). Un exemple de l'influence du milieu sur les emissions vocales des oiseaux: revolution de chants en forget equatoriale. *Terre et Vie*, **25**, 183–202.

Cherry, C. (1957). *On Human Communication*. New York: Wiley.

Clutton-Brock, T. H. & Albon, S. D. (1979). The roaring of red deer and the evolution of honest advertisement. *Behaviour*, **69**, 145–170.

Coss, R. G. & Goldthwaite, R. O. (1995). The persistence of old designs for perception. In N. S. Thompson, ed., *Perspectives in Ethology 11: Behavioral Design*. New York: Plenum Press, pp. 83–148.

Coss, R. G. & Owings, D. H. (1985). Restraints on ground squirrel antipredator behavior: adjustments over multiple time scales. In T. D. Johnston & A. T. Pietrewicz, eds., *Issues in the Ecological Study of Learning*. New York: Lawrence Erlbaum Associates, pp. 167–200.

Coss, R. G., McCowan, B. & Ramakrishnan, U. (2007). Threat-related acoustical differences in alarm calls by wild bonnet macaques (*Macaca radiata*) elicited by python and leopard models. *Ethology*, **113**, 352–367.

Daanje, A. (1950). On the locomotary movements of birds, and the intention movements derived from them. *Behaviour*, **3**, 48–98.

Daniels, F. (1935). Photons in chemistry and biology. *Science*, **81**, 523–528.

Davies, N. B. & Halliday, T. R. (1978). Deep croaks and fighting assessment in toads, *Bufo bufo*. *Nature*, **274**, 683–685.

Dawkins, R. & Krebs, J. R. (1978). Animal signals: information or manipulation? In J. R. Krebs & N. B. Davies, eds., *Behavioural Ecology: An Evolutionary Approach*. Oxford, Blackwell: pp. 282–309.

Deacon, T. W. (1997). *Symbolic Species: The Co-evolution of Language and the Brain*. Norton: New York and London.

Donald, M. (1991). *Origins of the Modern Mind: Three Stages in the Evolution of Culture and Cognition*. Cambridge, MA: Harvard University Press.

Ellinger, N. & Hödl, W. (2003). Habitat acoustics of a lowland tropical rainforest. *Bioacoustics*, **13**, 297–321.

Endler, J. E. (1993). Some general comments on the evolution and design of animal communication systems. *Philosophical Transactions of the Royal Society of London B*, **340**, 215–225.

Enquist, M., Arak, A., Ghirlanda, S. & Wachtmeister, C. A. (2002). Spectacular phenomena and limits to rationality in genetic and cultural evolution. *Philosophical Transactions of the Royal Society of London B*, **357**, 1585–1594.

Font, E. & Carazo, P. (2010). Animals in translation: why there is meaning (but probably no message) in animal communication. *Animal Behaviour*, **80**, e1–e6.

Fromkin, V., Rodman, R., Hyams, N. (2011). *An Introduction to Language*, 9th edn. Boston, MA: Wadsworth Cengage Learning.

Geary, J. (2011). *I is An Other: The Secret Life of Metaphor and How It Shapes the Way We See the World*. New York: Harper Collins.

Gibson, J. J. (1966). *The Senses Considered as Perceptual Systems*. Boston, MA: Houghton Mifflin.

Gil, D. & Gahr, M. (2002). The honesty of bird song: multiple constraints for multiple traits. *Trends in Ecology and Evolution*, **17**, 133–141.

Gish, S. & Morton, E. S. (1981). Structural adaptations to local habitat acoustics in Carolina wren songs. *Zeitschrift für Tierpsychologie*, **56**, 74–84.

Gleick, J. (2011). *The Information*. New York: Pantheon Books.

Guilford, T. & Dawkins, M. S. (1991). Receiver psychology and the evolution of animal signals. *Animal Behaviour*, **42**, 1–14.

Gurwitsch, A. A. (1988). A historical review of the problem of mitogenetic radiation. *Experientia*, **44**, 545.

Hansen, P. (1979). Vocal learning: its role in adapting song structures to long distance propagation, and a hypothesis on its evolution. *Animal Behaviour*, **27**, 1270–1271.

Hauser, M. D. (1996). *The Evolution of Communication*. Cambridge, MA: MIT Press.

Hennessy, D. F. (1980). Mobbing ecology: a 'threat' management model. Unpublished paper presented at the *Annual Meeting of the Animal Behavior Society*.

Hennessy, D. F., Owings, D. H., Rowe, M. P., Coss, R. G. & Leger, D. W. (1981). The information afforded by a variable signal: constraints on snake-elicited tail flagging by California ground squirrels. *Behaviour*, **78**, 188–226.

Holzer, B., Jacat, A. & Brinkoff, M. W. G. (2003). Condition-dependent signaling affects male sexual attractiveness in field crickets, *Gryllus campestris*. *Behavioral Ecology*, **14**, 353–359.

Hunter, M. L. & Krebs, J. R. (1979). Geographical variation in the song of the great tit (*Parus major*) in relation to ecological factors. *Journal of Animal Ecology*, **48**, 759–785.

Lakatos, I. (1970). Falsificationism and the methodology of scientific research programmes. In I. Lakatos & A. Musgrave, eds., *Criticism and the Growth of Knowledge*. Cambridge: Cambridge University Press, pp. 91–196.

Larson, S. G. (2009). Evolution of the hominid shoulder: Early Homo. *Vertebrate Paleobiology and Paleoanthropology*, **3**, 65–75.

López, P. & Martín, J. (2011). Male Iberian rock lizards may reduce the costs of fighting by scent matching of the resource holders. *Behavioral Ecology and Sociobiology*, **65**, 1891–1898.

Markl, H. (1983). Vibrational communication. In R. Huber & H. Markl, eds., *Neuroethology and Behavioral Physiology*. Berlin, Heidelberg, New York: Springer, pp. 332–353.

Marler, P. (1955). Characteristics of some animal calls. *Nature*, **176**, 6–8.

Marler, P. (1961). The logical analysis of animal communication. *Journal of Theoretical Biology*, **1**, 295–317.

Marler, P., Karakashian, S. & Gyger, M. (1991). Do animals have the option of withholding signals when communication is inappropriate? The audience effect. In C. A. Ristau, ed., *Cognitive Ethology: The Minds of Other Animals (Essays in Honor of Donald R. Griffin)*. Hillsdale, NJ: Lawrence Erlbaum Associates, pp. 243–273.

Marten, K. & Marler, P. (1977a). Sound transmission and its significance for animal vocalization. I. Temperate habitats. *Behavioral Ecology and Sociobiology*, **2**, 271–290.

Marten, K. & Marler, P. (1977b). Sound transmission and its significance for animal vocalization. II. Tropical forest habitats. *Behavioral Ecology and Sociobiology*, **2**, 291–302.

Maynard Smith, J. (1979). Game theory and the evolution of animal behavior. *Proceedings of the Royal Society of London Series: Biological Sciences*, **205**, 475–478.

Maynard Smith, J. & Harper, D. (2003). *Animal Signals*. Oxford: Oxford University Press.

Mayr, E. (1988). *Toward a New Philosophy of Biology: Observations of an Evolutionist*. Cambridge, MA: Harvard University Press.

Michelsen, A. (1978). Sound reception in different environments. In M. A. Ali, ed., *Sensory Ecology*. New York: Plenum Press, pp. 345–353.

Morton, E. S. (1975). Ecological sources of selection on avian sounds. *American Naturalist*, **109**, 17–34.

Morton, E. S. (1977). On the occurrence and significance of motivation-structural rules in some bird and mammal sounds. *American Naturalist*, **111**, 855–869.

Morton, E. S. (1986). Predictions from the ranging hypothesis for the evolution of long distance signals in birds. *Behaviour*, **99**, 65–86.

Morton, E. S. (1994). Sound symbolism and its role in non-human vertebrate communication. In L. Hinton, J. Ohala & J. Nichols, eds., *Sound Symbolism and Human Speech*. Cambridge: Cambridge University Press, pp. 348–365.

Morton, E. S. (1996). Why songbirds learn songs: an arms race over ranging? *Poultry and Avian Biology Reviews*, **7**, 65–71.

Morton, E. S. (2000). An evolutionary view of the origins and functions of avian vocal communication. *Japanese Journal of Ornithology*, **49**, 69–78.

Morton, E. S. (2012). Putting distance back into bird song with mirror neurons. *The Auk*, **129**, 1–5.

Morton, E. S. & Derrickson, K. C. (1996). Song ranging by the dusky antbird (*Cercomacra tyrannina*): ranging without song learning. *Behavioral Ecology and Sociobiology*, **39**, 195–201.

Moynihan, M. (1955). Remarks on the original sources of displays. *The Auk*, **72**, 240–246.

Nemeth, E., Winkler, H. & Dabelsteen, T. (2001). Differential degradation of antbird songs in a Neotropical rainforest: adaptation to perch height? *Journal of the Acoustical Society of America*, **110**, 3263–3274.

Nicholls, J. A. & Goldizen, A. W. (2006). Habitat type and density influence vocal signal design in satin bowerbirds. *Journal of Animal Ecology*, **75**, 549–558.

Overton, W. F. & Reese, H. W. (1981). Conceptual prerequisites for an understanding of stability–change and continuity–discontinuity. *International Journal of Behavioral Development*, **4**, 99–123.

Owings, D. & Hennessy, D. (1984). The importance of variation in sciurid visual and vocal communication. In J. O. Murie & G. R. Michener, eds., *Biology of Ground-dwelling Squirrels: Annual Cycles, Behavioral Ecology, and Sociality*. Lincoln, NE: University of Nebraska Press, pp. 322–347.

Owings, D. H. & Morton, E. S. (1997). The role of information in communication: an assessment/management approach. In D. H. Owings, M. D. Beecher & N. S. Thompson, eds., *Communication. Perspectives in Ethology*, Vol. 12. New York: Plenum Press, pp. 359–390.

Owings, D. H. & Morton, E. S. (1998). *Animal Vocal Communication: A New Approach*. Cambridge: Cambridge University Press.

Owren, M. J. & Rendall, D. (1997). An affect-conditioning model of non-human primate vocal signaling. In D. H. Owings, M. D. Beecher, & N. S. Thompson, eds., *Communication. Perspectives in Ethology*, Vol. 12. New York: Plenum Press, pp. 299–346.

Owren, M. J. & Rendall, D. (2001). Sound on the rebound: bringing form and function back to the forefront in understanding non-human primate vocal signaling. *Evolutionary Anthropology*, **10**, 58–71.

Parrish, J. K., Viscido, S. V. & Grünbaum, D. (2002). Self-organized fish schools: an examination of emergent properties. *Biological Bulletin*, **202**, 296–305.

Patricelli, G. L., Coleman, S. W. & Borgia, G. (2006). Male satin bowerbirds, *Ptilonorhynchus violaceous*, adjust their display intensity in response to female startling: an experiment with robotic females. *Animal Behaviour*, **71**, 49–59.

Pepper, S. C. (1942). *World Hypotheses: A Study in Evidence*. Berkeley, CA: University of California Press.

Pinker, S. & Bloom, P. (1990). Natural language and natural selection. *Brain and Behavioral Sciences*, **13**, 707–784.

Platt, J. R. (1964). Strong inference. *Science*, **146**, 347–353.

Powers, W. T. (1973). Feedback: beyond behaviorism. *Science*, **179**, 351–356.

Prum, R. O. (2010). The Lande–Kirkpatrick mechanism is the null model of evolution by intersexual selection: implications for meaning, honesty, and design in intersexual signals. *Evolution*, **64**, 3085–3100.

Rendall, D., Owren, M. J. & Ryan, M. J. (2009). What do animal signals mean? *Animal Behaviour*, **78**, 233–240.

Rundus, A. S., Owings, D. H., Joshi, S. S., Chinn, E. & Giannini, N. (2009). Ground squirrels use an infrared signal to deter rattlesnake predation. *Proceedings of the National Academy of Sciences USA*, **104**, 14372–14376.

Rowe, M. P. & Owings, D. H. (1990). Probing, assessment, and management during interactions between ground squirrels and rattlesnakes. Part 1: Risks related to rattlesnake size and body temperature. *Ethology*, **86**, 237–249.

Rowe, M. P. & Owings, D. H. (1996). Probing, assessment, and management during interactions between ground squirrels (Rodentia: Sciuridae) and rattlesnakes (Squamata: Viperidae). Part 2: Cues afforded by rattlesnake rattling. *Ethology*, **102**, 856–874.

Ryan, M. J. & Rand, A. S. (1990). The sensory basis of sexual selection for complex calls in the Tungara frog, *Physalaemus pustulosus* (sexual selection for sensory exploitation). *Evolution*, **44**, 305–314.

Ryan, M. J., Fox, J. H., Wilczynski, W. & Rand, A. S. (1990). Sexual selection for sensory exploitation in the frog *Physalaemus pustulosus*. *Nature*, **343**, 66–67.

Scherer, K. R. (1985). Vocal affect signaling: a comparative approach. In J. S. Rosenblatt, C. Beer, M.-C. Busnel & P. J. B. Slater, eds., *Advances in the Study of Behavior*, Vol. 15. New York: Academic Press, pp. 189–244.

Scott-Phillips, T. C. (2010). Animal communication: insights from linguistic pragmatics. *Animal Behaviour*, **79**, e1–e4.

Searcy, W. A. & Nowicki, S. (2005). *The Evolution of Animal Communication: Reliability and Deception in Signaling Systems*. Princeton, NJ: Princeton University Press.

Seddon, N. (2005). Ecological adaptation and species recognition drives vocal evolution in neotropical suboscine birds. *Evolution*, **59**, 200–215.

Seyfarth, R. M., Cheney, D. L., Bergman, T., Fischer, J. & Zuberbühler, K. (2010). The central importance of information in studies of animal communication. *Animal Behaviour*, **80**, 3–8.

Shannon, C. E. & Weaver, W. (1949). *The Mathematical Theory of Communication*. Urbana, IL: University of Illinois Press.

Slabbekoorn, H. & Smith, T. B. (2002). Habitat-dependent song divergence in the little greenbul: an analysis of environmental selection pressures on acoustic signals. *Evolution*, **56**, 1849–1858.

Smith, W. J. (1977). *The Behavior of Communicating: An Ethological Approach*. Cambridge, MA: Harvard University Press.

Stegmann, U. E. (2005). John Maynard Smith's notion of animal signals. *Biology and Philosophy*, **20**, 1011–1025.

Thuppil, V. & Coss, R. G. (2012). Mitigation of human–elephant conflict in India. *International Journal of Wildlife Law and Policy*, **15**, 167–185.

Tinbergen, N. (1952). 'Derived' activities, their causation, biological significance, origin and emancipation. *Quarterly Review of Biology*, **27**, 1–32.

Tobias, J. A., Aben, J., Brumfield, R. T. *et al.* (2010). Song divergence by sensory drive in Amazonian birds. *Evolution*, doi:10.1111/j.1558-5646.2010.01067.x.

Tubaro, P. L. & Lijtmaer, D. A. (2006). Environmental correlates of song structure in forest grosbeaks and saltators. *Condor*, **108**, 120–129.

VanWijk, R. (2001). Bio-photons and bio-communication. *Journal of Scientific Exploration*, **15**, 183–197.

Vehrencamp, S. L. (2000). Handicap, index, and conventional signal elements of bird song. In Y. Espmark, T. Amundsen & G. Rosenqvist, eds., *Animal Signals: Signalling and Signal Design in Animal Communication*. Trondheim: Tapir Academic Press, pp. 277–300.

Wagner, R. H. & Danchin, E. (2010). A taxonomy of biological information. *Oikos*, **119**, 203–209.

Waser, P. M. & Brown, C. H. (1984). Is there a 'sound window' for primate communication? *Behavioral Ecology and Sociobiology*, **15**, 73–75.

Weber, B. & Deacon, T. (2000). Thermodynamic cycles, developmental systems, and emergence. *Cybernetics and Human Knowing*, **7**, 1–23.

Wiley, R. H. & Richards, D. G. (1978). Physical constraints on acoustic communication in the atmosphere: implications for the evolution of animal vocalizations. *Behavioral Ecology and Sociobiology*, **3**, 69–94.

Wiley, R. H. & Richards, D. G. (1982). Adaptations for acoustic communication in birds: sound transmission and signal detection. In D. E. Kroodsma & E. H. Miller, eds., *Acoustic Communication in Birds*, Vol. 1. New York: Academic Press, pp. 132–182.

Zuberbühler, K., Jenny, D. & Bshary, R. (1999). The predator deterrence function of primate alarm calls. *Ethology*, **105**, 477–490.

Commentaries

A conclusion that "the process of perceiving signals produces information" exemplifies the position that information depends on the state of the receiver. As explained in my chapter, the alternative position ascribes information to the associations of signals. In the latter case, there is no question that the receiver has a substantial role in the *decoding* of information, but it has no role in the *encoding* of information. Any potential receiver responds to signals in accordance with its particular internal state and context, so the decoding of signals, the association of signals with responses, depends entirely on the receiver. The encoding of signals, the association of signals with the internal state or context of the signaller, depends entirely on the signaller. The *transmission* of information requires both encoding by a signaller and decoding by a receiver.

R. Haven Wiley

According to Morton and Coss (MC), it is wrong to infer that "there must be information in the signal" simply because "individuals that perceive . . . signals extract information from them". On their view, there is no such thing as information transmitted by signals. Thinking otherwise leads to placing "the sender in control of the evolution of communication because its transmitted information causes things". This reveals that MC are in the throes of the encoding–decoding model of information, which I have also rejected. But there is an alternative, perfectly respectable notion of information – predictive information – that puts the recipient in control of what information signals carry. See my commentary to Rendall and Owren for further discussion.

Andrea Scarantino

Viewing assessment as extracting natural information echoes Millikan's chapter in providing the very conceptual cashing out that mitogenic rays lacked. Form/function analysis has in fact thrived under the information approach, both in bird song (cf. Botero & de Kort, Ch. 11 of this volume) and nestling begging (Kilner & Hinde, 2008). Particularly for nestling begging, struggling with the concept of reliable information transfer has forced researchers to articulate what that information is, and what selective factors maintain it, even though we are all still arguing vehemently – and productively – over both issues (e.g. Mock, Dugas & Strickler, 2011).

Kilner, R. M. & Hinde, C. A. (2008). Information warfare and parent–offspring conflict. *Advances in the Study of Behavior*, **38**, 283–336.

Mock, D. W., Dugas, M. B. & Strickler, S. A. (2011). Honest begging: expanding from Signal of Need. *Behavioral Ecology*, **22**, 909–917.

Andrew G. Horn and Peter McGregor

Response

How clever of **Horn and McGregor** to ferret out the source of our example, information transmitted by begging nestlings, of how *not* to use information! Is begging a signal of need, of quality or of hunger? To remind you of the example:

> When we ask why gaping is performed we are interested in the information borne by this display and how the interests of sender and receiver are affected." We would ask: "Affected by what, the information?" We would answer: "No, it's the signal itself, its physical form and how its form relates to its function. You are *not* interested in the information but in the accomplishment of the communication.

We disagree with Horn and McGregor because we feel the 'debate' they point to progresses on an irresolvable course because of its focus on a search for honesty in transmitted information. Transmitted information is the issue at the centre of the controversy. The debate is founded upon the Procrustean assumption that information is transmitted and must be encoded and decoded.

We wonder why protagonists of Shannon's measure of information still weigh so heavily in animal communication (cf. Rendall & Owren, Ch. 6 of this volume). While we agree with **Wiley** that the process of perceiving produces information, we do not agree that it is worthwhile to continue with the concept of reliable information transfer, nor do we agree with his stance, based upon Shannon's information theory, that information is encoded and decoded. This is a concept of information stripped of its links to reference, meaning and significance, ignoring the representational aspect of information (Deacon, 2012, p. 372). Vigo (2011) sees Shannon information, its axioms of probability theory, as preventing the measure from capturing the impact that *context* has on events, and potentiates the subjective nature of probability judgements by human observers. Furthermore, the theory is formulated in terms of event uncertainty (and expectancy) and not in terms of the relational information that is present with certainty in a set of objects. Even Shannon (as cited in Luce, 2003) doubted that his information theory should be applied to fields outside of mathematical communication theory.

We agree with **Scarantino's** emphasis on the perceiver's strong role in 'extracting information', but we do not see a need to invoke the presence of information in the signal itself by virtue of what a potential recipient can predict upon receiving it. Instead, we prefer to focus on the natural history of communication by animals in the field. Only here can the non-arbitrary physical form (or pattern of delivery; cf. Botero & de Kort, Ch. 11 of this volume) of signals be couched in terms of selection based on accomplishment, i.e. the balance sheet of positive and negative selection on managers and assessors.

This balance brings to mind how the natural history of organisms affects their communication. Consider the talent of being a first-rate empirical theorist, using observation and experiment to produce understanding. You must know the natural history of your subject and be conceptually and constantly aware of the logic of natural selection. Starting here, you gather your observations to determine how your living subjects reflect homologous or convergent evolution, and how they are balancing constraints and contradictory sources of natural and sexual selection on traits, some of which are ancestral and often exapted for new functions, and some more recent (cf. Ryan, Ch. 9 of this volume). To be a first-rate empirical theorist takes a lifetime of devotion to learning to be observant, and a great amount of experience with fieldwork. As we mentioned in our chapter, this naturalist view is at odds with the notion that the analysis of behaviour can be achieved purely by the application of game theory (cf. Enquist *et al.*, 2002). The evolution of communication is out of equilibrium – it is an arms race – and so needs a revamping of concepts used to understand it (Owings & Morton, 1998).

Our hope is that those beginning a career in animal communication will realise that there are better ways to skin a cat, and, specifically, we feel the management and assessment view of communication is such a way. It describes the proximate and evolutionary interplay among communicants by incorporating insights from biology and by downplaying linguistics-based and game theoretic attempts at understanding it. One take-home message is that the perceiver's foundational role in animal communication should be elevated. This role will become clearly defined when the concept of transmitted information disappears.

Deacon, T. W. (2012). *Incomplete Nature: How Mind Emerged from Matter*. New York and London: W. W. Norton.

Enquist, M., Arak, A., Ghirlanda, S. & Wachtmeister, C. A. (2002). Spectacular phenomena and limits to rationality in genetic and cultural evolution. *Philosophical Transactions of the Royal Society of London B*, **357**, 1585–1594.

Luce, R. D. (2003). Whatever happened to information theory in psychology? *Review of General Psychology*, **7**, 183–188.

Owings, D. H. & Morton, E. S. (1998). *Animal Vocal Communication: A New Approach*. Cambridge: Cambridge University Press.

Vigo, R. (2011). Representational information: a new general notion and measure of information. *Information Sciences*, **181**, 4847–4859.

Eugene S. Morton and Richard G. Coss

9

The importance of integrative biology to sexual selection and communication

MICHAEL J. RYAN

9.1 Introduction

I am writing this adjacent to a tropical forest in Panama where I have worked for several decades. I continue to be struck by the number and diversity of organisms here, and how well they function in the world around them. How did all this happen? In this chapter I will focus this general question on the more specific topic of the evolution and mechanisms of sexual communication, and I will draw heavily on my own work and that of my colleagues on one of the inhabitants of this forest.

9.1.1 *A nocturnal serenade*

One of the animals in this forest of which I am most fond is the túngara frog (*Physalaemus = Engystomops pustulosus*). Like many animals with lek-like mating systems, male túngara frogs gather at breeding sites where they sexually advertise for females. Their call consists of a long frequency-modulated whine followed by up to seven short bursts of sound called chucks (Figure 9.1A). All males add chucks when they are in choruses and escalate chuck number during vocal competition. Females visit these sites and choose mates. Females prefer calls with chucks, so males that add chucks gain a benefit through sexual selection because they are more likely to mate. Frog-eating bats use the frog's call to locate their anuran prey, and the bats also prefer calls with chucks; thus the males incur a cost through natural selection when adding chucks to their calls. In addition, females are more likely to choose larger males as mates. Thus

Animal Communication Theory: Information and Influence, ed. Ulrich Stegmann. Published by Cambridge University Press.

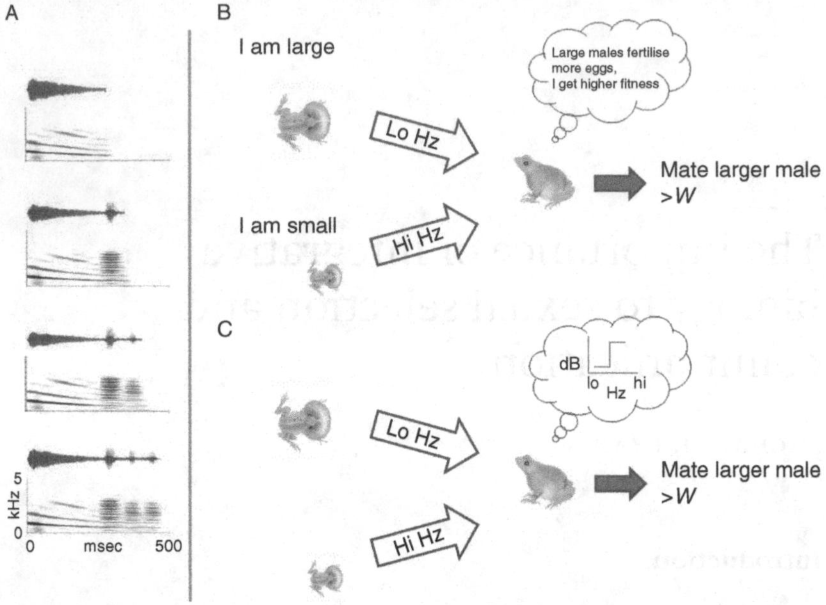

Figure 9.1 A, Waveforms (top of each call) and sonograms (bottom of each call) of mating calls of the túngara frog. From top to bottom a whine followed by 0, 1, 2 and 3 chucks is illustrated. B, C, Two narratives describing sexual selection in túngara frogs. > *W* refers to an increase in fitness.

larger males gain an additional fitness advantage via sexual selection. Larger males fertilise more of a female's eggs than do smaller males. Thus female choice of larger males accrues a fitness advantage to the females due to natural selection. These are the facts (Ryan, 1985, 2010). We can entertain two narratives of the underlying processes (Figure 9.1B, C).

Narrative one: Males *encode* information about their body size in the chuck's frequency; larger males have lower-frequency chucks. *Information* about male body size is transmitted to the female. The females *decode* this information in order to choose males that fertilise more eggs. In the past, selection has favoured the females who *decided* to mate with larger males since these males fertilise more eggs and these females experience greater reproductive success. Of course, for female choice to evolve there must be heritable variation in their mating decisions (Figure 9.1B).

Narrative two: For many animals, the frequency of a vocalisation is *correlated* with the size of the vibrating membrane that produces it. Larger males have larger larynges and thus lower-frequency chucks. In frogs, the *sensory organs* in the inner ear used in hearing are tuned to the frequency characteristics of the call. In túngara frogs, the low-frequency chucks of larger males *better match* the female's tuning than the higher-frequency chucks of smaller males. As larger males fertilise more eggs, selection favouring females to mate with larger males would cause females to evolve auditory tuning that would guide them towards lower-frequency calls. Of course, for female choice to evolve there must be heritable variation in auditory tuning (Figure 9.1C).

It is not unusual for science to adopt different narratives to explain the same phenomenon. In the visual sciences we discuss light as a wave to understand how it travels through the environment but as a particle to describe its interaction with photoreceptors (Bradbury & Vehrencamp, 2011). The first narrative about sexual selection in túngara frogs emphasises how information is encoded and decoded. The second emphasises how the structure and influence of signals are tied to morphology and sensory biology. One might consider these two interpretations as deriving from different levels of analysis: Narrative 1 is the ultimate explanation and Narrative 2 the proximate explanation. They both, however, offer an explanation of the specific mechanisms used in the communication system. One might then consider these two explanations functionally equivalent, that Narrative 1 might be a metaphor for the specific mechanisms outlined in Narrative 2.

I would disagree that these are equally accurate descriptions of the same phenomenon. Consider, for example, the fact that larger males have lower-frequency calls. Narrative 1 posits that males encode information about body size in their calls. In this case, 'encode' does not really refer to something that males do, but instead is a metaphor for a biophysical principle, in the same sense that the amplitude of the sound a rock produces when we drop it on the pavement 'encodes' information about the rock's size.

Narrative 2 specifies the relationship between size and frequency directly, and views it as a simple biophysical phenomenon that is generally applicable and not specific to the problem of communication. The fact that frequency is related to body size does not, of course, preclude its independent evolution.

Of the two narratives, the first might offer the more intuitive and generally appealing explanation, and would probably be more effective in communicating to students the scenario of sexual selection. But as Kennedy (1992) has emphasised, introducing metaphors into evolutionary explanations merely for the sake of convenient communication can be quite successful in capturing the imagination, but it carries the risk of obscuring the real biology of the phenomenon and can unintentionally promote a teleological view of evolution. This seems to be a real danger in studies of animal communication.

In addition to the use of metaphor, another issue in animal communication that requires some attention is the extrapolation from the present to the past, especially the far past. Each of the narratives above suggests how female preferences for chucks and lower-frequency chucks have evolved. The data, however, address the question of current maintenance and not necessarily past evolution. As I argue that sensory biology should be an important component of animal communication studies, so should phylogenetic comparisons. There are several ways to gain insights into the past; given the usual absence of fossils, comparative studies are among the more useful. When applied to the túngara frog system they lead to a not so obvious conclusion.

Anurans have two inner-ear organs that are sensitive to air-borne vibrations (Capranica, 1977; Wilczynski & Ryan, 2010). The amphibian papilla (AP) is more sensitive to lower-frequency sounds, <1500 Hz, and the basilar papilla (BP) is more sensitive to higher-frequency sounds, >1500 Hz. The tuning of the two end organs matches the distribution of spectral energy in the call. In some species only one of the inner-ear organs is recruited for communication, while in others, including túngara frogs, both sensory channels are used (Gerhardt & Schwartz, 2001). A combination of neurophysiological and behavioural studies of túngara frogs show that in the auditory periphery the whine is processed primarily by the AP and the chuck by the BP (Figure 9.1A), and the BP is more sensitive to the lower-frequency chucks of larger males than the higher-frequency chucks of smaller males (Ryan *et al.*, 1990; Wilczynski, Rand & Ryan, 1995). These data, combined with Narrative 2, would suggest that females evolved BP tuning to match the spectral characteristics of the chuck because of the advantage of mating with larger males. Comparative studies allow us to evaluate this hypothesis.

Most close relatives of *P. pustulosus* do not produce complex calls. They all have whines whose dominant frequencies match the tuning of their AP (Wilczynski, Rand & Ryan, 2001). Wilczynski *et al.* (2001) showed that among *P. pustulosus* and seven close relatives there is substantial variation in the tuning of the AP among species. But except for one species, *P. pustulatus*, the tuning of the BPs are almost identical. This suggests that BP tuning is a characteristic of a common ancestor that existed long before the chuck evolved, and there has been little evolution since. These results suggest that the chuck evolved to match the preexisting tuning of the female's BP rather than female tuning evolving to match this call component. Of course, frogs have brains, and we know a considerable amount as to how the signals that stimulate these two end organs are integrated in the túngara frog's central nervous system and interact to result in enhanced stimulation in the frog's main auditory nucleus (Hoke, 2004) and also to stimulate neural networks that are important in decision-making (Hoke, Ryan & Wilczynski, 2007). Some closely related frogs that lack chucks show a preference for their own calls with chucks (Ryan & Rand, 1993) while others do not (Tárano & Ryan, 2002; Ron, 2008). Thus stimulation of the BP seems to play an important part in the evolution of complex calls in the túngara frogs, but there seem to have been concomitant changes in the brain as well.

The details of how this one species of frog hears might seem idiosyncratic if not downright tedious. But the purpose of this chapter is to argue for an integrative approach to studying animal communication, and it is true that the devil is in the detail. In addition to knowledge of current fitness effects, we also need to address a broader understanding of where signals and responses to signals come from, and how the past evolutionary history and the animal's biology in other domains all have an important influence on how animals communicate. Integrative approaches in animal behaviour are becoming quite common (reviewed in Ryan & Wilczynski, 2011), and this has been a most fruitful approach in studies of animal communication (e.g. Gerhardt & Huber, 2002; Greenfield, 2002).

9.2 Sexual selection and aesthetic traits

9.2.1 *Darwinian aesthetics*

We are surrounded by beauty in the animal kingdom. Few can deny how spectacular are the serenades of nightingales, the bountiful colours of coral reef fishes and the flashing of fireflies across an open field. All of these traits have been fashioned by sexual selection. For many of us the assortment of avian plumages that have evolved for sexual signalling as a result of sexual selection is at least as awe-inspiring as the cunning fit of the beaks of Galapagos finches to their feeding ecology which has resulted from natural selection (Figure 9.2). Beauty is in the eyes, ears and nares of the beholder. The fact that we, as humans, find beauty in many of the same sexual traits that evolved because they were attractive to other animals might suggest some generalities in the appreciation of beauty.

The development of Darwin's theory of sexual selection has been well chronicled, especially by Cronin (1991; see also West-Eberhard, 1979). But I think there is something missing in those scenarios. Darwin offered this theory of sexual selection, first in *On the Origin of Species* (1859) and more fully developed in *The Descent of Man and Selection in Relation to Sex* (1871), as an addendum to his theory of natural selection. Natural selection, Darwin thought, was lacking in its ability to explain the evolution of one particular class of traits. These traits shared some commonalities: they were usually sexually dimorphic, often more elaborate in males than females; they were involved in reproduction, either as weapons or sexual signals; and they seemed to be maladaptive relative to survival. These traits were favoured by sexual selection, not because they

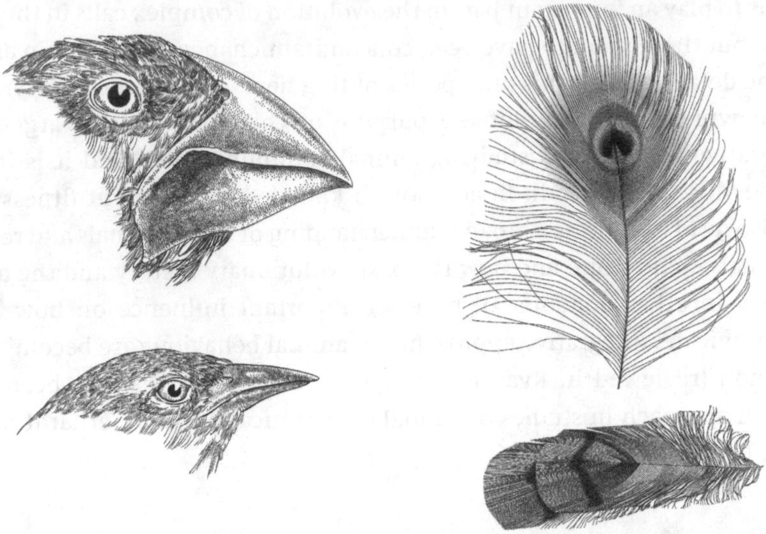

Figure 9.2 The beaks of two species of Galapagos finches that have evolved by natural selection, and two samples of bird feathers that have evolved under sexual selection. Redrawn from Ryan (2001) with permission from *Nature*.

promoted survival but because they promoted mating. Ryan and Keddy-Hector (1992) and Andersson (1994) gave hundreds of examples in which females prefer males with more elaborate traits, such as higher-amplitude calls, greater size, more intense colour, longer tails.

As elaborate sexual signals are more common in males than in females, Darwin phrased his arguments for sexual selection in terms of males competing for female mating partners. This generality seems to hold, although we now know that males and females can fill the opposite roles in different mating systems and that the two sexes can choose and compete with one another simultaneously (Arnqvist & Rowe, 2005; Clutton-Brock, 2007; Gowaty & Hubbell, 2009). Here, I am concerned with sexually selected traits that evolved as communication signals. Thus I will speak more generally of senders and receivers with the understanding that each sex can fill each role and need not be restricted to only one role.

The notion that weapons could evolve under sexual selection was not an issue with Darwin's contemporaries (Cronin, 1991). The problem was in understanding the evolution of the elaborate sexual signals. Darwin stated that females were more attracted to males with elaborate sexual traits. Just as Darwin relied on his analogy between artificial selection and natural selection, he made the same point about sexual selection. Artificial selection had been successful in increasing an animal's beauty to the eyes and ears of the human breeder. When one examines the traits that respond to artificial selection for beauty, they are almost always sexual signals: plumage in pigeons, songs in canaries, colours in guppies. The same response to sexual selection occurs in nature, Darwin argued. Mate choice generates selection on these traits, but why do females have these preferences for extreme and sometimes maladaptive traits in males? Darwin's response was that female animals had an aesthetic sense similar to that of the artificial breeder. Furthermore, Darwin argued that the aesthetic senses were grounded in the animal's sensory biology and these aesthetic senses could be shared widely among some species. Perhaps, then, this is why artificial selection for animals to evolve to become more attractive to humans seems to mimic the process of sexual selection that drives the evolution of traits attractive to that species' receiver.

The statement that females have an aesthetic sense seems like a definition and not an explanation of female preferences, and has been interpreted as Darwin's surrender to this thorny question of the origin of preferences (e.g. Cronin, 1991). I would suggest that perhaps that is not the case, and this is where something has gone missing in previous accounts. In *The Expression of the Emotions in Man and Animals* (1872) Darwin stated:

> When male animals utter sounds in order to please the females, they would naturally employ those which are sweet to the ears of the species; and it appears that the same sounds are often pleasing to widely different animals, owing to the similarity of their nervous systems.

Darwin is arguing that there is selection on senders to employ signals that are inherently attractive given the receivers' sensory, neural and cognitive mechanisms that are already in place. Darwin seemed to think that sexual signals were charming, alluring and seductive, and that they evolved to tickle the receiver's sensibilities. In some ways this echoes Marshall McLuhan's (1964) famous dictum that "the medium is the message". This view does not exclude the possibility that signals could have information relevant to female fitness, but the potency of a signal's interaction with the receiver's sensory biology is one component of the evolutionary process that has received less attention than the emphasis on information encoding and decoding of signals.

A similar point is made by Marler (1998; see also Hartshorne, 1956, 1973):

> The [bird] song functions as affective rather than symbolic symbols, and the variety is generated not to diversify meaning, but rather to maintain the interest of anyone who is listening.

There is an interesting congruence between Darwin's insight and the recent emphasis on the role of the receiver's sensory biology in explaining the diversity of sexual signals (Endler & McLellan, 1988; Ryan, 1990, 1998, 2011; Endler & Basolo, 1998; Endler *et al.* 2005; Grether, 2010). These hypotheses are known as latent preferences (Burley, 1986), sensory traps (West-Eberhard, 1979; Christy, 1995), sensory drive (Endler & McLellan, 1988) and sensory exploitation (Ryan, 1990; Ryan *et al.*, 1990). Endler and Basolo (1998) formalise this jargon, and emphasise that a prediction fundamental to all of these hypotheses is that senders are under selection to evolve sexual signals that coincide with latent or preexisting preferences of receivers. This seems to be exactly what Darwin was asserting.

An animal's sensory biology consists of components which receive, detect and perceive a signal, process and analyse the signal, and then make decisions by marshalling different behaviours in response to different signals. Nervous (peripheral end organs and the brain) and cognitive (analysis of and decisions based on perceived stimuli) systems share many similarities across taxa: these systems habituate; they exhibit heightened response to contrast and greater signal:noise ratio; and they often are more stimulated by signals of greater quantity. It should not be surprising, therefore, that across taxa and sensory modalities we seem to know a sexually selected trait when we see, hear or smell one. By not offering specific adaptive hypotheses as to why females have aesthetic preferences, Darwin might not have been throwing in the towel – he might have assumed he had solved the puzzle.

9.3 The evolution of the unexploited receiver

If senders evolve traits to exploit (*to make productive use of*, Merriam Webster Dictionary) a receiver's preexisting preferences, does it necessarily follow that the receiver incurs a fitness loss when they choose such a mate? Although there are a number of cases in which there is such a cost (Arnqvist & Rowe, 2005), there are some fundamental processes of signal reception that suggest there are inherent benefits as well.

Signal elaboration can increase the potency of any signal, endowing it with a larger active space, a longer active time, greater localisability and enhanced contrast with the background. All of these characteristics of signals should reduce search costs by receivers. There are several costs involved with searching, such as energy, time and predation. There is an energetic cost due to longer paths travelled to the source of the signal. Time is lost, and time is at a premium for external fertilisers, such as frogs, who ovulate at the breeding site and will drop their eggs if they do not find a mate. This explains why female túngara frogs become less selective as the night goes on (Lynch *et al.*, 2005). Another search cost is related to predation risk, and this might be the most important one for most animals. As Bonochea and Ryan (2011) point out, the presence of a predator can cause receivers to become less choosy or even reverse their mating preferences (Evans, Bisazza & Pilastro, 2004; Schwartz & Hendry, 2006), to change thresholds of attractiveness for mating (Demary, Michaelidis & Lewis, 2006; Su & Li, 2006; Vélez & Brockman, 2006) and to reduce the time spent searching for (Karino *et al.*, 2000; Kim, Christy & Choe, 2007) and sampling mates (Karino *et al.*, 2000). By matching a sexual signal to the female's sensory, neural and cognitive biases a male might be doing her a favour, increasing rather than decreasing her fitness, by making it easier and less costly for her to find him.

In cases in which sensory exploitation is suggested, it does not seem that females are behaving optimally, preferring the signal that has the greatest positive impact on their reproductive success. This is where it is crucial to remember two things: reproduction is only one component of fitness; and sensory systems can be subject to selection in numerous domains besides reproduction.

Pollinators make productive use of the pollen and nectar of flowers, but this is to the flower's advantage not its disadvantage. In an extreme example, some orchids exploit male bees that are either so sexually aroused or easily duped that they attempt to mate with the flower, pollinating it in the process. In this case the bee gets no reward of pollen or nectar (Darwin, 1890; Schiestl, 2005), but the cost of missed identification (mating with a flower) is lower than the cost of a missed opportunity (passing up a real, live female). The same calculus might explain how female hosts, such as reed warblers, are exploited by cuckoo parasites: shifting their recognition threshold might result in rejecting some of their own offspring (Kilner, Noble & Davies, 1999). The same explanation applies to model-mimicry systems: passing up a palatable butterfly might be a much better Darwinian decision than taking the risk of eating a poisonous one (Bates, 1862; Joron, 2008).

My point is that to understand why receivers respond as they do to a specific signal, we must understand how the mechanisms that generate this type of response influence the receiver's overall fitness, not just the fitness consequences of making a single mating decision. This is where understanding the neural and cognitive mechanisms underlying receiver responses becomes crucial. We can only examine the fitness effects of the receiver's mate choice when it chooses a mate, but by understanding the mechanisms that generate these responses we gain an appreciation of the more varied fitness effects that it entails. This becomes all the more clear when we consider pleiotropic effects of mechanisms involved in mate choice.

9.3.1 *Pleiotropy and domain specificity*

Central to notions of reliability and information in animal communication is the prediction that receivers should respond to signals only if there is on average a fitness advantage to doing so (e.g. Bradbury & Vehrencamp, 2000; Searcy & Nowicki, 2005). It is important to specify 'on average' because every interaction between a sender and a receiver does not result in an increase in fitness.

There is another concept of 'on average' that applies: the fitness effects of this 'response' also need to include the fitness consequences of all the underlying mechanisms that regulate it across all of its domains. This is a point that is lost on most studies of animal communication. Understanding the potential pleiotropic effects of receiver biases can be important to understanding why receivers respond as they do, and why senders evolve particular signals.

Animals see with their eyes, smell with their nares, hear with their ears and feel with their legs. Those are the sensory end organs that initiate processing of communication signals. It is worth remembering that in almost all cases these modalities did not evolve originally for communication. Once these end organs are stimulated, the processing of signals often continues in parts of the brain more or less dedicated to that modality. In the túngara frog, for example, the VIIIth cranial or auditory nerve communicates between the inner-ear organs and the brain. The neural activity in the brainstem is then transformed into sensory–motor interactions in the diencephalon, followed by motor-related activation in the telencephalon. Hearing the conspecific mating call increases correlations of neural activity between many of these anatomically distant brain divisions (Hoke *et al.*, 2007). The female's response to a sexual signal involves all of these aspects of the sensory system. Evolution of the female's preference for a call occurs somewhere in this circuit (Kimchi, Xu & Dulac, 2007; Hoke, Ryan & Wilczynski, 2008). But these circuits are not solely dedicated to sexual communication. The locomotion motor patterns triggered in the mate choice decision, such as movement away from an undesirable call, are also triggered by predators. The auditory system is exquisitely sensitive to conspecific calls, but it is also sensitive to calls of predatory frogs, rustling sounds made by predator movement (Ryan, Bernal & Rand, 2010; Bonachea & Ryan, 2011) and even the sounds of fire moving through savannas (Grafe, Döbler & Linsenmair, 2002). As with most aspects of an animal's phenotype, sensory systems evolve in response to multiple selection pressures, and the responses to selection are biased by its past evolutionary history. Regardless of why these sensory biases exist, they can have current effects on how receivers respond to signals.

Sexual communication brings the sexes together so they can mate. But sexual reproduction also requires coordination of the participants' physiology, and this is often accomplished by the interaction of mating signals and the animal's internal hormonal milieu. In many of the cases that have been documented, the male is the sender and the female is the receiver. Studies of hormones and behaviour have analysed how reproductive synchronisation between the sexes can be achieved through a series of actions in which the behaviour of one member of the pair influences both the partner's behaviour and its own behaviour. The behavioural interactions of the sexes that bring about reproductive synchrony are well known in a variety of animals. In songbirds, the male's song influences follicular development in the female. In rats, tactile stimulation of the female's flank and tail initiates a mating posture, lordosis, and a cascade of responses that eventually synchronises lordosis with ovulation. In addition, dewlap displays in anolis lizard, calling in green treefrogs, and exogenous hormonal steroids in fishes all influence the physiological or behavioural reproductive state of their conspecific partners (reviewed in Adkins-Regan, 2005; Nelson, 2011; Ryan & Wilczynski, 2011).

Interestingly, in most of these examples the signals of males that stimulate the female's reproductive axis are the same signals that are used by females when they choose a mate. In some cases the signal's influences on reproductive physiology and on mate choice are disassociated in time while in others they are nearly simultaneous. The signals are detected by the same sensory end organs, such as ears or eyes, and are then processed in the brain (Figure 9.3C). After sensory processing, however, the information is fed-forward to either a reproductive physiology axis (e.g. hypothalamus → pituitary → gonads and other endocrine glands) or mate choice axis (thalamus → telencephalon → descending to brainstem and spinal cord motor areas → musculoskeletal system), which then subsequently influences reproductive state or mating behaviour, respectively. On the one extreme, the two domains could be mechanistically dissociated. This would be true if they were stimulated by different signals and relied on different sensory channels and brain regions for processing (Figure 9.3A, B). Our review of the limited data available (Ryan & Wilczynski, 2011; see also Adkins-Regan, 2005; Nelson, 2011) suggests that in many vertebrate systems the same signals are used to stimulate both reproductive state and mating behaviour, and that at least early processing of sexual signals is accomplished by the same sensory channels and the same brain regions in both domains (Figure 9.3C). Thus we expect reproductive physiology and mating behaviours to be mechanistically associated to some degree. The evolution of signals and responses in one domain could influence other functions in other domains.

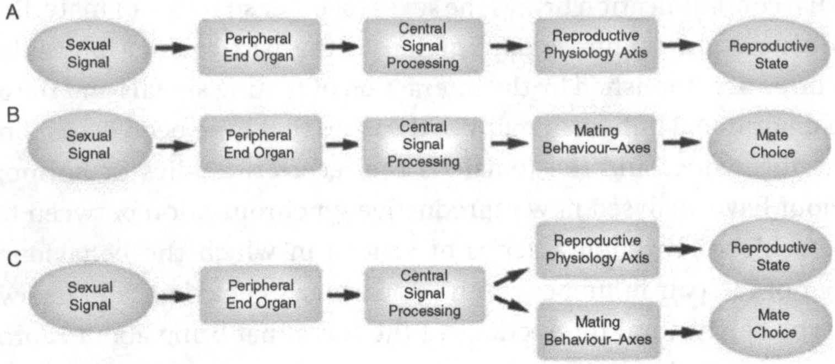

Figure 9.3 A–C, Various ways in which mating signals might influence activation of the reproductive physiology axis and mating behaviour axis.

Just as the need to stimulate the animal's nervous and physiological systems should exert strong selection on signal evolution, ecological selection can also play an important role. Morton (1975; Boncoraglio & Saino, 2007) pioneered the field of evolutionary habitat acoustic by showing how the environment favours the evolution of different acoustic structures, primarily bird song, in different habitats; for example, low frequencies and tones are favoured on the forest floor while high frequencies and high trill rates are more common in open fields (Figure 9.4; Hunter & Krebs, 1979; Wiley, 1991; Slabbekoorn & Smith, 2002; Podos, Huber & Taft, 2004). Senders can also adjust the frequency spectrum of their signals in response to anthropogenic noise (Slabbekoorn & Peet, 2003; Katti & Warren, 2004; Brumm & Slabbekoorn, 2005; Slabbekoorn & den Boer-Visser, 2006). All of these cases show that some primary components of acoustic signals evolve not, or at least not only, because they transmit information but because they enhance the active space of the signal, the area over which the signal can be detected and recognised.

An example of how ecological selection influences both senders and receivers engaged in sexual communication comes from several studies of visual communication in fishes. For example, Cummings (2007) showed that variation in sensitivity of photopigments among species of surf perch in the variable light environment of the Pacific kelp forest evolved in ways that enhance the visual contrast of one of their most common prey. Males, in turn, have evolved signals that match the female's photopigment sensitivity. Similar results have been found in sticklebacks by Boughman (2002) and cichlids by Seehausen, van Alphen & Witte, (1997). In all of these cases the photic environment is thought to influence visual sensitivity, and males, in turn, evolve signals that then match the female's visual sensitivity.

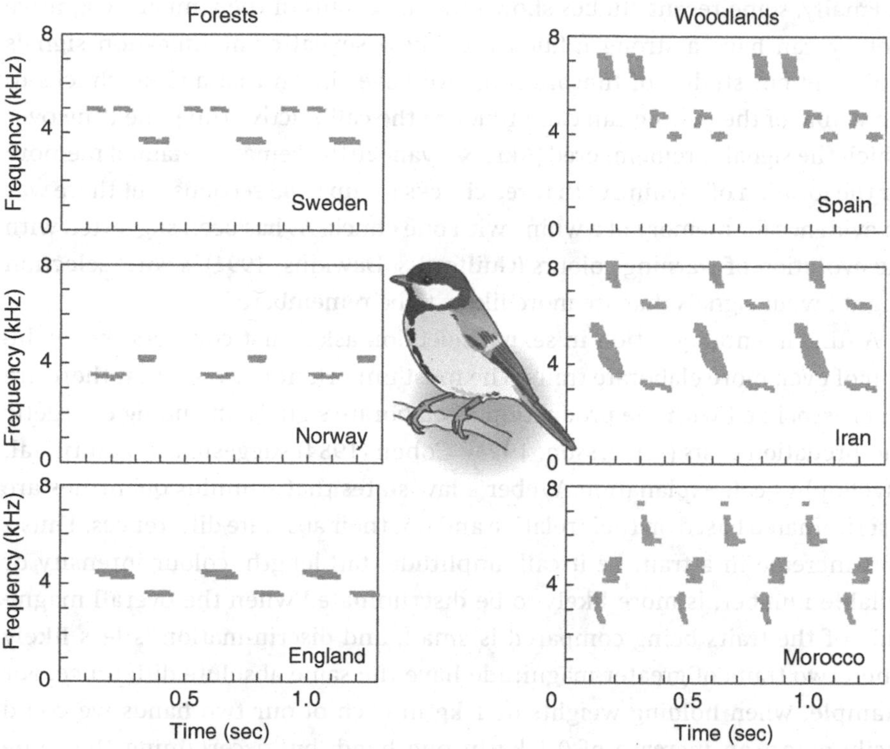

Figure 9.4 Convergence of song structure in great tits within similar habitats. Reprinted from Ryan and Wilczynski (2011) with permission from Cold Spring Harbor Laboratory Press.

A different ecological selection force that influences sexual selection in a fish has been suggested by Rodd *et al.* (2002). Guppies are well known for their extensive orange-pigment pattern variation in nature (Haskins *et al.*, 1961; Endler, 1980) and for female preference for males with more orange. Guppies are attracted to orange fruit in nature. Rodd *et al.* showed that a measure of a female's interest in orange disks, independent of the domains of both foraging and mate choice, was a significant predictor of the strength of her preference for orange coloration in males. The authors concluded that the female's preference for orange evolved in the domain of food preferences, and that males evolved their orange coloration in order to exploit this preference. In this case the evidence for cause and effect is less compelling than in other cases, but this research shows clearly how preferences might be shared across domains. Macias Garcia and Ramirez (2005) also offer convincing evidence that preferences for pigmentation on the caudal fin of some Goodeid fishes came about through the exploitation of female foraging responses.

Finally, some recent studies show how the details of the animal's cognitive biology can have a strong influence on how sexual communication signals evolve. In our studies of túngara frogs we have shown that adding chucks to the whine of the mating call can influence the call's active time, the time over which the signal is remembered (Akre & Ryan, 2010). Females retained memory for the location of a whine with three chucks for up to 45 seconds, but there was no evidence for memory of a whine with one chuck. As has been suggested with the evolution of warning colours (Guilford & Dawkins, 1991), sexual selection might favour signals that are more likely to be remembered.

A fundamental question in sexual selection asks what counters the evolution of even more elaborate traits. The most important reason is that there are costs associated with the production of elaborate signals, including energetic and predation costs (Andersson, 1994). Cohen (1984) suggested an additional, psychophysical, explanation. Weber's law states that stimulus quantities are discriminated based on their relative and not their absolute differences. Thus a unit increase in a trait, be it call amplitude, tail length, colour intensity or syllable number, is more likely to be discriminated when the overall magnitude of the traits being compared is small, and discrimination is less likely when two traits of greater magnitude have the same absolute difference. For example, when holding weights of 1 kg in each of our two hands we could easily detect an increase of 0.1 kg in one hand, but ascertaining the same absolute difference, 0.1 kg, would be less likely if we were holding 10 kg in each hand. We recently showed that the strength of preference for more versus fewer chucks in calls of túngara frogs follows Weber's law (Figure 9.5; Akre *et al.*, 2011). Females are much more likely, for example, to prefer a whine with two chucks versus a whine with one chuck than they are to show a preference between whines with six versus five chucks. Is this pattern of preference an adaptive response to the manner in which male quality scales to male signals? We were able to reject some predictions of this hypothesis. For example, there was no relationship between male relative condition and the number of chucks he produced. But it was impossible to test all possible adaptive hypotheses. To resolve this issue, we tested frog-eating bats with the same set of calls. These bats use the calls to localise male túngara frogs, one of their common prey items. The frogs and the bats use the same signals but for different reasons, a mate versus a meal; female frogs might want good genes but the bats are only concerned with good protein. As do females, the bats prefer calls with more chucks to fewer chucks. Also, the bat's preference for more versus fewer chucks followed a Weber function almost identical to that of the female túngara frogs (Figure 9.5). The most parsimonious interpretation of these data is that both túngara frogs and the bats that eat them perceive

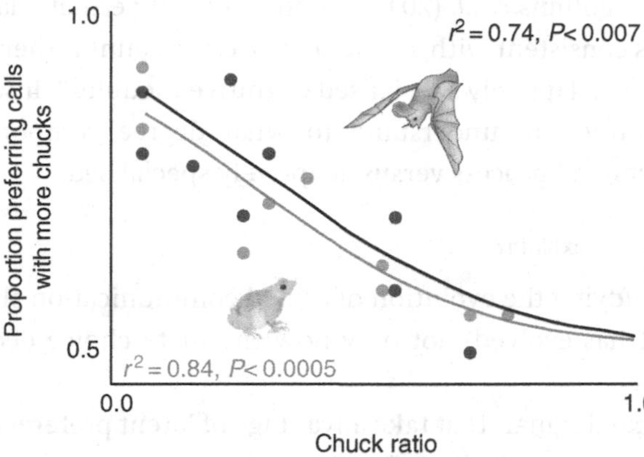

Figure 9.5 Preference for mating calls of túngara frogs that vary in the number of chucks by female frogs and frog-eating bats. The strength of the preference for the call with more chucks is predicted by the ratio in the number of chucks in each of the two stimulus calls being compared by the receiver. Curves are the least-squares fit of the psychometric function (Weber's law). Data are from Akre *et al.* (2011) and used with permission from *Science*.

stimulus quantity in similar ways, and these perceptions of stimulus quantity should influence the dynamics of evolution of complex calls.

This brief summary should make it clear that to understand why signals and receivers evolve one cannot merely focus on how a specific signal influences a specific receiver at a single point in time. As Darwin recognised, survivorship and mating success are two different components of fitness. Sensory systems often function in both of these general domains, and it is not expected that sensory systems can always be optimised for all tasks at hand.

This importance of pleiotropy in animal communication parallels a debate about evolutionary psychology. One of the edifices of evolutionary psychology is massive modularity, which posits that the mind consists of numerous cognitive modules that have evolved to solve different adaptive problems (Cosmides & Tooby, 1992, 1994). An alternative to this extreme domain specificity is the notion that there are domain-general features that influence numerous behaviours involved in different tasks and might be subject to different selection forces. Domain specificity versus domain generality is an empirical question; its resolution probably varies among tasks and taxa, and lies somewhere between the two extremes. Despite the importance that evolutionary psychologists place on massive modularity, Bolhuis *et al.* (2011; see also Bolhuis & Wynne, 2009) suggest that they "... rarely examine whether their hypotheses regarding evolved psychological mechanisms are supported by what is known about how the brain works". Bolhuis *et al.* (2011) go on to conclude that "data from animal experiments is consistent with a general-process account rather than an interpretation involving adaptively specialised cognitive modules". It would be an important contribution to understand to what degree components of receiver systems are general-process versus adaptively specialised.

9.3.2 *What do we want to explain?*

The goal of studying the evolution of sexual communication should be to understand how it has evolved, not only how the mate choice decision is adaptive to the receiver.

The evolution of sexual signals that take advantage of latent preferences does not exclude the subsequent evolution of preferences to ignore a signal if it on average decreases the receiver's fitness, or to favour even greater elaboration of the signal if it enhances the receiver's fitness (Ryan, 1997). Sensory biases do not prohibit receiver responses from evolving, and I have previously discussed how various forces in selection can act on a receiver (Ryan, 1997). Whether receivers prefer signals that indicate greater resource-holding potential, good genes or just being a conspecific, there are taxon-specific and ecological-specific factors that strongly influence signal evolution and the receivers' responses to them. A fish is not likely to use ultrasonic vocalisations to advertise its genetic quality – even if it could make such sounds, the receiver could not hear them. Even if red might indicate the sender's quality because it contains carotenoids, deep sea fish will not evolve such colours because long wavelengths are filtered out by the environment. If female frogs choose males that make energetically more expensive signals, as Welch, Semlitsch and Gerhardt, (1998) have shown, this can explain why these females attend to pulse duration, but it does not address the broader question of why females are attracted to other components of the call, why males make these types of calls and why frogs call instead of advertising with flashing bioluminescence. The point is that the evolution of communication is a larger question than the fitness consequences of mate choice in a single context.

The strength of selection on a receiver will vary depending on the type of benefits they receive. Benefits are often classified into direct or indirect. Direct benefits include those that have an immediate effect on fecundity. Choosing a mate that holds more resources or is a better parent is one type of direct benefit that could favour the evolution of certain response properties. Reducing search costs is another. When considering direct benefits, it is also important to take into account the fitness effects due to pleiotropy. For example, Cummings (2007) argued that a direct benefit of the mate preference of surf perch for certain colour patterns does not derive from the mating partner but from the foraging advantage that drives the evolution of photopigment sensitivity. The adaptive advantage of this 'response', or the underlying physiology that drives it, must be considered over more than one domain. Indirect benefits are those that deliver a genetic advantage to the offspring, and this can be due to passing on 'good genes' that enhance survivorship or result in more attractive mates owing to Fisherian runaway selection. Kirkpatrick and Barton (1997) have shown that, in general, selection for responses that result in direct benefits trumps selection for responses that result in indirect benefits.

Summary

The primary point of this chapter is that gaining a deep and thorough understanding of animal communication requires an integration of behaviour, neurobiology and evolution. Quantifying or theorising about the fitness advantages that occur when a receiver responds to a signal is an important component of this understanding, but only one. Only by studying communication as it is embedded in the environment that affects its signal transmission, how it is moulded by the underlying mechanisms that generate its signals and responses, and the details that influence its evolutionary history will we approach Darwin's notion of the grandeur in this view of life.

References

Adkins-Regan, E. (2005). *Hormones and Animal Social Behavior*. Princeton, NJ: Princeton University Press.

Akre, K. A. & Ryan, M. J. (2010). Complexity increases working memory for mating signals. *Current Biology*, **20**, 502–505.

Akre, K. L., Farris, H. E., Lea, A. M., Page, R. A. & Ryan, M. J. (2011). Signal perception in frogs and bats and the evolution of mating signals. *Science*, **333**, 751–752.

Andersson, M. (1994). *Sexual Selection*. Princeton, NJ: Princeton University Press.

Arnqvist, G. & Rowe, L. (2005). *Sexual Conflict*. Princeton, NJ: Princeton University Press.

Bates, H. W. (1862). Contributions to an insect fauna of the Amazon valley. Lepidoptera: Heliconidae. *Transactions of the Linnean Society of London*, **23**, 495–566.

Bolhuis, J. J. & Wynne, C. D. L. (2009). Can evolution explain how minds work? *Nature*, **458**, 832–833.

Bolhuis, J. J., Brown, G. R., Richardson, R. C. & Laland, K. N. (2011). Darwin in mind: new opportunities for evolutionary psychology. *PLoS Biol*, **9**, e1001109.

Bonachea, L. A. & Ryan, M. J. (2011). Simulated predation risk influences female choice in túngara frogs, *Physalaemus pustulosus*. *Ethology*, **117**, 400–407.

Boncoraglio, G. & Saino, N. (2007). Habitat structure and the evolution of bird song: a meta analysis of the evidence for the acoustic adaptation hypothesis. *Functional Ecology*, **21**, 134–142.

Boughman, J. W. (2002). How sensory drive can promote speciation. *Trends in Ecology and Evolution*, **17**, 571–577.

Bradbury, J. W. & Vehrencamp, S. L. (2011). *Principles of Animal Communication*, 2nd edn. Sunderland, MA: Sinauer Associates, Inc.

Bradbury, J. W. & Vehrencamp, S. L. (2000). Economic models of animal communication. *Animal Behaviour*, **59**, 259–268.

Brumm, H. & Slabbekoorn, H. (2005). Acoustic communication in noise. *Advances in the Study of Behavior*, **35**, 151–209.

Burley, N. (1986). Sexual selection for aesthetic traits in species with biparental care. *American Naturalist*, **127**, 415–445.

Capranica, R. R. (1977). Auditory processing in anurans. *Federation Proceedings*, **37**, 2324–2328.

Christy, J. H. (1995). Mimicry, mate choice, and the sensory trap hypothesis. *American Naturalist*, **146**, 171–181.

Clutton-Brock, T. (2007). Sexual selection in males and females. *Science*, **318**, 1882.

Cohen, J. (1984). Sexual selection and the psychophysics of female choice. *Zeitschrift für Tierpsychologie*, **64**, 1–8.

Cosmides, L. & Tooby, J. (1992). Cognitive adaptations for social exchange. In J. Barkow, L. Cosmides & J. Tooby, eds., *The Adapted Mind: Evolutionary Psychology and the Generation of Culture*. New York: Oxford University Press, pp. 163–228.

Cosmides, L. & Tooby, J. (1994). Origins of domain-specificity: the evolution of functional organization. In L. Hirschfeld & S. Gelman, eds., *Mapping the Mind: Domain-specificity in Cognition and Culture*. New York: Cambridge University Press, pp. 85–116.

Cronin, H. (1991). *The Ant and the Peacock: Altruism and Sexual Selection from Darwin to Today*. Cambridge: Cambridge University Press.

Cummings, M. E. (2007). Sensory trade-offs predict signal divergence in surfperch. *Evolution*, **61**, 530–545.

Darwin, C. (1859). *On the Origin of Species*. London: Murray.

Darwin, C. (1871). *The Descent of Man and Selection in Relation to Sex*. London: Murray.

Darwin, C. (1872). *The Expression of the Emotions in Man and Animals*. London: Murray.

Darwin, C. (1890). *The Various Contrivances by which Orchids are Fertilised by Insects*. London: Murray.

Demary, K., Michaelidis, C. I. & Lewis, S. M. (2006). Fire-fly courtship: behavioral and morphological predictors of male mating success in *Photinus greeni*. *Ethology*, **112**, 485–492.

Endler, J. A. (1980). Natural selection on color patterns in *Poecilia reticulata*. *Evolution*, **31**, 76–91.

Endler, J. A. & Basolo, A. L. (1998). Sensory ecology, receiver biases and sexual selection. *Trends in Ecology and Evolution*, **13**, 415–420.

Endler, J. A. & McLellan, T. (1988). The processes of evolution: towards a newer synthesis. *Annual Review of Ecology and Systematics*, **19**, 395–421.

Endler, J., Westcott, D., Madden, J. & Robson, T. (2005). Animal visual systems and the evolution of color patterns: sensory processing illuminates signal evolution. *Evolution*, **59**, 1795–1818.

Evans, J. P., Bisazza, A. & Pilastro, A. (2004). Female mating preferences for colorful males in a population of guppies subject to high predation. *Journal of Fish Biology*, **65**, 1154–1159.

Gerhardt, H. C. & Huber, F. (2002). *Acoustic Communication in Insects and Anurans*. Chicago, IL: University of Chicago Press.

Gerhardt, H. C. & Schwartz, J. J. (2001). Auditory tunings and frequency preferences in anurans. In M. J. Ryan, ed., *Anuran Communication*. Washington, DC: Smithsonian Institution Press, pp. 73–85.

Gowaty, P. A. & Hubbell, S. P. (2009). Reproductive decisions under ecological constraints: it's about time. *Proceedings of the National Academy of Sciences, USA*, **106**, 10017–10024.

Grafe, T. U., Döbler, S. & Linsenmair, K. E., (2002). Frogs flee from the sound of fire. *Proceedings of the Royal Society of London Series B*, **269**, 999–1003.

Greenfield, M. D. (2002). *Signalers and Receivers, Mechanisms and Evolution of Arthropod Communication*. Oxford: Oxford University Press.

Grether, G. F. (2010). The evolution of mate preferences, sensory biases, and indicator traits. *Advances in the Study of Behavior*, **41**, 35–76.

Guilford, T. & Dawkins, M. (1991). Receiver psychology and the evolution of animal signals. *Animal Behaviour*, **42**, 1–14.

Hartshorne, C. (1956). The monotony-threshold in singing birds. *The Auk*, **73**, 176–192.

Hartshorne, C. (1973). *Born to Sing*. Bloomington, IN: Indiana University Press.

Haskins, C., Haskins, E., McLaughlin, J. & Hewitt, R. (1961). Polymorphism and population structure in *Lebistes reticulatus*, an ecological study. In W. F. Blair, ed., *Vertebrate Speciation*. Austin, TX: University of Texas Press, pp. 320–395.

Hoke, K. L., Burmeister, S. S., Fernald, R. D. *et al.* (2004). Functional mapping of the auditory midbrain during mate call reception. *Journal of Neuroscience*, **24**, 11264–11272.

Hoke, K. L., Ryan, M. J. & Wilczynski, W. (2007). Integration of sensory and motor processing underlying social behaviour in túngara frogs. *Proceedings of the Royal Society of London Series B: Biological Sciences*, **274**, 641–649.

Hoke, K. L., Ryan, M. J. & Wilczynski, W. (2008). Candidate neural locus for sex differences in reproductive decisions. *Biology Letters*, **4**, 518–521.

Hunter, M. L. & Krebs, J. R. (1979). Geographical variation in the song of the great tit (*Parus major*) in relation to ecological factors. *Journal of Animal Ecology*, **48**, 759–785.

Joron, M. (2008). Batesian mimicry: can a leopard change its spots – and get them back? *Current Biology*, **18**, R476–R479.

Karino, K., Kuwamura, T., Nakashima, Y. & Sakai, Y. (2000). Predation risk and the opportunity for mate choice in a coral reef fish. *Journal of Ethology*, **18**, 109–114.

Katti, M. & Warren, P. S. (2004). Tits, noise and urban bioacoustics. *Trends in Ecology and Evolution*, **19**, 109–110.

Kennedy, J. (1992). *The New Anthropomorphism*. Cambridge: Cambridge University Press.

Kilner, R. M., Noble, D. G. & Davies, N. B. (1999). Signals of need in parent–offspring communication and their exploitation by the common cuckoo. *Nature*, **397**, 667–672.

Kim, T. W., Christy, J. H. & Choe, J. C. (2007). A preference for a sexual signal keeps females safe. *PLoS ONE*, **2**, e422.

Kimchi, T., Xu, J. & Dulac, C. (2007). A functional circuit underlying male sexual behaviour in the female mouse brain. *Nature*, **448**, 1009–1014.

Kirkpatrick, M. & Barton, N. (1997). The strength of indirect selection on female mating preferences. *Proceedings of the National Academy of Sciences USA*, **94**, 1282–1286.

Lynch, K. S., Rand, A. S., Ryan, M. J. & Wilczynski, W. (2005). Reproductive state influences female plasticity in mate choice. *Animal Behaviour*, **69**, 689–699.

Macias-Garcia, C. M. & Elvia Ramirez, E. (2005). Evidence that sensory traps can evolve into honest signals. *Nature*, **434**, 501–505.

Marler, P. (1998). Animal communication and human language. *Memoirs of the California Academy of Sciences*, **24**, 1–19.

McLuhan. M. (1964). *Understanding Media: The Extensions of Man*. New York: Mentor.

Morton, E. S. (1975). Ecological sources of selection on avian sounds. *American Naturalist*, **109**, 17–34.

Nelson, R. J. (2011). *An Introduction to Behavioral Endocrinology*. Sunderland, MA: Sinauer Associates.

Podos, J., Huber, S. K. & Taft, B. (2004). Bird song: the interface of evolution and mechanism. *Annual Review of Ecology, Evolution and Systematics*, **35**, 55–87.

Rodd, F. H., Hughes, K. A., Grether, G. F. & Baril, C. T. (2002). A possible non-sexual origin of mate preference: are male guppies mimicking fruit? *Proceedings of the Royal Society of London Series B*, **269**, 475–481.

Ron, S. R. (2008). The evolution of female mate choice for complex calls in túngara frogs. *Animal Behaviour*, **76**, 1783–1794.

Ryan, M. J. (1985). *The Túngara Frog, A Study in Sexual Selection and Communication*. Chicago, IL: University of Chicago Press.

Ryan, M. J. (1990). Sensory systems, sexual selection, and sensory exploitation. *Oxford Surveys in Evolutionary Biology*, **7**, 157–195.

Ryan, M. J. (1997). Sexual selection and mate choice. In J. R. Krebs & N. B. Davies, eds., *Behavioural Ecology, An Evolutionary Approach*. Oxford: Blackwell, pp. 179–202.

Ryan, M. J. (1998). Receiver biases, sexual selection and the evolution of sex differences. *Science*, **281**, 1999–2003.

Ryan, M. J. (2001). Food, song and speciation. *Nature*, **409**, 139–140.

Ryan, M. J. (2010). The túngara frog: a model for sexual selection and communication. In M. D. Breed & J. Moore, eds., *Encyclopedia of Animal Behavior*. Oxford: Academic Press, pp. 453–461.

Ryan, M. J. (2011). The brain as a source of selection on the social niche: examples from the psychophysics of mate choice in túngara frogs. *Integrative and Comparative Biology*, **51**, 756–770.

Ryan, M. J. & Keddy-Hector, A. (1992). Directional patterns of female mate choice and the role of sensory biases. *American Naturalist*, **139**, S4–S35.

Ryan, M. J. & Rand, A. S. (1993). Sexual selection and signal evolution: the ghost of biases past. *Philosophical Transactions of the Royal Society Series B*, **340**, 187–195.

Ryan, M. J. & Wilczynski, W. (2011). *An Introduction to Animal Behavior: An Integrative Approach*. Cold Springs Harbor, New York: Cold Springs Harbor Laboratory Press.

Ryan, M. J., Bernal, X. E. & Rand, A. S. (2010). Female mate choice and the potential for ornament evolution in the túngara frog *Physalaemus pustulosus*. *Current Zoology*, **56**, 343–357.

Ryan, M. J., Fox, J. H., Wilczynski, W. & Rand, A. S. (1990). Sexual selection for sensory exploitation in the frog *Physalaemus pustulosus*. *Nature*, **343**, 66–67.

Schiestl, F. P. (2005). On the success of a swindle: pollination by deception in orchids. *Naturwissenschaften*, **92**, 255–264.

Schwartz, A. K. & Hendry, A. P. (2006). Sexual selection and the detection of ecological speciation. *Evoutionary Ecology Research*, **8**, 399–413.

Searcy, W. & Nowicki, S. (2005). *The Evolution of Animal Communication: Reliability and Deception in Signaling Systems*. Princeton, NJ: Princeton University Press.

Seehausen, O., van Alphen, J. M. & Witte, F. (1997). Cichlid fish diversity threatened by eutrophication that curbs sexual selection. *Science*, **277**, 1808–1811.

Slabbekoorn, H. & den Boer-Visser, A. (2006). Cities change the songs of birds. *Current Biology*, **16**, 2326–2331.

Slabbekoorn, H. & Peet, M. (2003). Birds sing at a higher pitch in urban noise. *Nature*, **424**, 267.

Slabbekoorn, H. & Smith, T. B. (2002). Habitat dependent song divergence in the little greenbul: an analysis of environmental selection pressures on acoustic signals. *Evolution*, **56**, 1849–1858.

Su, K. F. Y. & Li, D. (2006). Female-biased predation risk and its differential effect on the male and female courtship behavior of jumping spiders. *Animal Behaviour*, **71**, 531–537.

Tárano, Z. & Ryan, M. J. (2002). No preexisting biases for heterospecific call traits in the frog *Physalaemus enesefae*. *Animal Behaviour*, **64**, 599–607.

Vélez, M. J. & Brockman, H. J. (2006). Seasonal variation in female response to male calling song in the field cricket, *Gryllus rubens*. *Ethology* **112**, 1041–1049.

Welch, A. M., Semlitsch, R. D. & Gerhardt, H. C. (1998). Call duration as an indicator of genetic quality in male gray tree frogs. *Science*, **280**, 1928–1930.

West-Eberhard, M. J. (1979). Sexual selection, social competition, and evolution. *Proceedings of the American Philosophical Society*, **123**, 222–234.

Wilczynski, W. & Ryan, M. J. (2010). The behavioral neural science of acoustic processing in anurans. *Current Opinion in Neurobiology*, **20**, 754–763.

Wilczynski, W., Rand, A. S. & Ryan, M. J. (1995). The processing of spectral cues by the call analysis system of the túngara frog, *Physalaemus pustulosus*. *Animal Behaviour*, **49**, 911–929.

Wilczynski, W., Rand, A. S. & Ryan, M. J. (2001). Evolution of calls and auditory tuning in the *Physalaemus pustulosus* species group. *Brain, Behavior and Evolution*, **58**, 137–151.

Wiley, R. H. (1991). Associations of song properties with habitats for territorial oscine birds of eastern North America. *American Naturalist*, **138**, 973–993.

Commentary

Narrative 1 is not just metaphor. It's a shorthand explanation, just like function and adaptation (spelled out, for example, in Millikan, Ch. 5 of this volume). We see no contentious issue here. We, too, endorse integrative studies of animal communication. Ryan's chapter beautifully illustrates the integrative approach, and explains how it followed from avoiding information constructs. However, Botero and de Kort's chapter (Ch. 11) is a beautiful example, too, yet stemmed from an information approach. Informational approaches are certainly problematic, but they don't hold back research.

Andrew G. Horn and Peter McGregor

Response

Regardless of whether Narrative 1 is a metaphor (as it would seem to be according to Kennedy (1992)) or a shorthand explanation, it does not provide the reader with the information about the actual biology that is taking place. For the uninitiated, Narrative 1 can confuse a population-based understanding of selection with a teleological one, it could suggest cognitive abilities in animals that might not exist, and it robs the reader of the grandeur in Darwin's view of life and replaces it with a comic-book version. Why would we want to do this?

Michael J. Ryan

PART III CASE STUDIES

10

Animal signals: always influence, sometimes information

CLAIRE HORISK AND REGINALD B. COCROFT

Because signals evolve to influence the behaviour of receivers, we believe the term 'influence' provides the basis for a general definition of animal signals. We will argue that the reason a receiver's behaviour is influenced by signals is often, but by no means always, because the receiver gains information as a result of attending to the signals. We suggest that definitions of information that focus on what the receiver gains by assessing signals are the most useful, allowing an organism's response to signals to be discussed in the same framework as its responses to other important aspects of its environment, rather than setting communication apart from the rest of behavioural and evolutionary ecology. Our view of signals, then, is that they evolve to influence the behaviour of receivers, and that the information gained by receivers is one possible means by which signallers exert their influence. We make our case by discussing four examples, some of which are new to this literature.

10.1 Introduction

Owren, Rendall and Ryan have challenged definitions of animal signalling in terms of information. For example, they reject definitions of animal signalling "as a process in which evolutionarily specialised morphology or behaviour in a signaller is used to encode and convey information to a perceiver, who in turn relies on evolved neural and perceptual processes to decode and recover the information" (Owren *et al.*, 2010, p. 758). They prefer to define

Animal Communication Theory: Information and Influence, ed. Ulrich Stegmann. Published by Cambridge University Press.

animal signalling as "the use of specialized, species-typical morphology or behaviour to influence the current or future behaviour of another individual" (p. 771). We agree that a definition of signalling that is based on 'influence' should extend to all examples of animal communication. If signals do not influence the behaviour of receivers in a way that benefits the signaller, on average, it will not pay animals to signal, and communication would not be maintained by selection. We also agree that there are animal signals that influence without providing information; we give an example of this below. However, we believe that animals can be influenced by signals because of the information they gain from them; again, we give an example below. Although we believe that animals can gain information from signals, like Owren *et al.* we are uncomfortable with the idea that when animal signals are informative, there must be a signaller encoding the information and a receiver decoding that same information; a third example, described below, makes this point. We think that receivers can gain information even if senders do not intend to provide information, and we discuss below a fourth example, of human language users who cannot fully identify other people's informational needs.

We adopt the position that receivers sometimes gain information from signals, in the same sense that they gain information about other aspects of the environment by sampling the environment with their sensory systems (Dall *et al.*, 2005; Wagner & Danchin, 2010). Given that signals evolve to influence the decisions of other individuals, one useful definition of information based on statistical decision theory is "the change in a receiver's estimated probabilities that a given condition is currently true" (Bradbury & Vehrencamp, 2011). Some of those arguing against the 'information perspective' are in agreement that receivers at least sometimes gain information by attending to signals. For example, Morton and Coss (this volume) state that "information or content is just whatever the signal is correlated with and what perceivers infer or 'make' of the signal given their own private information, context, age, sex etc". Information in this sense is not the 'phlogiston' invoked by Rendall and Owren (Ch. 6 of this volume), or the 'transmitted information' that Morton and Coss (Ch. 8 of this volume) do not find in signals; as noted by Bradbury and Vehrencamp (2011), it does not 'flow' between signaller and receiver. In Bradbury and Vehrencamp's sense, animal decisions are based on information about relevant aspects of the environment, which sometimes include signals. For example, a butterfly gains information about host plants from the shape of their leaves (Parmesan, Singer & Harmis, 1995). But animals can also gain information from signals, as when a honeybee learns the location of a foraging site from the dances of a nestmate (Seeley, 1995).

10.2 Signals that reduce information

In this section, we describe an example of communication during mate localisation by insects. We focus on a signal produced by competing males, which influences receivers not because it allows them to gain information, but because it interferes with their perception of other signals. We think the utility of this example for the information-versus-influence debate is that both sides can agree that the signal does not provide information. Instead, the question is whether it should be considered a signal at all. We will argue that a common function of signalling is to reduce the information a receiver can obtain from other signallers, and that excluding this function from the definition of 'signal' would be counterproductive.

In many insects, mate choice involves an ongoing back-and-forth alternation of signals, or 'duet' between male and female (Bailey, 2003). Duetting occurs in some fireflies, katydids, grasshoppers and cicadas, and is especially common in insects such as leafhoppers that communicate with substrate-borne vibrations (Bailey, 2003). In most cases, it is the female who remains stationary while the male searches. During the duet, the female signals immediately after the male's advertisement signals, and the male finds the female by attending to directional cues provided by her signal.

Duetting systems are vulnerable to eavesdropping by competing males, and a variety of specialised signals have evolved in this competitive context (Bailey, 2003). In general, signals produced by the duetting male reduce the benefit of eavesdropping (e.g. by preventing a listening male from detecting the female's response; Hammond & Bailey, 2003), and signals produced by the eavesdropping male either disrupt the ongoing duet (Cooley & Marshall, 2001; Mazzoni *et al.*, 2009a, 2009b) or cause the female to respond preferentially to the eavesdropper (Bailey & Field, 2000). Here we focus on an example from the research of one of the authors, which involves signal masking that occurs during mate-searching when more than one male is present.

The treehopper *Tylopelta gibbera* is a small, sap-feeding insect whose signals are transmitted as substrate-borne vibrations through the stems and leaves of its herbaceous host plants (Legendre, Marting & Cocroft, 2012). Males search for females by producing two-part advertisement signals (Figure 10.1A): the first part is a whistle-like downsweep (the 'whine'), and the second is a higher-pitched series of pulses. If an unmated female finds the signal sufficiently attractive, she produces a vibrational signal of her own, a low-pitched drone rich in harmonics (Figure 10.1A). The male then engages in a localised search, walking along the stem and up side branches, stopping every few centimetres to produce a bout of one to five advertisement signals, each of which usually elicits a female reply.

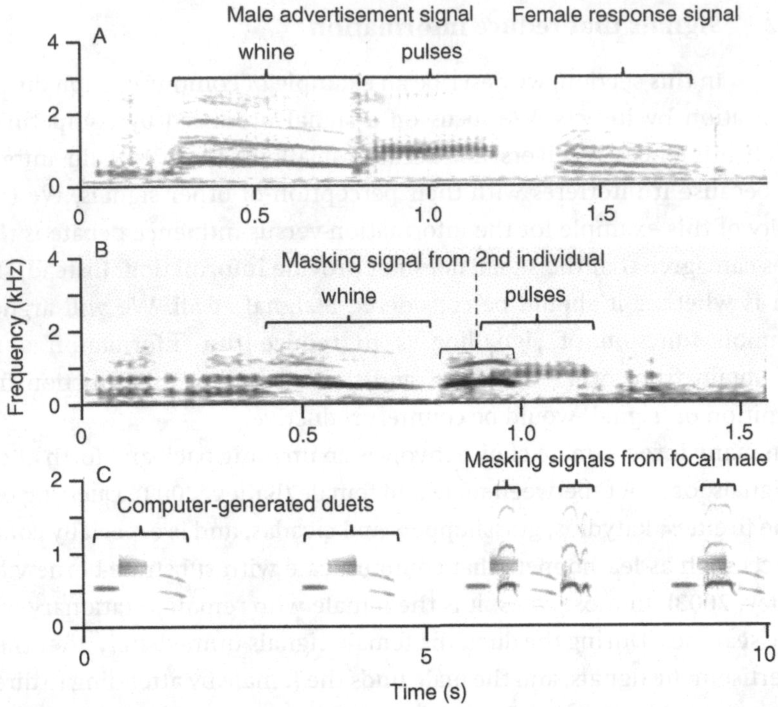

Figure 10.1 Spectrograms of the vibrational signals of duetting *Tylopelta gibbera* treehoppers. **A**, Male advertisement signal and female response. **B**, Masking signal overlapping the pulses of a competitor's advertisement signal. **C**, Playback to a male *T. gibbera* of four computer-generated duets, with three masks produced by the focal male; the first and third masks overlap with the virtual male's pulses, while the second follows closely after the virtual female response.

If a second male is on the same plant with a duetting pair, he immediately begins producing advertisement signals. The female replies to both males, producing her signal immediately after the signals of first one male, then the other. She mates with the first male to arrive. Tellingly, mate localisation takes longer when more than one male is present (Legendre *et al.*, 2012). Each male produces not only advertisement signals, but also a new kind of signal, carefully timed to overlap with the pulses of the other male's advertisement signal (Figure 10.1B, 10.1C). The masking signal impedes localisation by suppressing female responses: masked advertisement signals are only about one-third as likely to evoke a female reply. Masking benefits the signaller because when the female does not respond to a rival, the rival fails to gain information on whether the female's signals are arriving from ahead or behind, and from what distance. Duetting between a female and each of two males results in a series of complex, fast-paced acoustic interactions as each male alternately produces advertisement signals (which may be masked by its rival), masks any advertisement signals of the rival male and moves to a new signalling location.

Our working hypothesis is that the psychophysical basis of the reduction in female responses lies in signal masking (Legendre *et al.*, 2012). That is, the overlapping signal masks the pulses produced by the first male, where 'masking' is defined as an increase in the threshold for detecting one stimulus, caused by the presence of a second stimulus (Gelfand, 2010). Consistent with the interpretation that masking signals interfere with the female's perception of the pulses, females seldom reply to playback of signals lacking any pulses after the whine (P. R. Marting & R. B. Cocroft, unpublished data). We do not argue that no receiver can gain any information from the presence of masking signals (e.g. that there is more than one male present), but that the reduction in female responses to masked advertisement signals results directly from decreased audibility of the pulses. It is not simply a consequence of the female's perception that there is a second male present, because during experimental playbacks of unmasked signals from more than one male, females typically reply to almost every signal (Marting & Cocroft, unpublished data). In our view, masking signals are an example of signalling that is best understood on the influence, rather than the information, definition.

Our argument in favour of an influence definition of communication in *T. gibbera* rests on the claim that the masking vibrations produced by competing males are signals. However, someone committed to an information account could simply counter that if the masking vibrations do not provide information, they are by definition not signals.[1] We argue below that this solution has undesirable consequences. The main issue is that reducing the information that receivers can obtain from rivals is a common function of signals, sometimes involving specialised signals, and sometimes involving the timing of an individual's mating signals relative to those of neighbours. Excluding from consideration as signals all cases in which information is decreased, rather than increased, would require arbitrary distinctions, and separate out phenomena that are best considered under the same theoretical umbrella.

The masking vibration of *T. gibbera* is only one of many examples of signals whose function is to interfere with communication. Masking signals have been found, for example, in some species of katydids (Bailey, MacLeay & Gordon, 2006; Bailey & Field, 2000), periodical cicadas (Cooley & Marshall, 2001) and

[1] We thank Ruth Millikan, Ulrich Stegmann and an anonymous reviewer for pressing this point.

leafhoppers (Mazzoni *et al.*, 2009 b).[2] Because duetting is widespread in vibrational communication systems, an under-studied modality (Cocroft & Rodriguez, 2005), there are probably many more examples of vibrational 'interference' signals remaining to be described (e.g. Miranda, 2006).

In addition to the use of specialised masking sounds or vibrations, individuals in many species use their advertisement signals to mask those of competitors. In choruses of acoustic frogs and insects, the timing of a male's signals relative to those of its neighbours can have a profound effect on attractiveness. For example, when one advertisement signal follows closely after another, females in many species prefer the leading signal (Greenfield, 2005). This 'leader preference' can result from a number of mechanisms including the precedence effect, which is thought to be an adaptation for enhanced signal detection in the presence of echoes: when the same sound arrives from two directions, separated by a short time delay, the listener will detect both but only localise the first (Gelfand, 2010). Although males cannot lead all other signallers in a chorus, they can attend to the signal timing of their closest neighbours, and adjust their own timing accordingly (Snedden, Greenfield & Jang, 1998); males likewise attempt to initiate their signals at times outside the 'forbidden interval' after the start of a rival's signal (Höbel, 2011). A male that signals just before a rival reduces the information a listener can obtain from the rival's signal. There is a clear parallel with the masking vibrations of *T. gibbera*, which likewise reduce the female's information about the rival's signal, albeit through a different psychoacoustic mechanism. In the case of chorusing species there has been no specialisation of functions into one signal that provides information and another that reduces information; instead, the advertisement signal has both functions, with the interference function depending entirely on signal timing.

Because communication often occurs in a competitive context, it is not surprising that a common function of signals is to interfere with the signals of

[2] In some Australian katydids, competing males have a complex repertoire of signals used during competitive mate localisation. Duetting males may produce loud series of clicks immediately after a female reply, preventing eavesdroppers from detecting the female (Bailey *et al.*, 2006); eavesdropping males may 'over-sing' a rival's advertisement signal, preventing a female reply (Bailey *et al.*, 2006), or they may produce a short series of clicks during the rival's signal, causing some females (which approach the signalling male in that species) to localise the eavesdropper instead of the duetting male (Bailey & Field, 2000). When a duetting periodical cicada male detects the arrival of a second male, it produces a 'buzz' during a key portion of the rival's mating song, preventing the female from replying to the rival (Cooley & Marshall, 2001). In a leafhopper, males that detect a male–female vibrational duet produce a series of rattling pulses, timed to overlap with the male signal or the female response (Mazzoni *et al.*, 2009a); so effective is this signal at disrupting courtship that playback of artificial 'disruptive signals' can prevent reproduction in these grapevine pests (Mazzoni *et al.*, 2009b).

rivals. Currently, the literature on animal communication treats the examples of competitive masking and other forms of interference as signals (using terms such as 'masking signals' or 'disturbance signals'). Likewise, the issue of signal timing within choruses is simply treated as a general issue in communication, of when a signal should be produced to maximise its effectiveness (Greenfield, 2002). But if the response of an 'information' proponent to the masking signals of *T. gibbera* is to argue that they are not signals, then this response also requires the development of a new classification scheme, separating out signals from other signal-like behaviours. Ultimately the distinction would have to rely on function: if the function of a signal-like behaviour is to interfere with communication, then it is not a signal. In operational terms, this will depend largely on timing. For *T. gibbera*, the whine component of the advertisement signal and the masking signal are both sinusoidal vibrations with a fundamental frequency around 500 Hz. If a male *T. gibbera* produces a 500-Hz vibration that is followed by a series of pulses, and does not overlap with the pulses of another male, it is a signal; if it overlaps with the pulses of another male and is not itself followed by a series of pulses, it is a non-signal. For chorusing species, a mating song produced in isolation is a signal, but one produced immediately before the mating song of a rival has both signal and non-signal functions.

We suggest that it would be arbitrary to exclude 'interference' from the list of possible signal functions, or to classify similar phenotypes into signals and non-signals based on their timing relative to the signals of competitors. A strict information view would seem to require this approach. In contrast, the view that signals evolve to influence the behaviour of receivers allows us to view all of these phenomena as signals under one theoretical umbrella, and in so doing better reflects the complexity of communicative interactions.

10.3 An informative signal

In this section, we briefly review the honeybee waggle dance, one of the most widely known examples of animal signalling. We discuss it here because we think that it provides a particularly clear instance of the utility of the term 'information' in explanations of animal signalling.

Honeybee scouts that return to the colony after foraging in a flower patch may advertise their find with a waggle dance, performed on the vertical surface of the comb. The dance is a 'miniaturised reenactment' (Seeley, 2010) of the trip to the patch of flowers, with the direction and distance to the patch reflected in the dance. The dance consists of a series of straight waggle runs, during which the dancer runs forward for a few centimetres while vibrating its body from side to side and buzzing, then circles around to the beginning (von Frisch, 1967). The direction of the waggle runs relative to vertical is correlated with the direction to the flower patch with respect to the Sun; for example, when the dance is oriented straight up, the patch is directly in line with the Sun. The duration of the waggle runs is correlated with the distance to the patch (Seeley, 1995). During a dance, one or more potential recruits follow closely behind the dancing forager (von Frisch, 1967).

For a human observer, the dance contains enough information to plot the colony's foraging locations on a map. The information is obtained not only by human observers, but also by bees. When dance followers were captured upon leaving the hive and released some distance away, their flight paths took them straight to what would have been the location of the experimental feeder (Riley *et al.*, 2005). Importantly, dance followers sample the odour present on the dancing forager (Díaz, Grüter & Farina, 2007), and they engage in a localised search for flowers with that odour once they have arrived at the target location (Seeley, 1995). Dance followers are flexible in how they integrate the information from floral cues and waggle run angle and duration; individuals that had previously foraged at flowers with a similar odour, but at a different location, may disregard the vector information from the dance and leave the hive to forage at the familiar location (Grüter, Balbuena & Farina, 2008).

Dancing bees influence the behaviour of their nestmates; and in addition to any motivational effect of their dancing on dance followers, it would be difficult to provide an account of the evolution of the dance language without reference to the information receivers gain about the location of the flower patch and the scent of the floral resource. Accordingly, while the lesson we drew from the duetting example was that the term 'information' should not be required in all accounts of animal signals, the lesson we draw from this one is that neither should we exclude information from all accounts of animal signals.

10.4 Informative signals from uninformed signallers

Our third example illustrates that the idea that an animal can gain information from a signal does not require the assumption that animals *send* information in signals (Morton & Coss, Ch. 8 of this volume; Bradbury & Vehrencamp, 2011).

The example we focus on here is collective signalling by broods of offspring of the thornbug treehopper, *Umbonia crassicornis*. Female thornbugs lay a single clutch of eggs on a host-plant stem, and then remain on that stem for the rest of their lives, caring for their offspring (Wood, 1983). After hatching, the offspring cluster together around the stem, feeding through incisions in the bark made by the female. The nymphs are frequently attacked by invertebrate predators such as wasps and stink bugs, and their only defence is the mother's active protection (Wood, 1976; Cocroft, 2002).

Immature thornbugs solicit the mother's protection with collective signals. When a predator approaches, the nearest individuals produce signals with two components. One is a substrate-borne vibrational 'chirp' (Cocroft, 1996); the other is a tactile signal consisting of a side-to-side movement of the abdomen (Borduin *et al.*, 2008). Signals of the first individuals initiate a wave of signalling that sweeps through the group. Although the vibrational chirps are transmitted within a millisecond or two throughout the 10–20-cm-long aggregation, the wave of signalling takes up to half a second to reach the other end of the group; the spread of signalling within the group depends largely on the transmission of tactile signalling behaviour from each individual to its immediate neighbours (Borduin *et al.*, 2008; Cocroft *et al.*, in preparation). The result of this spread of signalling across a group is a collective, group signal that is longer and higher in amplitude than the individual signals; indeed, individual signals can no longer be distinguished within the group signal, except for one or two that occur at the beginning or end (Figure 10.2A). Alarmed groups produce collective signals every 1–2 seconds (Cocroft, 1999). Note that only the few initiators of the collective signal are responding directly to perception of a predator; most of the individuals producing the signal are responding only to the behaviour of their neighbours.

Female thornbugs are normally sedentary, facing their offspring from a few cm away (Figure 10.2B). In response to collective signals, a female will walk into the brood and attempt to locate the predator. The female must approach the predator closely, because her defences (wing-buzzing and kicking) work only at very close range (Wood, 1976). The farther an attacked nymph is from the female, the longer it takes the female to arrive and the less likely the nymph is to survive the attack (Cocroft, 2002). Because the female must approach the predator to drive it away, and because her movement is relatively slow, there is a premium on efficient localisation of the predator. If the female can see the predator from a distance she will move directly towards it, but with small, inconspicuous predators such as stink bugs, the female relies on the offspring signals for clues to the predator's location. Almost all predator attacks occur on one of the two ends of the cylindrical aggregations (Cocroft, 2002), so the female's main problem is to determine which end has been attacked.

Females use the offspring's collective signals to locate the predator (Ramaswamy & Cocroft, 2009). How is this possible, given that most of the offspring have no personal information about the predator's presence or location? First, females respond only to collective signals, and not to single or uncoordinated signals (Cocroft, 1996). And given the dynamics of how collective

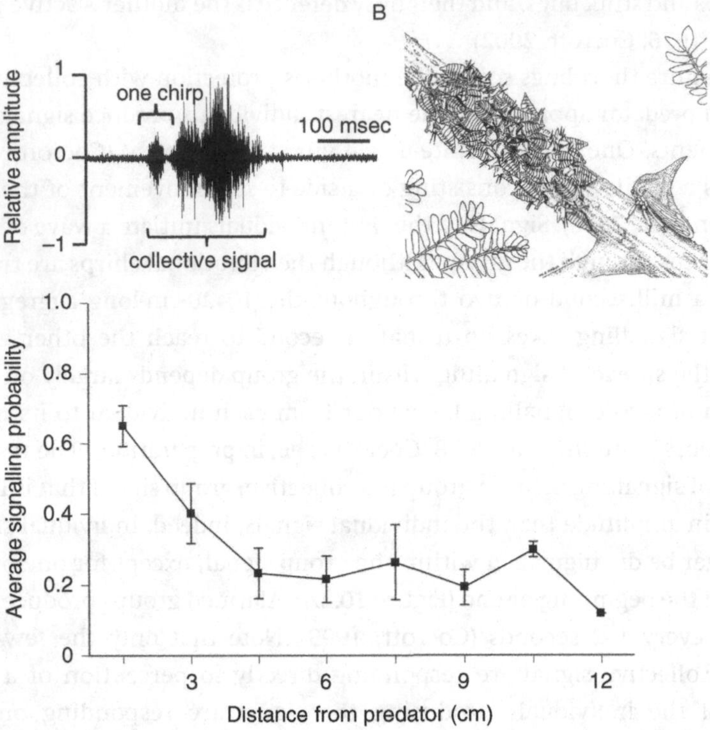

Figure 10.2 Collective communication in *Umbonia crassicornis*. **A**, Waveform of the vibrational component of a collective signal produced by a brood responding to the approach of a predatory wasp. A single chirp from the initiating individual can be seen, as well as the collective vibration resulting from the spread of signalling across the group. **B**, Female and her brood on a host-plant stem. **C**, Participation in the group signal decreases with distance from the site of initiation, creating a signal gradient that contains information about the predator's location. For a female within the aggregation, there will be more signal energy in the direction of the predator.

signals are generated, the properties of the overall signal reveal the predator's location within the brood (Ramaswamy & Cocroft, 2009). A number of aspects of the collective signals are correlated with the predator's location, one of which is a signalling gradient. Because there is a process of attrition as the signalling behaviour is transmitted across the brood, individuals closer to the predator are more likely to participate in a given collective signal (Figure 10.2C; Ramaswamy & Cocroft, 2009). In the absence of any cues apart from the offspring signals, females can locate a 'virtual predator' using this signalling gradient (K. Ramaswamy & R. B. Cocroft, unpublished data).

Female thornbugs, then, gain information about the existence of a predator, and about its location, from the signalling behaviour of their offspring. On the

Bradbury and Vehrencamp account of information, there is a change in the female's estimated probability that there is a predator, and a change in her estimated probability of the location of the predator. However, there are many signallers rather than one, and the feature(s) of the signal that reveal the predator's location are a property of the collective signal, not the individual signals. Although one could argue that the 'information' account works here if one considers the collective signal rather than the individual signallers, it remains true that the signal giving the female information about predator presence and location is not sent by a signaller who possesses that information; there is no signaller that has the information, encodes it and sends it along to the female. Very few of the signalling nymphs can see the predator; the rest are signalling either in response to the chirping and tactile signalling of a neighbour, or to the chirping of many individuals in the group. It is the signalling of the group as a whole that provides information to the mother; the signalling of those few nymphs who know of the existence and location of the predator is not enough. So there is no signaller who sends or encodes the information that is gained by the mother.

10.5 Human language and mental state attribution

Some participants in this debate think that differences between animal and human communication are relevant to whether we can speak of animal signalling in terms of information. In this section we focus on one purported difference, that humans intend to provide needed information whereas animals do not. Rendall, Owren & Ryan (2009) say that "the failure of calling animals to take account of the informational needs of listeners corroborates a growing literature showing that non-human primates show little of the perspective-taking and mental state attribution abilities considered to be foundational to the referential quality of human language" (p. 235). We do not believe it has been established that perspective-taking and mental state attribution abilities are foundational to the referential quality of human language, and we do not think that the failure of animals to take into account the informational needs of listeners provides evidence that can be used to determine whether we can speak of animal signalling in terms of information. In our opinion, there is evidence that some human language users – speakers with Autism Spectrum Disorder (ASD) – have limited ability to attribute mental states, and thus limited ability to identify what information is needed by a listener, and yet use referential language. Our final example makes this point. Furthermore, we believe that it remains to be seen to what extent non-human primates can take the perspective of another, or attribute mental states to another. We conclude that there is as yet no reason to think that this particular difference between typical humans and animals is relevant to the question of whether animals gain information from signals.

Rendall *et al.* (2009) argue that animals do not have the mental capacities that underlie human communication; they argue that a series of studies have shown an "absence of the intent to inform by calling animals (D. Cheney & Seyfarth 1990; D. L. Cheney *et al.* 1996; D. Rendall *et al.* 2000)" and that "callers prove to be fundamentally unaware of the informational value of their own signals" (p. 235). Owren *et al.* (2010) argue that

> [Human] communication shows intentionality. In other words, humans routinely taking [sic] the beliefs, motivations, and knowledge of listeners into account when speaking to them, thereby communicating more effectively and efficiently. (pp. 768–769)

In contrast,

> non-human primates have limited understanding of the mental states of others – an ability considered fundamental in using language. (p. 769)

Similarly, Cheney and Seyfarth (2005) argue that

> If, as Grice (1957) and others have argued, true linguistic communication cannot occur unless both speaker and listener take into account each other's state of mind, then monkeys cannot be said to communicate unless they use calls like contact barks with the intent to provide information to others. (p. 138)

Cheney and Seyfarth go on to argue that baboons do not communicate with contact barks; their evidence is that female baboons answer contact barks from a relative only when the answerer is separated from the group, not when the answerer is herself at no risk of becoming lost. Thus both proponents of signalling as influence and proponents of signalling as information have a shared assumption about human communication – that it requires the capacity to take into account the state of mind of the listener, and thus take into account what information he or she needs. Furthermore, humans, but not animals, have the intent to provide needed information.

Both Rendall *et al.* and Cheney and Seyfarth are motivated in part by Grice, who held that for a person to mean something by what she says, she must have communicative intentions towards her audience (Grice, 1989). But the Gricean account is far from accepted doctrine. Human conversation is a highly complex form of behaviour. To participate fully and smoothly in a conversation, a speaker must grasp the syntax and semantics of a language, and have substantial pragmatic ability; she must be capable of assessing how much or little to say, when to say it, how to say it and so on. Competence with pragmatics clearly requires the ability to consider what another believes or knows. But we have little reason to suppose that the ability to represent the state of mind of a listener is a prerequisite for the acquisition of the syntax and semantics of a natural language; so we do not have the evidence required to support the thesis that having communicative intentions towards an audience is necessary for what one says to mean something.

One line of evidence against the Gricean account comes from language development in young children. On the Gricean account, in order to mean something, a speaker must intend that a listener form a belief, and furthermore, she must intend that the listener form that belief because he recognises that the speaker intends that he form that belief. This is a complex intention, and it has been argued that young children become competent with syntax and semantics before they become capable of having such a complex intention (Risjord, 1996). A second line of evidence comes from research on language development in speakers with ASD, which suggests that syntax and semantics can be acquired without at least some elements of the capacity that typically developed adults have to represent the state of mind of a listener. This is the example we focus on here. Competence with syntax and semantics is sufficient to provide information, even though it is not sufficient to provide the most apt information. So while we agree with Rendall *et al.* that effective and efficient human communication seems to depend on a rich ability to attribute mental states to others, that is not to say that we cannot glean information from speakers who are not fully sensitive to the mental states of others.

ASD is a developmental disorder with onset before the age of three; it is characterised by qualitative impairment in social interaction, qualitative impairment in communication, and restricted, repetitive and stereotyped patterns of behaviour, interests and activities (American Psychiatric Association, 2000). There are two features of ASD that are of particular interest here, mind-blindness and impairment in communication.

Baron-Cohen, Leslie and Frith (1985) first proposed that children with autism lack a theory of mind; to have a theory of mind is to be able to ascribe psychological or mental states such as beliefs and desires to themselves and others (Premack & Woodruff, 1978). Someone who lacks a theory of mind cannot use beliefs and desires to predict and explain the behaviour of others (Baron-Cohen *et al.*, 1985). Baron-Cohen *et al.* held that to be capable of attributing a belief, one must be capable of attributing a false belief, so on their view, the inability to attribute a false belief indicates the lack of a theory of mind. In Baron-Cohen *et al.*'s study, 85% of neurotypical children could attribute a false belief to others or to themselves, as could 86% of children with Down's syndrome, but only 20% of children with ASD could do this.

With regard to communication, people with ASD exhibit a broad range of ability with language, as DeVilliers *et al.* explain:

> Though some individuals with ASD, especially those with Asperger's syndrome, are able to develop typical speech and language abilities, many speakers with ASD have immense trouble understanding metaphor, irony, sarcasm, indirect speech acts[3], and conversational implicature[4]. In contrast, even these pragmatically challenged speakers often exhibit surprising competence when it comes to abilities that are widely assumed to be properly linguistic, for example, complex syntax, phonology, and compositional semantics. They may exhibit some difficulties, specifically flat intonation and some highly idiosyncratic meanings for lexical items. Notoriously as well, many speakers with ASD exhibit delays in acquiring language. However, for the most part, the language-related difficulties of so-called high functioning individuals with autism do not lie on the 'encoding/decoding' side; instead, they have to do with appropriate use. (DeVilliers, Stainton & Szatmari 2007, p. 296)[5]

3 An example of an indirect speech act is "Can you pass the salt?" which has the sentence structure of a question but is usually meant as a request. More generally, indirect speech acts are speech acts where the force of the speech act is not encoded by a performative verb in the sentence (such as 'order', 'ask', 'inform') or by a sentence type (the three major sentence types in English being the imperative, interrogative and declarative). See Levinson (1983).

4 A speaker conversationally implicates that q by saying p by exploiting conversational maxims (Grice, 1989). For example, it is a maxim that one should be as informative as is required. Failing to follow this maxim can communicate information. For instance, if Grice is asked to provide a recommendation letter for an applicant for an academic job, and the letter says only that the applicant has good handwriting, he fails to follow the maxim and conversationally implicates that the applicant is not a good candidate for the job.

5 At the time of writing, DSM-IV is the most recent edition of the American Psychological Association's diagnostic manual for psychiatric disorders. The diagnostic criteria for ASD in DSM-IV require that there be at least one of the following impairments: (a) delay in, or total lack of, the development of spoken language (not accompanied by an attempt to compensate through alternative modes of communication such as gesture or mime); (b) in individuals with adequate speech, marked impairment in the ability to initiate or sustain a conversation with others; (c) stereotyped and repetitive use of language or idiosyncratic language; (d) lack of varied, spontaneous make-believe play or social imitative play appropriate to developmental level (p. 75). The diagnostic criteria for ASD are expected to be modified for DSM-V, which has an anticipated publication date of 2013.

The individuals with ASD who are of interest to the current topic are people whose syntax, phonology and compositional semantics are complete. Glüer and Pagin (2003) review the literature and show that there are individuals with ASD with intact syntax, phonology and compositional semantics who are incapable of attributing false beliefs to others; i.e. they do not have all the capacities of non-ASD human beings to take into consideration the state of mind of another, yet become competent with representational aspects of human language (Happé, 1993, 1995; Baron Cohen, 1997). They can judge sentences as right or wrong, and distinguish between what is said to be the case and what is the case (Baron-Cohen, 1997), "thus indicating an understanding of the representational character of the utterances" (Glüer & Pagin, 2003, p. 33). Thus, contra Rendall *et al.*, these speakers are competent with the referential qualities of human language, but have atypical ability to take someone else's perspective, or attribute mental states to someone else. They may find it difficult to interpret metaphor (Happé, 1993), identify a joke (Baron-Cohen, 1997), comprehend irony (Filippova & Astington, 2008) or contribute appropriately to a conversation. In short, speakers with ASD cannot fully take into account the informational needs of others; yet we can gain information from what they say. Thus we believe that the fact that animal signallers do not take into account the informational needs of others has no bearing on the question of whether animals can gain information from animal signals.

More recently, Wellman and Liu (2004) argue that theory of mind has a number of elements that develop in stages; typically developing children first understand that different people may want different things, then that different people may have different beliefs about the same thing, then that not seeing leads to not knowing, then they understand false belief, and then they understand that people can feel a different emotion from the one that they display. Peterson, Wellman & Slaughter (2012) found that the last two stages were reversed for ASD children. Thus passing the false belief task that played a key role for Baron-Cohen *et al.* (1985) is a relatively complex task, and an autistic speaker who cannot pass this task may nevertheless have a more limited theory of mind. One might speculate that the mental state attribution and perspective-taking that comes along with recognising diverse beliefs and with understanding that not seeing leads to not knowing would be enough to underpin the referential qualities of language that concern Rendall, Owren and Ryan.

However, this more nuanced conception of what constitutes a theory of mind does not undermine our main point, that there is no reason to suppose that the intent to provide needed information is relevant to the question of whether animal signals should be understood in terms of information. We have two reasons for thinking this. The first is that Peterson *et al.* (2012) controlled statistically for individual differences in language ability, and showed that the development of theory of mind represents conceptual developments other than increasing language competence; so their study does not support the idea that language development and theory of mind somehow develop in lockstep. Second, Kaminski, Call & Tomasello (2008) and Hare, Call & Tomasello (2001) have evidence suggesting that chimpanzees recognise that not seeing leads to not knowing, the step on the Wellman and Liu scale that in typically developing children falls right below false belief, and that chimpanzees recognise that different chimpanzees have different beliefs depending on what they have seen. If these are the abilities that are required for referential language, then at least some non-human primates may have what it takes.

We wish to emphasise that we do not maintain that animals have the same abilities in perspective-taking and mental state attribution as we do; and we do not maintain that perspective-taking and mental state attribution are completely irrelevant to the development of human language in children. Furthermore, we do not maintain that human language could have evolved as it has if humans did not have a rich theory of mind. Rather, we think that it has not been established that perspective-taking and mental state attribution are required in order for human language to have its referential properties. The evidence that would be needed to support the thesis that the intent to provide needed information is a marker that distinguishes animal communication and human communication is currently unavailable.

10.6 Conclusion

The strength of the 'information' approach is that, if we avoid assuming that higher cognitive processes are necessary and use a clear definition that focuses on what receivers can gain from signals, it allows us to talk about how receivers assess signals in the same terms we use to talk about how they assess other stimuli in their environment. Furthermore, for cases such as the honeybee waggle dance, insisting on avoidance of the term 'information' would unnecessarily constrain our ability to describe the behaviour and its function in the life of the colony. Animals can gain information from signals even if that information is not packaged up by senders, as the collective signalling of treehopper nymphs shows, and even if the sender cannot assess what information is required by the receiver, as the case of human speakers with ASD shows. The strength of the 'influence' approach is its fruitful emphasis on the mechanisms and evolutionary history of signal production and perception. Because only signals that influence receivers will be maintained by selection, a definition of communication based on 'influence' should extend to all examples of communication. Furthermore, there are clear examples of animal signals, such as the masking signal of treehoppers, which influence the behaviour of receivers, but from which the receiver does not gain information. On the whole, then, we believe that the 'influence' approach provides a strong framework for understanding animal communication, but that it would be incomplete without the acknowledgement that providing information is one way that signallers can influence receivers.[6]

References

American Psychiatric Association (2000). *Diagnostic and Statistical Manual of Mental Disorders: DSM-IV-TR*, 4th edn. Washington, DC: American Psychiatric Publishing, Inc.

Bailey, W. J. (2003). Insect duets: underlying mechanisms and their evolution. *Physiological Entomology*, **28**, 157–174.

Bailey, W. J. & Field, G. (2000). Acoustic satellite behaviour in the Australian bushcricket *Elephantodeta nobilis* (Phaneropterinae, Tettigoniidae, Orthoptera). *Animal Behaviour*, **59**, 361–369.

Bailey, W., MacLeay, C. & Gordon, T. (2006). Acoustic mimicry and disruptive alternative calling tactics in an Australian bushcricket (Caedicia; Phaneropterinae; Tettigoniidae; Orthoptera): does mating influence male calling tactic? *Physiological Entomology*, **31**, 201–210.

Baron-Cohen, S. (1997). Hey! It was just a joke! Understanding propositions and propositional attitudes by normally developing children and children with autism. *Israel Journal of Psychiatry and Related Sciences*, **34**, 174–178.

Baron-Cohen, S., Leslie, A. M. & Frith, U. (1985). Does the autistic child have a 'theory of mind'? *Cognition*, **21**, 37–46.

Borduin, R., Ramaswamy, K., Mohan, A. *et al.* (2008). Modeling the rapid transmission of information within a social group of insects: emergent patterns in the antipredator signals. *American Society of Mechanical Engineers Dynamic Systems and Control Conference Proceedings DSCC2008–2298*, 1441–1447.

Bradbury, J. W. & Vehrencamp, S. L. (2011). *Web Topic 1.2: Information and Communication. Principles of Animal Communication*, 2nd edn companion website. http://sites.sinauer.com/animalcommunication2e.

Cheney, D. & Seyfarth, R. (1990). Attending to behaviour versus attending to knowledge: examining monkeys' attribution of mental states. *Animal Behaviour*, **40**, 742–753.

Cheney, D. L. & Seyfarth, R. M. (2005). Constraints and preadaptations in the earliest stages of language evolution. *Linguistic Review*, **22**, 135–159.

Cheney, D. L., Seyfarth, R. M. & Palombit, R. (1996). The function and mechanisms underlying baboon 'contact' barks. *Animal Behaviour*, **52**, 507–518.

[6] We thank Ulrich Stegmann, Ruth Millikan and two anonymous reviewers for comments.

Cocroft, R. B. (1996). Insect vibrational defence signals. *Nature*, **382**, 679–680.

Cocroft, R. B. (1999). Parent–offspring communication in response to predators in a subsocial treehopper (Hemiptera: Membracidae: *Umbonia crassicornis*). *Ethology*, **105**, 553–568.

Cocroft, R. B. (2002). Maternal defense as a limited resource: unequal predation risk in broods of an insect with maternal care. *Behavioral Ecology*, **13**, 125–133.

Cocroft, R. B. & Rodríguez, R. L. (2005). The behavioral ecology of insect vibrational communication. *BioScience*, **55**, 323–334.

Cooley, J. R. & Marshall, D. C. (2001). Sexual signaling in periodical cicadas, *Magicicada* spp (Hemiptera: Cicadidae). *Behaviour*, **138**, 827–855.

Dall, S. R. X., Giraldeau, L. A., Olsson, O. *et al.* (2005). Information and its use by animals in evolutionary ecology. *Trends in Ecology and Evolution*, **20**, 187–193.

De Villiers, J., Stainton, R. J. & Szatmari, P. (2007). Pragmatic abilities in autism spectrum disorder: a case study in philosophy and the empirical. *Midwest Studies in Philosophy*, **31**, 292–317.

Díaz, P. C., Grüter, C. & Farina, W. M. (2007). Floral scents affect the distribution of hive bees around dancers. *Behavioral Ecology and Sociobiology*, **61**, 1589–1597.

Filippova, E. & Astington, J. W. (2008). Further development in social reasoning revealed in discourse irony understanding. *Child Development*, **79**, 126–138.

Gelfand, S. A. (2010). *Hearing: An Introduction to Psychological and Physiological Acoustics*, 5th edn. London: Informa Healthcare.

Glüer, K. & Pagin, P. (2003). Meaning theory and autistic speakers. *Mind and Language*, **18**, 23–51.

Greenfield, M. D. (2002). *Signalers and Receivers: Mechanisms and Evolution of Arthropod Communication*. Oxford: Oxford University Press.

Greenfield, M. D. (2005). Mechanisms and evolution of communal sexual displays in arthropods and anurans. *Advances in the Study of Behavior*, **35**, 1–62.

Grice, H. P. (1957). Meaning. *Philosophical Review*, **66**, 377–388.

Grice, H. P. (1989). *Studies in the Way of Words*. Cambridge, MA: Harvard University Press.

Grüter, C., Balbuena, M. & Farina, W. M. (2008). Informational conflicts created by the waggle dance. *Proceedings of the Royal Society of London B: Biological Sciences*, **275**, 1321.

Hammond, T. J. & Bailey, W. J. (2003). Eavesdropping and defensive auditory masking in an Australian bushcricket, Caedicia (Phaneropterinae: Tettigoniidae: Orthoptera). *Behaviour*, **140**, 79–95.

Happé, F. G. E. (1993). Communicative competence and theory of mind in autism: a test of relevance theory. *Cognition*, **48**, 101–119.

Happé, F. G. E. (1995). The role of age and verbal ability in the theory of mind task performance of subjects with autism. *Child Development*, **66**, 843–855.

Hare, B., Call, J. & Tomasello, M. (2001). Do chimpanzees know what conspecifics know? *Animal Behaviour*, **61**, 139–151.

Höbel, G. (2011). Variation in signal timing behavior: implications for male attractiveness and sexual selection. *Behavioral Ecology and Sociobiology*, **65**, 1283–1294.

Kaminski, J., Call, J. & Tomasello, M. (2008). Chimpanzees know what others know, but not what they believe. *Cognition*, **109**, 224–234.

Legendre, F., Marting, P. R. & Cocroft, R. B. (2012). Competitive masking of vibrational signals during mate searching in a treehopper. *Animal Behaviour*, **83**, 361–368.

Levinson, S. C. (1983). *Pragmatics*. Cambridge: Cambridge University Press.

Mazzoni, V., Lucchi, A., Čokl, A. *et al.* (2009a). Disruption of the reproductive behaviour of *Scaphoideus titanus* by playback of vibrational signals. *Entomologia Experimentalis et Applicata*, **133**, 174–185.

Mazzoni, V., Presern, J., Lucchi, A. & Virant-Doberlet, M. (2009b). Reproductive strategy of the Nearctic leafhopper *Scaphoideus titanus* Ball (Hemiptera: Cicadellidae). *Bulletin of Entomological Research*, **99**, 401–413.

Miranda, X. (2006). Substrate-borne signal repertoire and courtship jamming by adults of *Ennya chrysura* (Hemiptera: Membracidae). *Annals of the Entomological Society of America*, **99**, 374–386.

Owren, M. J., Rendall, D. & Ryan, M. J. (2010). Redefining animal signaling: influence versus information in communication. *Biology and Philosophy*, **25**, 755–780.

Parmesan, C., Singer, M. C. & Harris, I. (1995). Absence of adaptive learning from the oviposition foraging behaviour of a checkerspot butterfly. *Animal Behaviour*, **50**, 161–175.

Peterson, C. C., Wellman, H. M. & Slaughter, V. (2012). The mind behind the message: advancing theory-of-mind scales for typically developing children, and those with deafness, autism, or Asperger Syndrome. *Child Development*, **83**, 469–485.

Premack, D. & Woodruff, G. (1978). Does the chimpanzee have a theory of mind? *Behavioural and Brain Sciences*, **1**, 515–526.

Ramaswamy, K. & Cocroft, R. B. (2009). Collective signals in treehopper broods provide predator localization cues to the defending mother. *Animal Behaviour*, **78**, 697–704.

Rendall, D., Cheney, D. L. & Seyfarth, R. M. (2000). Proximate factors mediating 'contact' calls in adult female baboons (*Papio cynocephalus ursinus*) and their infants. *Journal of Comparative Psychology*, **114**, 36.

Rendall, D., Owren, M. J. & Ryan, M. J. (2009). What do animal signals mean? *Animal Behaviour*, **78**, 233–240.

Riley, J. R., Greggers, U., Smith, A. D. *et al.* (2005). The flight paths of honeybees recruited by the waggle dance. *Nature*, **435**, 205–207.

Risjord, M. (1996). Meaning, belief, and language acquisition. *Philosophical Psychology*, **9**, 465–475.

Seeley, T. D. (1995). *The Wisdom of the Hive: The Social Physiology of Honey Bee Colonies*. Cambridge, MA: Harvard University Press.

Seeley, T. D. (2010). *Honeybee Democracy*. Princeton, NJ: Princeton University Press.

Snedden, W. A., Greenfield, M. D. & Jang, Y. (1998). Mechanisms of selective attention in grasshopper choruses: who listens to whom? *Behavioral Ecology and Sociobiology*, **43**, 59–66.

von Frisch, K. (1967). *The Dance Language and Orientation of Bees*. Cambridge, MA: Harvard University Press.

Wagner, R. H. & Danchin, É. (2010). A taxonomy of biological information. *Oikos*, **119**, 203–209.

Wellman, H. M. & Liu, D. (2004). Scaling of theory-of-mind tasks. *Child Development*, **75**, 523–541.

Wood, T. K. (1976). Alarm behavior of brooding female *Umbonia crassicornis* (Homoptera: Membracidae). *Annals of the Entomological Society of America*, **69**, 340–344.

Wood, T. K. (1983). Brooding and aggregating behavior of the treehopper, *Umbonia crassicornis*. *National Geographic Society Research Reports*, **15**, 753–758.

Commentary

Horisk and Cocroft's chapter offers us some fascinating examples of insect behaviour. I wonder, however, whether its central engagement is more than a verbal dispute. If every time you try to whisper sweet nothings in your darling's ear, I screech so loud that she can't hear you, is my screech a 'signal'? It seems that you can use the word 'signal' that way if you want to. But in more usual cases there exists an answer to the question, what is the signal signalling? What is it a signal of, or a signal that?

Ruth G. Millikan

Response

We agree with **Millikan** that it is not unreasonable to consider a behaviour that interferes with signals as not itself being a signal. Furthermore, we are sympathetic to the idea that the choice to describe a phenomenon as a signal may be driven by the theoretical interests of the researcher more than by a robust reality to be found in the natural world. In that sense, this may be a verbal dispute. But the theoretical interests of researchers are legitimate considerations. Treating 'interference' as one of the possible functions of signals would bring a range of similar phenomena under the same theoretical umbrella. For example, in many chorusing species, individuals time their mating signals to interfere with those of others, and disrupting others' signals contributes to mating success. Our approach allows one to consider interference to be one of the ways in which the mating signals enhance fitness, rather than requiring one to separate out the ways in which the behaviour is a signal and the ways in which it is not. In the insect example we described, there has been specialisation within the signal repertoire, such that some signals have evolved to be effective at interference, without the need to also be attractive to mates. These masking vibrations are similar to the mating vibrations in frequency, duration and amplitude, with the most striking difference being their timing relative to the rival's mating signals. We prefer not to have to consider some of the vibrations as signals and others as non-signals, but instead to treat all of them as signals that differ in the means by which they influence fitness. One consequence of this view is that some signals exist that do not inform.

As to the question of what this is a signal of or a signal that, perhaps it is not a signal of or that anything. We wonder what is gained by considering the signals of organisms such as insects, frogs, fish or cellular slime moulds as signals of something or signals that something occurs; we suspect those terms are conversational conveniences for biologists. In general, with possible exceptions like the vervet alarm calls, we are not convinced that it is usual for signals to be of, or that, something. On an influence approach, there is no need for signals to have that representational component.

Reginald Cocroft and Claire Horisk

11

Learned signals and consistency of delivery: a case against receiver manipulation in animal communication

CARLOS A. BOTERO AND SELVINO R. DE KORT

11.1 Introduction

It was recently suggested that concepts such as 'information' and 'encoding' should be dropped from usage because they are not clearly defined when applied to animal communication (Rendall, Owren & Ryan, 2009; Owren, Rendall & Ryan, 2010). We disagree with that assessment and note that the utility of these concepts is firmly based on principles of statistical decision theory, probability monitoring, alternative coding schemes and Bayesian updating (reviewed in Bradbury & Vehrencamp, 2011). Nevertheless, we acknowledge that there remains a valid debate about how often and how much selection should favour the provision of information during animal communication.

One of the arguments used in support of the view that animal signals do not contain information is the observation that some signals trigger reflexive responses that startle receivers, capture their attention and/or elicit direct physiological changes within them (Rendall *et al.*, 2009). For example, the spectral structure of alarm calls in many species appears to be optimally designed to stimulate areas of the brain that regulate arousal and activation. Such design features imply that direct sensory stimulation may be a more parsimonious explanation for why receivers respond to alarm calls than the acquisition of 'information' about imminent dangers in the environment (see Rendall *et al.*, 2009). Nevertheless, examples abound of animal signals that are reasonably well

Animal Communication Theory: Information and Influence, ed. Ulrich Stegmann. Published by Cambridge University Press.

correlated with aspects of the world that are unknown to receivers but important for their fitness (Andersson, 1994; Maynard Smith & Harper, 2003; Searcy & Nowicki, 2005; Bradbury & Vehrencamp, 2011). In these systems, information is said to be 'encoded' as a general association between certain stimuli types (i.e. the different signal types or signal intensities) and alternative world states allowing the evolution of adaptive responses that are tailored to specific situations (for explicit theoretical formulations of these ideas see Bradbury & Vehrencamp, 2000; Botero *et al.*, 2010). For example, the tail length of male long-tailed widowbirds (*Euplectes progne*) contains information about individual quality that is useful in mate choice and male–male competition because, on average, individuals with longer tails show a slower decline in condition under intense physical activity (Pryke & Andersson, 2005). Details on the mechanisms that maintain such correlation over time and thereby promote the evolution of 'honest' signalling systems can be found elsewhere (e.g. Maynard Smith & Harper, 2003; Searcy & Nowicki, 2005; Bradbury & Vehrencamp, 2011).

Put simply, the current debate on the nature of animal communication appears to be concerned with whether receiver responses are strictly the product of (1) direct sensory stimulation, or (2) the acquisition of new relevant information. However, we think that the two suggested views are not mutually exclusive 'alternatives' and that this debate reflects some confusion about proximate and ultimate levels of analysis (*sensu* Tinbergen, 1963). Specifically, proponents of the non-informational view of communication have focused on proximate mechanisms of how signals work, whereas defendants of the informational view have mainly emphasised ultimate causation (see Guilford & Dawkins, 1991, for a review of similar issues). Furthermore, the idea that animal signals are optimally designed to excite perceptual mechanisms in receivers is not incongruent with an informational view of communication. The question is therefore not which view of animal communication is correct, but rather to what extent proximate and ultimate considerations provide a better understanding of signalling systems.

In our opinion, disregarding altogether the possibility of information transfer in animal communication is problematic and potentially short-sighted. Although reflexive attention-stimulation signals are by definition highly effective in eliciting responses, they are also easily exploited by senders and can therefore lead to maladaptive responses in receivers that will eventually promote selection against communication (Seyfarth *et al.*, 2010). We therefore expect such signalling systems to be highly unstable or to persist only when being 'manipulated' is somehow advantageous to receivers or when ignoring misleading stimuli is simply too costly. In contrast, signalling systems based on the provision of information are likely to be stable under a broader range of conditions because they allow receivers a choice and, therefore, a greater chance of benefiting from the exchange (Maynard Smith & Harper, 2003; Searcy & Nowicki, 2005; Bradbury & Vehrencamp, 2011).

To explore these issues, we review in this chapter recently discovered links between song learning ability in oscine birds and various aspects of individual quality that are relevant to potential receivers (Byers, 2007; Botero *et al.*, 2009b; de Kort *et al.*, 2009b). More specifically, we examine the evidence that song consistency, or the ability to produce virtually identical repetitions of any given song component, is a signal that does not conform with the expected demands of reflexive attention-stimulation of receivers. We argue that in this type of communication system, the stimulus that elicits the strongest neurological response (i.e. a deviant song) is precisely what senders should try to avoid in order to be perceived as attractive by females or intimidating by rivals. Thus, selection acts against signal structures that startle or otherwise produce a neurological response in receivers (i.e. less consistent song) not because these stimuli are more costly to produce but because they are associated with less attractive or less intimidating senders. Senders are unable to manipulate receivers in this system because consistency cannot be exaggerated and because their only alternative (i.e. to produce less consistent songs) could lower their own fitness. We conclude that the use of song consistency as a signal cannot be explained without reference to information transfer, and suggest that the basic principles discussed in this chapter may also apply to other signalling systems in which displays require practice or learning.

11.2 Information content of song learning

The acoustic structure of bird songs, like that of many other animal signals, is shaped through sexual selection via mate choice and the competition for mates. Song is a channel of communication in which a variety of parameters can be set, each potentially correlated with different sender attributes and exposed to different pressures of selection. For example, the rate at which songs are produced may be correlated with a sender's condition, whereas the number of song types it sings (i.e. its repertoire size) may correlate with its immunocompetence or resource-holding potential (Vehrencamp, 2000). Playback experiments have repeatedly demonstrated that receivers not only respond to variation in many of these subtle parameters but also that they do so in a way that is consistent with the idea of adaptive information provision. For example, females tend to mate preferentially with males with more elaborate song displays, and rivals tend to avoid them (Collins, 2004). What truly sets bird songs apart from most other sexually selected signals is that their production, at least in oscines, hummingbirds and parrots, requires learning (Farries, 2001; Beecher & Brenowitz, 2005).

Because learning to sing and storing learned songs in memory bear many similarities with other cognitive processes (Nowicki & Searcy, 2011), it has been suggested that bird songs can provide information on general cognitive ability (Nowicki *et al.*, 2000; Boogert, Giraldeau & Lefebvre, 2008; Botero *et al.*, 2009a; Boogert *et al.*, 2011). Recent experimental studies have provided preliminary, yet not unconditional support for this hypothesis. For example, captive male zebra finches, *Taeniopygia guttata*, with more complex songs show a faster learning curve when mastering a novel foraging task than individuals with simpler songs (Boogert *et al.*, 2008), and wild male song sparrows, *Melospiza melodia*, with larger song repertoires learn more quickly to reach around rather than to peck directly at mealworms presented behind clear Plexiglas (detour-reaching task; see Boogert *et al.*, 2011). These results indicate that by evaluating an individual's song learning abilities, receivers may gain information about the singer's ability to learn in other contexts or to solve certain types of problems. But how general is that information? Should we expect better singers to be generally smarter and song learning to reflect an individual's ability to acquire, store and process information in every other context? Although this question is an active area of research (see Nowicki & Searcy, 2011), the preliminary answer appears to be no. For example, a variety of studies have shown that selection on specific cognitive tasks may promote localised changes in areas of the brain related to the performance of those tasks rather than general cognitive improvements (e.g. Pravosudov & Clayton, 2002; Shettleworth, 2003; Garamszegi & Eens, 2004; Healy, de Kort & Clayton, 2005; Sherry, 2006). In addition, in some species there appears to be no correlation among individual performances in different cognitive tasks (Boogert *et al.*, 2011; Keagy, Savard & Borgia, 2011). These results suggest that cognition, just as song, may be more properly viewed as a multidimensional entity, at least in birds, rather than a single trait, and that different features of song learning may relate to very different cognitive abilities (see Shettleworth, 2010).

One cognitive trait with promising links to the evolution of bird song is the ability to copy or learn complex motor patterns. Motor control areas in the avian brain show remarkable anatomical and topographic similarities with the song control system (Jarvis, 2004; Finlay, Cheung & Darlington, 2005; Feenders *et al.*, 2008). In particular, there are striking parallels between the neural control of feeding and singing, perhaps because both of these activities rely on the movement of some of the same head, beak and tongue muscles (Dubbeldam, 1997). Besides being located in areas immediately adjacent to the song system, more general motor control areas in the bird brain are also organised into anterior and posterior pathways, and there appears to be a similar distinction between nuclei in charge of movement and nuclei involved in fine-tuning the motor patterns during learning (Feenders *et al.*, 2008). In addition, recent evidence suggests that two important nuclei in the song system (HVC and RA) are active during the learning and sequencing of feeding movements and food-related associative tasks (Tokarev *et al.*, 2011). Taken together, these studies indicate that a singer's ability to learn songs is likely to reflect its ability to learn and reproduce certain other complex motor patterns, especially those involving the head, beak and tongue (see Sakata & Vehrencamp, 2012 for a review). Because such movements are relevant for survival, feeding, fighting and predator avoidance, the information provided by song is therefore likely to have generalised adaptive value in the context of sexual selection.

A relevant distinction at this point is the difference between quantity and quality metrics of song learning. Quantity metrics include the number of different song types an individual can learn (i.e. its repertoire size) and the variety with which these types are presented to receivers (e.g. song versatility; see Derrickson, 1988). Quality metrics, on the other hand, include measures of the ability to sing demanding song types (e.g. song complexity or trill performance; see Podos, 1997), and the ability to copy song models accurately (Nowicki, Peters & Podos, 2002; Holveck *et al.*, 2008). Based on this distinction, we propose that quantity-related metrics of song learning should reflect an individual's ability to process and commit to memory a number of motor patterns, whereas quality-related metrics should more closely indicate its ability to acquire and reproduce these patterns in an accurate and consistent fashion.

The acoustic similarity between renditions of a given song type or syllable type within a song, also known as song consistency (Byers, 2007; Botero *et al.*, 2009b; de Kort *et al.*, 2009b), has recently received an increased amount of attention as a non-subjective measurement of the quality of song learning. A number of studies have shown that song consistency is related to the singer's fitness. In the tropical mockingbird, *Mimus gilvus*, males with greater song consistency have higher reproductive success and enjoy higher dominance ranks (Botero *et al.*, 2009b). Similarly, male black-capped chickadees, *Poecile atricapillus*, with more consistent frequency jumps between the two notes of their fee-bee song tend to achieve higher dominance ranks than less consistent rivals (Christie, Mennill & Ratcliffe, 2004). In the great tit, *Parus major*, older individuals are able to maintain more consistent inter-song intervals than inexperienced males (Lambrechts & Dhondt, 1988; Rivera-Gutierrez, Pinxten & Eens, 2010, 2011). A similar association between age and the ability to produce more consistent repetitions of each song type has been recorded in the banded wren, *Thryophilus pleurostictus* (de Kort *et al.*, 2009b), the tropical mockingbird (Botero *et al.*, 2009b) and the great reed warbler, *Acrocephalus arundinaceus* (Wegrzyn, Leniowski & Osiejuk, 2010). Male zebra finches from smaller broods also tend to produce more consistent song motifs than those from larger broods (Holveck *et al.*, 2008), highlighting the importance of early-life conditions for the development of song learning (Nowicki, Peters & Podos, 1998).

In addition to the various studies supporting a correlation between male quality and song consistency, several lines of evidence indicate that this aspect of song learning is perceived by receivers and used in sexual selection. In the blue tit, *Parus caeruleus*, females mated to individuals with more consistent inter-song intervals produce larger clutches (Poesel, Foerster & Kempenaers, 2001), and in the chestnut-sided warbler, *Dendroica pensylvanica* (Byers, 2007), and the banded wren, *T. pleurostictus* (Cramer *et al.*, 2011), females prefer extra-pair mates with more consistent songs than their current social partners. Additionally, male receivers in both the banded wren and the great tit respond differentially to playback stimuli that vary only in song consistency (de Kort *et al.*, 2009b; Rivera-Gutierrez *et al.*, 2011).

The observed relationship between age and song consistency (Jones, Ten Cate & Slater, 1996; de Kort *et al.*, 2009b; Rivera-Gutierrez *et al.*, 2010) suggests that the ability to repeat each song type in a consistent fashion may be an acquired trait that improves with practice. This possibility is important because practice cannot be cheated, indicating a potential for song consistency to act as an honest indicator of experience. Although it is not clear what exactly needs to be practised, spectral analysis of the songs of the banded wren may give an indication. In this species, the individual notes in a trill are the units of repetition subject to selection for consistency. These trill notes of the banded wren show a bimodal distribution in amplitude (see Figure 11.1), similar to that observed in the notes of the northern cardinal, *Cardinalis cardinalis*. In the latter species, the temporary reduction in power at the middle of a trill note is associated with a transition from using the left versus the right syrinx to produce the different portions of the frequency sweep (Suthers & Goller, 1997; Suthers,Goller & Pytte, 1999). Young banded wrens often show a disconnection between the higher and lower frequency portions of a trill note, suggesting that they are not yet able to coordinate appropriately the movement of these two sound sources. In addition, both adult and young banded wrens sometimes show a distinct transition between singing narrow and broad bandwidth trills, possibly due to the cessation of sound production with one of the syrinxes (see Figure 11.2). Consistency in reproduction of trill notes is therefore likely to be achieved, at least in some cases, by improving the neuromuscular coordination of the left and right syrinx (see Suthers, 2004).

In conclusion, the current evidence is consistent with the hypotheses that song consistency is associated with multiple aspects of male quality, particularly those related to motor ability, and that receivers make use of this parameter during mate choice and agonistic behaviour. We now turn our

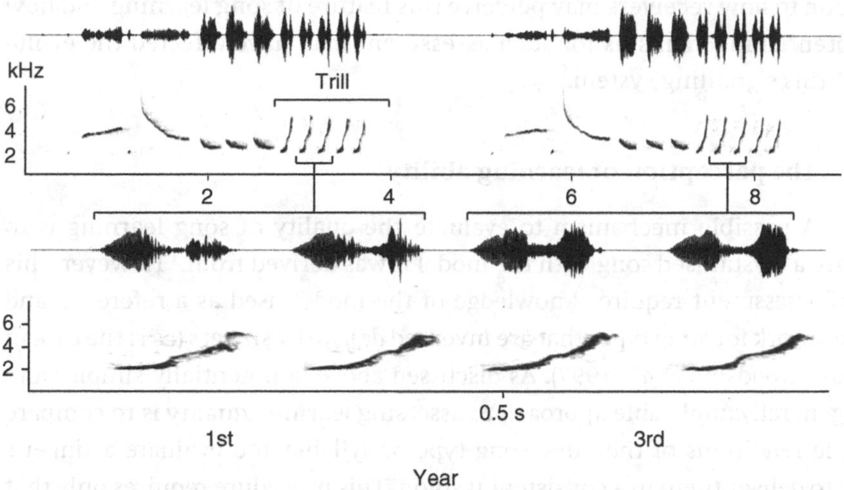

Figure 11.1 A waveform and spectrogram of a song type sung by a banded wren in its first breeding season (left) and the same song type sung by the same male in its third breeding season (top panel). Trill notes are enlarged in the bottom panel. Note in the waveform that each trill note shows two peaks in amplitude. Spectrogram settings: FFT (fast Fourier transform) size: 512 Hz, Hamming window, time resolution = 2.67 ms, frequency resolution = 94 Hz.

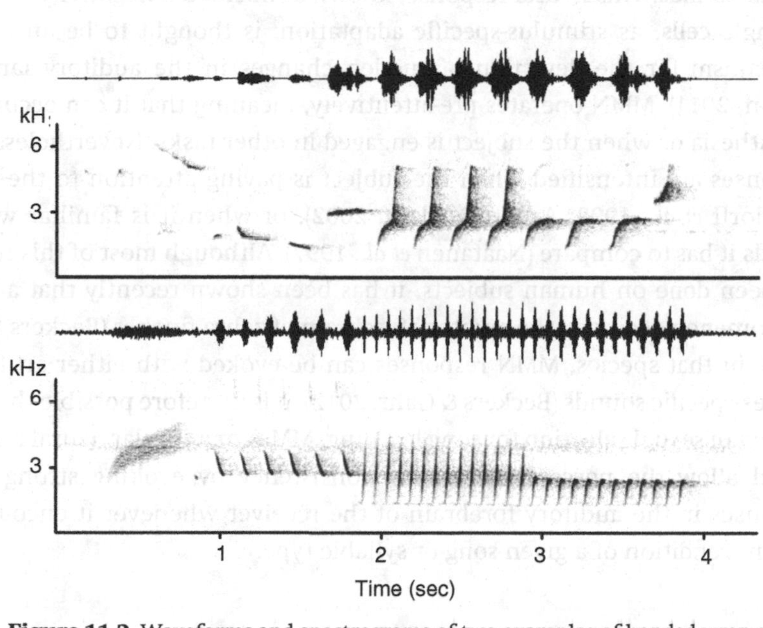

Figure 11.2 Waveforms and spectrograms of two examples of banded wren songs that show a discrete transition between wide and narrow frequency bandwidth use in the trill (latter) part of the song.

attention to how receivers may perceive this feature of song learning and how the potential mechanisms for such assessment may have affected the evolution of this signalling system.

11.3 The perception of learning ability

A possible mechanism to evaluate the quality of song learning is to compare a crystallised song with the model it was derived from.[1] However, this type of assessment requires knowledge of the model used as a reference and does not work for song types that are invented *de novo* by singers (as is the case in catbirds; Kroodsma *et al.*, 1997). As discussed above, a potentially simpler and more generally applicable approach to assessing learning quality is to compare multiple renditions of the same song type or syllable and evaluate a singer's ability to deliver them in a consistent fashion. This procedure requires only that each song type or syllable is repeated multiple times within the sampling period and does not rely on prior experience with a given song type or syllable or a common exposure to a reference model.

But can receivers perceive the subtle differences that are involved in the comparison of highly similar sounds? Auditory neurons in a variety of organisms exhibit responses to deviant stimuli that are presented within a string of similar sounds. This neural response, known as mismatch negativity (MMN) or, in single cells, as stimulus-specific adaptation, is thought to be an adaptive mechanism for the detection of sudden changes in the auditory landscape (Picton, 2011). MMN operates pre-attentively, meaning that it can occur under anaesthesia or when the subject is engaged in other tasks. Nevertheless, MMN responses are intensified when the subject is paying attention to the stimuli (Woldorff *et al.*, 1998; Arnott & Alain, 2002), or when it is familiar with the sounds it has to compare (Näätanen *et al.*, 1997). Although most of this research has been done on human subjects, it has been shown recently that a similar phenomenon occurs in the auditory forebrain of zebra finches (Beckers & Gahr, 2010). In that species, MMN responses can be evoked with either artificial or species-specific sounds (Beckers & Gahr, 2012). It is therefore possible that in the context of sexual selection for song learning, MMN, or a similar neural response, would allow the perception of song consistency by evoking strong neural responses in the auditory forebrain of the receiver whenever it encounters a deviant rendition of a given song or syllable type.

[1] Songs are called 'crystallised' if they have already been learned by the individual and can no longer be changed.

Regardless of the actual neural mechanism involved, a communication system based on the detection of slightly deviant repeats in a train of similar sounds is not conducive to receiver manipulation and is therefore inconsistent with the strictly non-informational view of animal communication (see Rendall *et al.*, 2009; Owren *et al.*, 2010). Specifically, contrary to the suggestion that signals per se should have a structure that is arousing and attention getting, the stimulus that most captures the receivers' attention in this type of communication system (i.e. a deviant song) is precisely what senders should try to avoid in order to appear attractive to females or intimidating to rivals. Moreover, the detection of deviant exemplars in a train of repeated stimuli appears to be independent of the acoustic structure of the song types being repeated because MMN responses can be triggered by very different acoustic stimuli in birds (Beckers & Gahr, 2010, 2012). Furthermore, the fact that MMN responses do not occur after a single presentation of a stimulus (see Sams *et al.*, 1985; Cowan *et al.*, 1993) indicates that what matters in this case is not the acoustic structure of the sound type itself but rather the similarity among repetitions of any given sound.

In a signalling system based on song consistency, selection is likely to favour not only the receiver's ability to perceive subtle differences between similar sounds but also the sender's behaviours that could potentially facilitate this task. Results from auditory testing in the Eurasian starling, *Sturnus vulgaris*, suggest that quick repetition of signals is crucial for the assessment of song consistency. Zokoll, Klump & Langemann (2007, 2008) exposed subjects to a sample stimulus followed by a silent interval and then a test stimulus. The subjects were required to indicate whether sample and test stimuli were the same and were subsequently rewarded if correct, or punished if not. These experiments showed that starlings have an auditory memory in these circumstances of roughly 20 s for spectral parameters and 12 s for temporal parameters, and that memory retention can increase with a greater number of repetitions of sample stimuli. Consistent with these observations, all species that have been evaluated with respect to song consistency tend to repeat syllable or song types in close temporal proximity (a behaviour that is common among many songbirds). Furthermore, most of these species repeat a single syllable type multiple times before switching to another one, either as part of a trill or within a syllable bout. In species exposed to strong selection for repertoire size, such as mockingbirds or wrens, this type of short-term repetition is surprising because such species are expected to maximise vocal versatility and therefore should not repeat any signal at all (see Collins, 2004). Thus, short-term repetitiveness is likely to have arisen from selection for behaviours that facilitate the assessment of song consistency, especially in cases in which quantifying repertoire size is too time-consuming or prohibitively demanding on the receiver's cognitive abilities (Botero *et al.*, 2008). In addition, consecutive repetition could also be a target of selection by receivers because it can induce exhaustion in the singer and is therefore difficult to cheat (Lambrechts & Dhondt, 1986; but see Brumm *et al.*, 2009). In great tits, song consistency decreases towards the end of a singing bout, and individual quality is related to the number and consistency of consecutive repetitions of a single phrase type (Lambrechts & Dhondt, 1986).

The assessment of learning ability appears to be facilitated through slightly different behaviours in the context of intra-sexual competition. In particular, rival songbirds often engage in counter-singing interactions during which both parties match each other's songs (Krebs, Ashcroft & Vanorsdol, 1981; Whitney & Miller, 1983; Falls, 1985; Stoddard *et al.*, 1992; Shackleton & Ratcliffe, 1994; Beecher *et al.*, 2000; Vehrencamp, 2001; Mennill & Ratcliffe, 2004). By reproducing a common motor programme in close temporal proximity, song matching could facilitate the comparison of rivals' performance levels, motor control and learning abilities (Logue & Forstmeier, 2008). Interestingly, matching may sometimes be restricted to the most demanding elements of a song. For example, male banded wrens sing songs composed of a versatile introduction and a repetitive trill, but during counter-singing, they only match the trilled portion of the song (de Kort *et al.*, 2009a).

11.4 Concluding remarks

There is ample and growing evidence that consistency in singing is a signal of learning ability in several species of songbirds. This metric of learning ability is (a) correlated with different aspects of individual quality such as age, fecundity and social dominance, and (b) correlated with receiver behaviour in both field observations and playback experiments. In addition, circumstantial evidence indicates that the display of song consistency is an evolved signal rather than a cue (see the introduction to this volume) because unlike in cues, senders are not obliged to display consistency in songs. Instead they may choose to sing or not, and to repeat or not each song type in close temporal proximity. The latter is especially apparent in species that facilitate the assessment of consistency via short-term repetition in spite of experiencing concurrent selection for high vocal versatility.

The idiosyncrasies of this communication system are particularly relevant to the current debate about the information content (or lack thereof) of animal signals. First, song consistency relies on properly functioning motor control areas in the brain and appears to be achieved through practice, meaning that it is likely to be an honest indicator of the learning abilities of the singer (an 'index' signal *sensu* Vehrencamp, 2000; Bradbury & Vehrencamp, 2011). Second, this signalling system appears to be based on the perception of signalling states (i.e. deviant renditions of a given song or syllable type) that should be actively avoided by the sender. Given these two features, it is unlikely that senders can exploit receiver sensitivities to manipulate them in any sense. The best a singer can do is to perform at the best of his ability because any deviation from such standard will negatively affect his fitness by rendering him less attractive to females or less intimidating to rivals. Therefore, the hypothesis that animal sounds are designed to elicit a neural response in the receiver regardless of sender correlates (Rendall *et al.*, 2009; Owren *et al.*, 2010) does not appear to hold in this particular case.

The issues described here may also apply more generally to any communication system that relies on ritualisation. In a stimulating essay, Zahavi (1980) pointed out that standardised displays can improve a receiver's ability to compare senders. Furthermore, he pointed out that variation among multiple renditions of a ritualised movement can provide information about the reliability of the signal itself. In other words, an occasional good display may be a matter of luck but a set of consistently good displays can only be achieved by high-quality senders. These ideas closely match the arguments developed above for song consistency and song matching. For example, the visual perception of variability in movement displays is likely to be subject to similar principles to the acoustic perception of consistency because in both cases, receivers must detect deviations from a general pattern (or a standard). Similarly, in both situations receivers benefit from sampling the same behaviour multiple times in short periods of time. Not surprisingly, ritualised movements are also often repeated in close temporal proximity (e.g. Jordao, Curto & Oliveira, 2007).

In conclusion, regardless of the signalling modality employed, we propose that senders should be unable to manipulate receivers whenever repeatability itself is the signal under consideration. Taken together, the arguments we have developed in this chapter suggest that receiver manipulation, one of the basic premises of the non-informational view of animal communication, may not be possible in many visual or acoustic ritualised displays. We therefore advocate the continued use of the concept of information in animal communication and suggest that the issues raised in the non-informational debate are more relevant to the possible origin of signals than to the issue of their evolutionary stability.

Acknowledgements

We would like to express our gratitude to Gabriël Beckers, Jack Bradbury, Sarah Collins, Karolina Kluk-de Kort, William Searcy and Sandra

Vehrencamp for discussion and comments on earlier versions of this chapter and Ulrich Stegmann for inviting us to contribute to this volume and for being an excellent editor.

References

Andersson, M. (1994). *Sexual Selection*. Princeton, NJ: Princeton University Press.

Arnott, S. R. & Alain, C. (2002). Stepping out of the spotlight: MMN attenuation as a function of distance from the attended location. *Neuroreport*, **13**, 2209–2212.

Beckers, G. J. L. & Gahr, M. (2010). Neural processing of short-term recurrence in songbird vocal communication. *PLoS ONE*, **5**, e11129.

Beckers, G. J. L. & Gahr, M. (2012). Large-scale synchronized activity during vocal deviance detection in the zebra finch auditory forebrain. *Journal of Neuroscience*, **32**, 10594–10608.

Beecher, M. D. & Brenowitz, E. A. (2005). Functional aspects of song learning in birds. *Trends in Ecology and Evolution*, **20**, 143–149.

Beecher, M. D., Campbell, S. E., Burt, J. M., Hill, C. E. & Nordby, J. C. (2000). Song-type matching between neighbouring song sparrows. *Animal Behaviour*, **59**, 21–27.

Boogert, N., Giraldeau, L. A. & Lefebvre, L. (2008). Song complexity correlates with learning ability in zebra finch males. *Animal Behaviour*, **76**, 1735–1741.

Boogert, N. J., Anderson, R. C., Peters, S., Searcy, W. A. & Nowicki, S. (2011). Song repertoire size in male song sparrows correlates with detour reaching, but not with other cognitive measures. *Animal Behaviour*, **81**, 1209–1216.

Botero, C. A., Boogert, N. J., Vehrencamp, S. L. & Lovette, I. J. (2009a). Climatic patterns predict the elaboration of song displays in mockingbirds. *Current Biology*, **19**, 1151–1155.

Botero, C. A., Mudge, A. E., Koltz, A. M., Hochachka, W. M. & Vehrencamp, S. L. (2008). How reliable are the methods for estimating repertoire size? *Ethology*, **114**, 1227–1238.

Botero, C. A., Pen, I., Komdeur, J. & Weissing, F. J. (2010). The evolution of individual variation in communication strategies. *Evolution*, **64**, 3123–3133.

Botero, C. A., Rossman, R. J., Caro, L. M. *et al.* (2009b). Syllable type consistency is related to age, social status, and reproductive success in the tropical mockingbird. *Animal Behaviour*, **77**, 701–706.

Bradbury, J. W. & Vehrencamp, S. L. (2000). Economic models of animal communication. *Animal Behaviour*, **59**, 259–268.

Bradbury, J. W. & Vehrencamp, S. L. (2011). *The Principles of Animal Communication*, 2nd edn. Sunderland, MA: Sinauer Associates.

Brumm, H., Lachlan, R. F., Riebel, K. & Slater, P. B. J. (2009). On the function of song type repertoires: testing the 'antiexhaustion hypothesis' in chaffinches. *Animal Behaviour*, **77**, 37–42.

Byers, B. E. (2007). Extrapair paternity in chestnut-sided warblers is correlated with consistent vocal performance. *Behavioral Ecology*, **18**, 130–136.

Christie, P. J., Mennill, D. J. & Ratcliffe, L. M. (2004). Pitch shifts and song structure indicate male quality in the dawn chorus of black-capped chickadees. *Behavioral Ecology and Sociobiology*, **55**, 341–348.

Collins, S. (2004). Vocal fighting and flirting: the functions of birdsong. In P. Marler & H. Slabbekoorn, eds., *Nature's Music, the Science of Birdsong*. San Diego, CA: Elsevier Academic Press.

Cowan, N., Winkler, I., Teder, W. & Naatanen, R. (1993). Memory prerequisites of the mismatch negativity in the auditory event-related potential (ERP). *Journal of Experimental Psychology: Human Perception and Performance*, **19**, 909–921.

Cramer, E. R., Hall, M. L., de Kort, S. R., Lovette, I. J. & Vehrencamp, S. L. (2011). Infrequent extra pair paternity in banded wrens, synchronously tropical passerines. *Condor*, **113**, 637–645.

de Kort, S. R., Eldermire, E. R. B., Cramer, E. R. A. & Vehrencamp, S. L. (2009a). The deterrent effect of bird song in territory defense. *Behavioral Ecology*, **20**, 200–206.

de Kort, S. R., Eldermire, E. R. B., Valderrama, S., Botero, C. A. & Vehrencamp, S. L. (2009b). Trill consistency is an age-related assessment signal in banded wrens. *Proceedings of the Royal Society of London Series B: Biological Sciences*, **276**, 2315–2321.

Derrickson, K. C. (1988). Variation in repertoire presentation in northern mockingbirds. *Condor*, **90**, 592–606.

Dubbeldam, J. L. (1997). Intratelencephalic sensorimotor circuits in birds – what have feeding and vocalization in common? *Netherlands Journal of Zoology*, **48**(3), 199–212.

Falls, J. B. (1985). Song matching in western meadowlarks. *Canadian Journal of Zoology Revue Canadienne de Zoologie*, **63**, 2520–2524.

Farries, M. A. (2001). The oscine song system considered in the context of the avian brain: lessons learned from comparative neurobiology. *Brain Behavior and Evolution*, **58**, 80–100.

Feenders, G., Liedvogel, M., Rivas, M. *et al.* (2008). Molecular mapping of movement-associated areas in the avian brain: a motor theory for vocal learning origin. *PLoS ONE*, **3**, e1768.

Finlay, B., Cheung, D. & Darlington, R. (2005). Developmental constraints on or developmental structure in brain evolution? In Y. Munakata & M. Johnson, eds., *Attention and Performance XXI. Process of Change in Brain and Cognitive Development*. Oxford: Oxford University Press, pp. 131–162.

Garamszegi, L. Z. & Eens, M. (2004). Brain space for a learned task: strong intraspecific evidence for neural correlates of singing behavior in songbirds. *Brain Research Reviews*, **44**, 187–193.

Guilford, T. & Dawkins, M. S. (1991). Receiver psychology and the evolution of animal signals. *Animal Behaviour*, **42**, 1–14.

Healy, S. D., de Kort, S. R. & Clayton, N. S. (2005). The hippocampus, spatial memory and food hoarding: a puzzle revisited. *Trends in Ecology and Evolution*, **20**, 17–22.

Holveck, M. J., de Castro, A. C. V., Lachlan, R. F., ten Cate, C. & Riebel, K. (2008). Accuracy of song syntax learning and singing consistency signal early condition in zebra finches. *Behavioral Ecology*, **19**, 1267–1281.

Jarvis, E. D. (2004). Learned birdsong and the neurobiology of human language. *Annals of the New York Academy of Sciences*, **1016**, 749–777.

Jones, A. E., ten Cate, C. & Slater, P. J. B. (1996). Early experience and plasticity of song in adult male zebra finches (*Taeniopygia guttata*). *Journal of Comparative Psychology*, **110**, 354–369.

Jordao, J. M., Curto, A. F. & Oliveira, R. F. (2007). Stereotypy and variation in the claw waving display of the fiddler crab *Uca tangeri*. *Acta Ethologica*, **10**, 55–62.

Keagy, J., Savard, J.-F. & Borgia, G. (2011). Complex relationship between multiple measures of cognitive ability and male mating success in satin bowerbirds, *Ptilonorhynchus violaceus*. *Animal Behaviour*, **81**, 1063–1070.

Krebs, J. R., Ashcroft, R. & Vanorsdol, K. (1981). Song matching in the great tit *Parus major L*. *Animal Behaviour*, **29**, 918–923.

Kroodsma, D. E., Houlihan, P. W., Fallon, P. A. & Wells, J. A. (1997). Song development by grey catbirds. *Animal Behaviour*, **54**, 457–464.

Lambrechts, M. & Dhondt, A. A. (1986). Male quality, reproduction, and survival in the great tit (*Parus major*). *Behavioral Ecology and Sociobiology*, **19**, 57–63.

Lambrechts, M. & Dhondt, A. A. (1988). The anti-exhaustion hypothesis – a new hypothesis to explain song performance and song switching in the great tit. *Animal Behaviour*, **36**, 327–334.

Logue, D. M. & Forstmeier, W. (2008). Constrained performance in a communication network: implications for the function of song-type matching and for the evolution of multiple ornaments. *American Naturalist*, **172**, 34–41.

Maynard Smith, J. & Harper, D. (2003). *Animal Signals*. Oxford: Oxford University Press.

Mennill, D. J. & Ratcliffe, L. M. (2004). Overlapping and matching in the song contests of black-capped chickadees. *Animal Behaviour*, **67**, 441–450.

Näätanen, R., Lehtokoski, A., Lennes, M. *et al.* (1997). Language-specific phoneme representations revealed by electric and magnetic brain responses. *Nature*, **385**, 432–434.

Nowicki, S. & Searcy, W. A. (2011). Are better singers smarter? *Behavioral Ecology*, **22**, 10–11.

Nowicki, S., Hasselquist, D., Bensch, S. & Peters, S. (2000). Nestling growth and song repertoire sire in great reed warblers: evidence for song learning as an indicator mechanism in mate choice. *Proceedings of the Royal Society of London Series B: Biological Sciences*, **267**, 2419–2424.

Nowicki, S., Peters, S. & Podos, J. (1998). Song learning, early nutrition and sexual selection in songbirds. *American Zoologist*, **38**, 179–190.

Nowicki, S., Searcy, W. A. & Peters, S. (2002). Quality of song learning affects female response to male bird song. *Proceedings of the Royal Society of London Series B: Biological Sciences*, **269**, 1949–1954.

Owren, M. J., Rendall, D. & Ryan, M. J. (2010). Redefining animal signaling: influence versus information in communication. *Biology and Philosophy*, **25**, 755–780.

Picton, T. W. (2011). *Human Auditory Evoked Potentials*. San Diego, CA: Plural Publishing.

Podos, J. (1997). A performance constraint on the evolution of trilled vocalizations in a songbird family (Passeriformes: Emberizidae). *Evolution*, **51**(2), 537–551.

Poesel, A., Foerster, K. & Kempenaers, B. (2001). The dawn song of the blue tit *Parus caeruleus* and its role in sexual selection. *Ethology*, **107**, 521–531.

Pravosudov, V. V. & Clayton, N. S. (2002). A test of the adaptive specialization hypothesis: population differences in caching, memory, and the hippocampus in black-capped chickadees (*Poecile atricapilla*). *Behavioral Neuroscience*, **116**, 515–522.

Pryke, S. R. & Andersson, S. (2005). Experimental evidence for female choice and energetic costs of male tail elongation in red-collared widowbirds. *Biological Journal of the Linnean Society*, **86**, 35–43.

Rendall, D., Owren, M. J. & Ryan, M. J. (2009). What do animal signals mean? *Animal Behaviour*, **78**, 233–240.

Rivera-Gutierrez, H. F., Pinxten, R. & Eens, M. (2010). Multiple signals for multiple messages: great tit, *Parus major*, song signals age and survival. *Animal Behaviour*, **80**, 451–459.

Rivera-Gutierrez, H. F., Pinxten, R. & Eens, M. (2011). Songs differing in consistency elicit differential aggressive response in territorial birds. *Biology Letters*, **7**, 339–342.

Sakata, J. T. & Vehrencamp, S. L. (2012). Integrating perspectives on vocal performance and consistency. *Journal of Experimental Biology*, **215**, 201–209.

Sams, M., Hamalainen, M., Antervo, A. *et al.* (1985). Cerebral neuromagnetic responses evoked by short auditory stimuli. *Clinical Neurophysiology*, **61**, 254–266.

Searcy, W. A. & Nowicki, S. (2005). *The Evolution of Animal Communication. Reliability and Deception in Signaling Systems.* Princeton, NJ: Princeton University Press.

Seyfarth, R. M., Cheney, D. L., Bergman, T., Fischer, J., Zuberbuehler, K. & Hammerschmidt, K. (2010). The central importance of information in studies of animal communication. *Animal Behaviour*, **80**, 3–8.

Shackleton, S. A. & Ratcliffe, L. (1994). Matched counter-singing signals escalation of aggression in black-capped chickadees (*Parus atricapillus*). *Ethology*, **97**, 310–316.

Sherry, D. F. (2006). Neuroecology. *Annual Review of Psychology*, **57**, 167–197.

Shettleworth, S. (2010). *Cognition, Evolution, and Behavior.* New York: Oxford University Press.

Shettleworth, S. J. (2003). Memory and hippocampal specialization in food-storing birds: challenges for research on comparative cognition. *Brain Behavior and Evolution*, **62**, 108–116.

Stoddard, P. K., Beecher, M. D., Campbell, S. E. & Horning, C. L. (1992). Song-type matching in the song sparrow. *Canadian Journal of Zoology Revue Canadienne de Zoologie*, **70**, 1440–1444.

Suthers, R. A. (2004). How birds sing and why it matters. In P. Marler & H. Slabbekoorn, eds., *Nature's Music: The Science of Birdsong*. San Diego, CA: Elsevier Academic Press.

Suthers, R. A. & Goller, F. (1997). Motor correlates of vocal diversity. In V. Nolan, E. Ketterson & C. F. Thompson, eds., *Current Ornithology*. New York: Plenum Press.

Suthers, R. A., Goller, F. & Pytte, C. (1999). The neuromuscular control of bird song. *Philosophical Transactions of the Royal Society of London Series B: Biological Sciences*, **354**, 927–939.

Tinbergen, N. (1963). On aims and methods in ethology. *Zeitschrift für Tierpsychologie*, **20**, 410–433.

Tokarev, K., Tiunova, A., Scharff, C. & Anokhin, K. (2011). Food for song: expression of C-Fos and ZENK in the zebra finch song nuclei during food aversion learning. *PLoS ONE*, **6**(6), e21157.

Vehrencamp, S. L. (2000). Handicap, index and conventional signal elements of bird song. In Y. O. Espmark, T. Amundsen & G. Rosenqvist, eds., *Animal Signals: Signaling and Signal Design in Animal Communication*. Trondheim, Norway: Tapir Academic Press, pp. 277–300.

Vehrencamp, S. L. (2001). Is song-type matching a conventional signal of aggressive intentions? *Proceedings of the Royal Society of London Series B: Biological Sciences*, **268**, 1637–1642.

Wegrzyn, E., Leniowski, K. & Osiejuk, T. S. (2010). Whistle duration and consistency reflect philopatry and harem size in great reed warblers. *Animal Behaviour*, **79**, 1363–1372.

Whitney, C. L. & Miller, J. (1983). Song matching in the wood thrush (*Hylocichla mustelina*): a function of song dissimilarity. *Animal Behaviour*, **31**, 457–461.

Woldorff, M. G., Hillyard, S. A., Gallen, C. C., Hampson, S. R. & Bloom, F. E. (1998). Magnetoencephalographic recordings demonstrate attentional modulation of mismatch-related neural activity in human auditory cortex. *Psychophysiology*, **35**, 283–292.

Zahavi, A. (1980). Ritualization and the evolution of movement signals. *Behaviour*, **72**, 77–81.

Zokoll, M. A., Klump, G. M. & Langemann, U. (2007). Auditory short-term memory persistence for tonal signals in a songbird. *Journal of the Acoustical Society of America*, **121**, 2842–2851.

Zokoll, M. A., Klump, G. M. & Langemann, U. (2008). Auditory memory for temporal characteristics of sound. *Journal of Comparative Physiology A: Neuroethology Sensory Neural and Behavioral Physiology*, **194**, 457–467.

12

Information, inference and meaning in primate vocal behaviour

JULIA FISCHER

12.1 Introduction

It is a beautiful day in the Okavango delta in Botswana. A troop of baboons is assembling after their midday rest to cross one of the large flood plains. All of a sudden, fierce screams of a female baboon can be heard from behind some shrubs. One of the adult males jumps up and runs into the thickets, looking for the caller. The male is Wanda, and he has heard the screams of the female baboon Hannah. They have spent a great deal of time together in the last weeks since the birth of Hannah's infant Hecuba. Wanda was her consort male when she conceived, and it is very likely that he fathered the infant. What do Hannah's screams mean? Do they provide or contain information? And how can we best understand primate vocal communication anyway?

The last few years have seen a revival of the interest in the key concepts applied to the study of animal communication. Three major issues have emerged, namely how to explain signal evolution (e.g. Scott-Phillips, 2008; Skyrms, 2010), whether the concept of information is useful at all (Rendall, Owren & Ryan, 2009; Scarantino, 2010; Seyfarth *et al.*, 2010; Ruxton & Schaefer, 2011) and whether linguistic approaches (see Zuberbühler, 2006; Fischer, 2010; Fitch, 2010 for some recent reviews) generate valuable insights into primate (vocal) communication.

Building on previous work (specifically Fischer, 2011), I here expand my consideration of the information content of primate vocalisations. I will argue that the concept of information is valuable and well suited to capture many aspects of primate vocal communication. Applying Skyrms' (2010) conception

Animal Communication Theory: Information and Influence, ed. Ulrich Stegmann. Published by Cambridge University Press.

of information content and the value of information, I will discuss the importance of sampling regime on the assessment of production specificity and will address the problems of identifying information content when dealing with graded signal repertoires, which can be found in many primate (and terrestrial mammal) taxa. I will then consider the implications of these insights for our understanding of 'referential signalling' (Marler, Evans & Hanset, 1992), one of the dominant topics in vocal communication studies in the past decades.

12.2 Methodological considerations in the study of meaning

The staple method of elucidating animals' responses to calls is the use of playback experiments, in which select vocalisations are broadcast and responses are recorded. Incidentally, when Wanda came running to the site where the calls came from, all he encountered were two researchers nearby – Ryne Palombit and his field assistant Mokupi Mokupi. Palombit and colleagues compared male responses to calls from their female associates as well as to the screams of other females. A control condition consisted of playing back the calls of Hannah, for instance, to another male with whom she was not affiliated. Males consistently responded more strongly to the calls of their female associates than to other females' calls; and likewise, males did not respond much to the playbacks of other males' associates (Palombit, Seyfarth & Cheney, 1997). The authors concluded that the close associations between males and particular females – as long as these have a young infant – presumably contribute to the reproductive success of the male. But what else can we learn from these results? And how are the findings related to the debate laid out in this book?

First, the results imply that the screams carry individual specific signatures that allow listeners to infer who is calling. Of course, a detailed acoustic analysis would be needed to identify which combination of features contributes to these individual differences, but it would certainly be difficult to explain these results if there were no cues to individual identity. In principle, individual differences could be detected in the spectral characteristics of the calls, the temporal succession of the calls within a bout of screaming or both. In any case, the results strongly suggest that individual recognition takes place, as males responded specifically to their female friend's calls. Further, the results suggest that the males not only inferred who was calling but also had learned under which context screams occur – namely when females have been attacked. So far, all that is required is a combination of associative learning and simple inferential reasoning. Accordingly, the meaning of Hannah's screams to her group mates is that it is she who is screaming and that she has probably been attacked.

A more controversial issue is whether it is appropriate to assume that Hannah's screams transmitted information.

12.3 Animal communication as information transmission?

The idea that communication can be characterised as the transfer of information from the signaller to the recipient has repeatedly led to vivid debate (Krebs & Dawkins, 1984). More recently, the concept of information was considered useful as a by-product at best (Scott-Phillips, 2008) or not at all (Rendall *et al.*, 2009). Others, however, have argued that "information is a crucial currency" (Dall *et al.*, 2005, p. 187) in behaviour and evolution, with implications for adaptation to changes in environmental conditions (Dall *et al.*, 2005). Information plays a central role in genetics (e.g. Jablonka & Lamb, 2005; Wagner & Danchin, 2010) as well as neuroscience (e.g. Koch, 1999), and it thus seems puzzling to shun this concept in studies of animal communication. As I have argued in more detail elsewhere (Fischer, 2011), I think that 'information' is essential to understand communication, although some specific issues may warrant further clarification.

Information theory was initially developed to study the processes of encryption and subsequent retrieval of information in technical systems (Shannon & Weaver, 1949). Information is quantified in terms of entropy, which provides a measure of the uncertainty in predicting the outcome of an event. One may argue that there is a fundamental difference between Shannon information and biological information, but following Wagner and Danchin (2010), I would define biological information as that part of all the possible information that "can affect the phenotype in ways that may influence fitness" (Wagner & Danchin, 2010, p. 204). Moreover, conceiving information as a reduction of uncertainty (or an increase in predictability) provides a strong link to animal behaviour (Seyfarth & Cheney, 2003a). As Krebs and Dawkins (1984) noted, animals benefit from predicting the future behaviour of other animals in their world. There is ample evidence that signals in particular can be used to predict signallers' subsequent behaviour (Bauers, 1991; Hesler & Fischer, 2007) and upcoming events more generally (Seyfarth, Cheney & Marler, 1980; Zuberbühler, 2000). More recently, Dall and colleagues (2005) provided an explicit model of information use by animals, using statistical decision theory as the framework. While their model attempts to explain under which conditions animals should collect further information, it does not explicitly integrate the processing of signals.

Conceiving information as uncertainty reduction ties the definition of information tightly to the recipient. Thus I have argued that, in the very strict sense, animal communication does not consist of information transmission, and animal signals do not contain information (Fischer, 2011). Instead, I have proposed that information is generated by the recipient. Accordingly, statistical regularities in the environment are potentially informative, and signals contain *potential* information. Wagner and Danchin made a similar point: they noted that "a fact only becomes information after an organism detects it" (Wagner & Danchin, 2010, p. 207). They distinguish between potential and realised information, akin to the distinction between potential and realised energy. Yet, I believe that a more relaxed use of the term information is also acceptable, as long as one is aware that the definition of information in the sense of uncertainty reduction always requires a certain vantage point – somebody has to measure the statistical regularities in the environment and has to determine whether or not they can be used to predict the future or to extract the information content from a given signal. I will thus continue to speak of the 'information content' of specific signals (e.g. Pfefferle *et al.*, 2011) in studies of the correlation of acoustic signals with specific factors such as contextual or physiological variables.

At the centre of the recent debate (Rendall *et al.*, 2009; Seyfarth *et al.*, 2010) is the question of whether signallers indeed 'provide information'. The critics of the informational stance take up an earlier view according to which communication should be understood as manipulation, where senders benefit from influencing others to behave in a way that is in their own interest (Dawkins & Krebs, 1978; Rendall *et al.*, 2009). Certainly, Hannah the baboon does not 'provide information' in the caricature sense that she wraps the information into a little package to transmit it to the listener in order to change his knowledge state. Based on what we know, non-human primates have only a rudimentary understanding of other subjects' mental states (at best), so it seems very unlikely that Hannah calls to alter Wanda's knowledge state. It seems possible, though, that she calls with the intention to alter his behaviour, because she has learned from the past that her calling will lead him to come running. This is equivalent to the assumption that monkeys have first- but not second-order intentionality (Dennett, 1971) – that is, they behave in a way to change others' behaviour but not their mental states. The simplest explanation, however, would be that Hannah's screams are just an expression of internal state, such as her fear and arousal, or the degree of aversion she experiences (Fichtel, Hammerschmidt & Jürgens, 2001).

12.4 Signal design and information content

Scholars of primate vocal communication have attempted to map the structure of calls to various internal and external driving forces. At the same

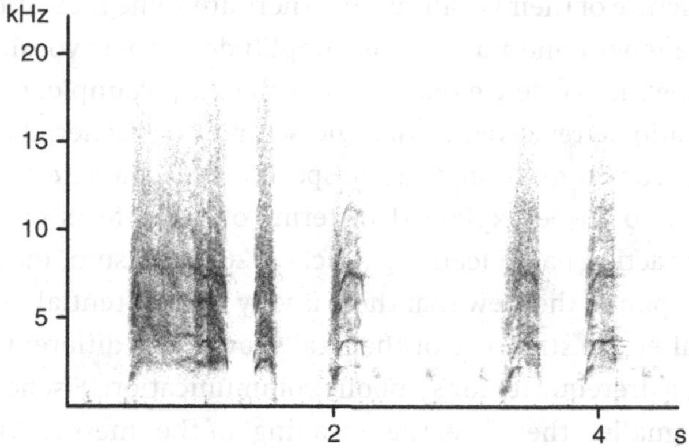

Figure 12.1 Spectrograms of female chacma baboon screams. Sampling frequency: 44.1 kHz, overlap 75%.

time, we have learned a great deal about the physics of sound production (Fitch & Hauser, 1995; Fitch, Neubauer & Herzel, 2002). These frameworks offer explanations for the signal design of Hannah's screams at different levels. Baboon screams, like those of many primates, are typically noisy and exhibit a sharp amplitude onset (Figure 12.1). In squirrel monkeys, calls vary with the degree of aversion and intensity (Fichtel *et al.*, 2001): that is, some variables change with the severity of aversion while others vary with intensity independently of whether the call is given in what an observer judges to be an aversive or hedonistic situation. Possibly, the structure of the screams is also influenced by the physiological stress response, specifically increased glucocorticoid levels. Another – non-mutually exclusive – explanation is that the structure of the calls is a by-product of the specifics of sound production when animals are threatened. Screams are produced with considerable air pressure, which leads to non-linear phenomena in the structure of the calls, such as sudden frequency shifts, additional spectral bands ('sub-harmonics') and deterministic chaos (Fitch *et al.*, 2002). At the same time, they reflect the degree of aversion. Recipients, however, also exert selective pressures on signallers. According to Owren and Rendall, such frequency characteristics have been selected because they have a direct effect on the physiology of the listener (Owren & Rendall, 1997, 2001). In other words, screams have taken the form they do because they achieve the desired effects, namely to repel the aggressor. To sum up, there are a number of possible non-mutually exclusive explanations for Hannah's calling, but it is difficult to rule out any of the possible assumptions with certainty.

In terms of the neural basis of vocal production in non-human primates, a large body of evidence suggests that non-human primates have little voluntary control over the structure of their vocalisations. There are some indications that they can control the length and possibly the amplitude of their vocalisations, but there is no compelling evidence that they are able, for example, to imitate each other's vocalisations (reviewed in Hammerschmidt & Fischer, 2008). The occurrence of vocal convergence and group-specific call characteristics that have been described could be explained in terms of the effects of sensory-motor integration or action-based learning (Fischer, 2008). In sum, most of the available evidence supports the view that there is very little potential for signallers to voluntarily alter the structure of their calls, or to use different calls in different situations, a prerequisite for symbolic communication (Fischer, 2010). At the level of the signaller, therefore, the 'meaning' of the 'message' remains rather elusive.

12.5 Problems inherent in the inference of meaning

Thanks to our ability to observe listeners' responses, we are able to deduce what the calls may mean *to the listeners*. A number of authors assume that the responses and the meaning are equivalent. I believe that it is important to distinguish between the two. Take the example of Hannah's screaming. As I have explained above, the meaning could be defined as the information (more on that later) the receiver obtains by recognising Hannah's identity and concluding that she must have been attacked. Empirically though, the meaning can only be inferred from the responses. Now let us assume that all the males in the group are able to recognise the caller and make an informed guess as to why she must be screaming. Yet, not all of them take action. How do we define the 'meaning' of the calls in such circumstances? Is the meaning of the calls for all the listeners in the group the same, namely something akin to "Hannah is being attacked", and do they then independently decide whether to take action or not? Or, alternatively, do the calls have no meaning to those that do not respond, while only for Wanda, the meaning would be, "She needs support"? It is next to impossible to know what goes on in the minds of animals that are not responding at all (and still difficult for those that do), but I would like to distinguish between the mental operations underlying the extraction of information and generation of meaning on the one hand and those that underpin overt responses on the other (Figure 12.2). Distinguishing between the two also facilitates the analysis of decision-making. For instance, some months later, when Hannah's infant has been weaned, her screaming may evoke only a simple head-turn from Wanda. He would still know who was calling and why – that is, he would retrieve the same amount of information from the signal – but there would be no need for him to come running to her aid. My

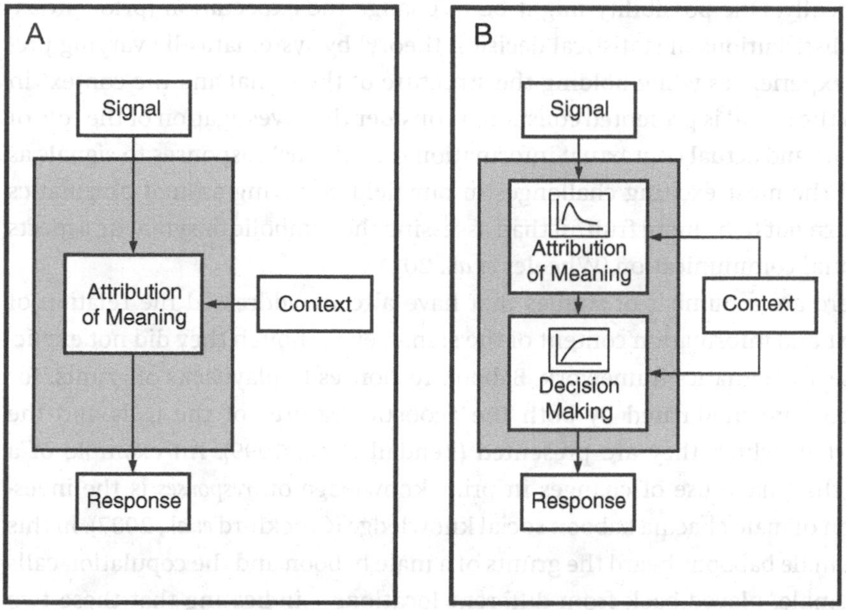

Figure 12.2 Two models to conceptualise the influence of signal and context in the attribution of meaning and the selection of responses to signals. **A**, According to Smith (1977), signals attain meaning by a combination of their features and the context in which they occur. **B**, In this model, attribution of meaning and decision-making are conceived as two different processes that are both affected by the context. The context may shift prior probabilities in response to previous experiences and current expectations; and it may affect cost–benefit ratios attributed to different types of responses.

view thus differs from Smith's (1977) argument that signals attain meaning by a combined assessment of signal features and the context in which they are given. I would instead argue that responses are chosen on the basis of signal information as well as contextual information (Fischer, 2011).

The importance of contextual information, however, should vary depending on the degree of production specificity, being more important for calls with low degrees of specificity. For instance, chacma baboon 'clear barks' are given when an individual has lost contact with the group or some specific individual, while 'harsh barks' are given in response to predators. Intermediate versions also occur (Fischer *et al.*, 2001a). Upon hearing such intermediate variants, animals may possibly rely on contextual information to classify the call. In sum, I suggest that one must distinguish between the influence the context may have on disambiguation on the one hand and the setting of the response criterion on the other, although I am aware of the difficulty in disentangling the two empirically. One possibility might be to change the expectation (prior probability distributions in statistical decision theory) by systematically varying previous experiences while holding the structure of the signal and the context in which the signal is presented constant. I consider the investigation of the role of previous and actual contextual information on animals' responses to signals as one of the most exciting challenges in our field. Studying animal pragmatics may turn out to be more fruitful than assessing the symbolic or syntactic aspects of animal communication (Wheeler *et al.*, 2011).

There are a number of studies that have already addressed the relation of context and information content of the signal, even though they did not explicitly use a pragmatics framework. Baboon responses to playbacks of grunts, for instance, are modulated by both the acoustic features of the calls and the context in which they are presented (Rendall *et al.*, 1999). An example of a study that made use of changes in prior knowledge on *responses* is the investigation of male chacma baboon social knowledge (Crockford *et al.*, 2007). In this study, male baboons heard the grunts of a male baboon and the copulation calls of a female, played back from different locations – indicating that these two subjects were not together. There were two conditions that are relevant for the issue at stake here: in the first, the female and male whose calls were played were actually in consort. In the control condition, the same two calls were presented, but now the consort was already terminated. Thus, in the first experiment, the listeners should be surprised to hear that the two individuals were apart, while the second condition should not evoke a strong response, as the sequence of events was compatible with the previous experience that the consort had broken up. Indeed, male listeners responded more strongly in the first condition (Crockford *et al.*, 2007), although all that was different was their prior experience or assumption about the state of the consort pair. What is still missing – at least to my knowledge – is a study that assesses the influence of prior knowledge on the classification of calls. Studies that use functional magnetic resonance imaging (fMRI) might provide a glimpse into the processing of stimuli independently from the overt responses.

Matters become even more complicated if we acknowledge that prior experiences shape the perception of social information. In humans, subjects' beliefs about whether someone else is actually able to see something affected reflexive gaze shifts (Teufel, Fletcher & Davis, 2010). Given that we do not grant a full-blown theory of mind to animals, such high-level modulation of perceptual processes seems unlikely; yet we should consider the idea that previous experiences might in principle change low-level perceptual processes. For instance, a lactating female might perceive infant screams in a different fashion than when she is in oestrus. This is a matter for empirical investigation.

12.6 Quantifying information content

Skyrms (2010) suggested that "the natural way to measure the information in a signal is to measure the extent that the use of that particular signal changes probabilities" (p. 8). He distinguished between the informational content of a signal and the quantity of information in a signal. Specifically, he suggested that "the informational content of a signal consists in how the signal affects probabilities", while the "quantity of information in a signal is measured by how far it moves probabilities" (Skyrms, 2010, p. 34). Skyrms goes on to explain this using a scenario with two states, both initially equiprobable. In this scenario, "signal A moves the probabilities to 9/10 for state 1 and 1/10 for state 2, and ... signal B moves the probabilities in exactly the opposite way: 1/10 for state 1 and 9/10 for state 2" (Skyrms, 2010, p. 34). Even when it is unclear how the quantity of information would be measured, one would conclude that these two signals contain the same amount of information. As Skyrms explains: "They move the initial probabilities by the same amount. But they do not have the same information content, because they move the initial probabilities in different directions" (Skyrms, 2010, p. 34).

An example might be the alarm calls of Barbary macaques, *Macaca sylvanus*. Barbary macaques utter high-frequency shrill barks in response to threatening stimuli and disturbances in the surroundings. An acoustic analysis revealed significant differences in relation to the stimulus that evoked the calling, in this particular analysis dogs versus human observers (Fischer, Hammerschmidt & Todt, 1995). *A priori*, the occurrence of dogs and threatening humans has the same probability. After hearing a 'dog' alarm though, the likelihood that a dog is indeed present is much higher; conversely, the likelihood that a 'human observer' is present is increased after hearing an 'observer' alarm call. In this study, we used a discriminant function analysis (DFA) to identify the combination of variables that best distinguished between calls given in the two contexts. The DFA provides a classification procedure that ascribes calls to the respective contexts based on the previously established discriminant functions. In the classification procedure, 3.4% of all calls given in response to the observer were misclassified as being given to a dog, while 5.3% of 'dog' alarm calls were classified as being given to the observer (data from Fischer *et al.*, 1995). Even though the relationships are not entirely symmetrical, let us assume that they are. In this case, we would conclude that both 'dog' and 'observer' alarms have the same information value, because they move probabilities (more or less) by the same amount, but not the same information content, because the signals map onto different context.

An example for a system where there is an asymmetric value of information can be found in those species that produce rather specific aerial alarm calls, and more general terrestrial alarm calls. Red-fronted lemurs (*Eulemur fulvus rufus*) and Verreaux's sifakas, *Propithecus verreauxi verreauxi*, for instance, both produce highly specific alarm calls in response to raptors, while they use different calls in response to terrestrial predators as well as in a variety of situations characterised by high arousal (Fichtel & Kappeler, 2002). Thus, aerial alarms move the probability for state A (raptor present) to perhaps 9/10, while probabilities for any specific event B, such as 'fossa present', that falls under the broader category 'terrestrial disturbance' is maybe only 2/10. So in this case, we would have two calls with differing information value and information content.

There is one feature of primate vocal behaviour that considerably complicates the issue though. Most Old World primates produce highly graded calls; that is, there is considerable variation not only between but also within types. Using a cluster analysis to identify call types on the basis of their acoustic features instead of their functional significance or the contexts in which they were uttered, Hammerschmidt and Fischer (1998) aimed to characterise the structure of the vocal repertoire of Barbary macaques. There was no single cluster solution that emerged as superior to all others; solutions with 7 or 16 clusters found the best support. The detailed analysis of the Barbary macaques' alarm calls supported the view that intermediate calls also exist in this domain (Fischer *et al.*, 1995). DFA resulted in a discriminant score for each call, as well as an assignment probability for each context. These assignment probabilities correspond in a non-linear fashion to the discriminant scores. Calls at the far ends of the distribution reveal a high assignment probability (>0.99), whereas calls in the overlapping region have lower assignment probabilities (Figure 12.3). In other words, not all calls given in a certain context move the probabilities equally far – some are more indicative than others, because they reveal higher production specificity. Yet, recipients may be equipped with perceptual mechanisms to categorise this graded variation into different call types (Fischer, 2006). Whether and in which way listeners categorise calls can be tested in the field with the habituation-recovery paradigm, in which a series of calls of one category is played back to a subject until it ceases to respond (or until the response is greatly diminished). Then, a call from the other category is presented. A recovery of the response suggests that this call exemplar is placed into a different category from the call exemplars used for habituation. Such experiments showed that Barbary macaques did indeed place their alarm calls into two different categories and that their categorical boundary closely matched that of the statistical analysis (Fischer, 1998). Thus, the calls fulfilled the criterion for functional reference (Fischer & Hammerschmidt, 2001). Chacma baboons, in contrast, which were tested in a similar study, were relatively insensitive to small changes in acoustic structure and only responded to

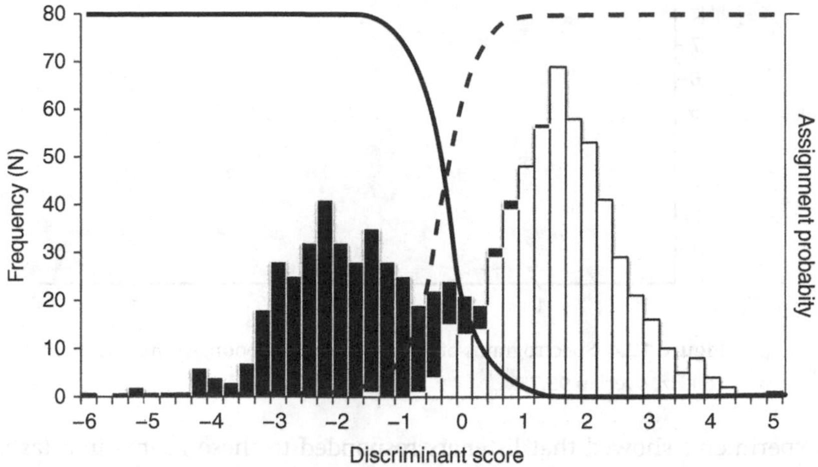

Figure 12.3 Frequency distribution of Barbary macaque shrill barks given in two contexts, and corresponding assignment probability functions (black and dashed lines) as derived from a discriminant function analysis. Original data from Fischer *et al.* (1995).

typical exemplars of their alarm calls, while they ignored intermediate variants (Fischer *et al.*, 2001b). We assumed that the Chacma baboons paid more attention to context than to acoustic variation, but further studies that shed light on the integration of information from different sources are clearly needed.

12.7 Assessing production specificity

Determining production specificity is not a trivial endeavour. Take the example of the Barbary macaque alarm calls. Here, calls given in only two contexts were recorded and subjected to acoustic analysis. Possibly, calls given in response to an observer may also be given in response to other disturbances in the surroundings. This would clearly affect the information value of the calls.

To explore the influence of the sampling regime on the assessment of production specificity, we conducted an acoustic analysis of baboon grunts (Meise *et al.*, 2011). Grunts are the most common short-distance vocalisations in the vocal repertoire of chacma baboons (*Papio ursinus*) (Cheney, Seyfarth & Silk, 1995). They are tonal, harmonically rich calls uttered in a variety of contexts (Rendall *et al.*, 1999) (Figure 12.4). Owren and colleagues (1997) distinguished between two acoustically different grunt types. The first type is given in move contexts when group members initiate a movement; the second when group members interact with infants or mothers. These calls are termed ‘infant grunts’. Playback

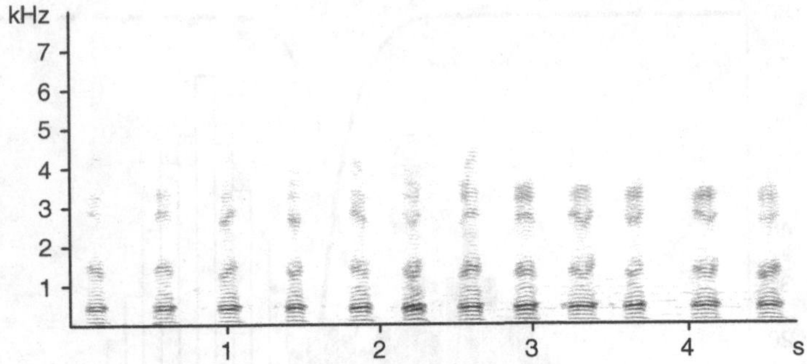

Figure 12.4 Spectrograms of female chacma baboon grunts. Sampling frequency: 16 kHz, overlap 93.75%.

experiments showed that listeners responded to these grunts in a fashion that took into account both the acoustic variation and the situation in which the calls were presented (Rendall *et al.*, 1999). Because only two contexts were sampled, however, the effective production specificity remained unclear.

We recorded vocalisations from adult female chacma baboons ranging in the Tsaobis National Park. Kristine Meise, the lead author of the study, followed the baboon troop from dawn to dusk, and recorded all grunt bouts occurring within 10 m distance. She noted the individual identity and the behavioural context. There were two 'social contexts', namely calls given to subjects with infants ('infant grunts'), or to other individuals while approaching ('social grunts'), and two 'non-social contexts', namely foraging and moving. For the latter two contexts, Kristine noted whether the calls were directed towards another individual or whether the individual was alone. Grunts uttered in the infant-handling and social-interaction contexts were by definition always directed to a receiver, either an infant and its mother or a social partner. Grunts from other, less frequent, contexts were excluded from the analysis because of insufficient sample size. We ran our staple acoustic analysis, in which a suite of acoustic variables was calculated from spectrograms using the software tool LMA developed by Kurt Hammerschmidt (Fischer *et al.*, 1995; Hammerschmidt & Todt, 1995; Hammerschmidt & Fischer, 1998). In addition, we conducted linear predictive coding (LPC) analyses (Owren & Bernacki, 1998). The resulting variables were finally submitted to DFA. For all DFAs, we calculated the error reduction as: ((classification results – chance level) / chance level) × 100 (Meise *et al.*, 2011). The classification results of the DFA revealed that grunts were more often assigned to the behavioural context in which the call occurred than to any other behavioural context. There were no obvious differences between undirected calls and directed calls. Therefore, we pooled directed and undirected grunts of the same context for the remaining analyses.

When we compared only infant-handling and move grunts, we found a classification accuracy of 78.7%, which corresponds to an error reduction of 57.4%. When we included the other two contexts as well, the error reduction decreased to 38.5%. The influence of the number of contexts on misclassification became particularly evident when we compared the error reduction rates of the move and infant-handling contexts in the two analyses (using two and four contexts, respectively). When comparing between two contexts, the DFA error-reduction rate for the move context was 62.8%, but it declined to 22.9% when four contexts were considered. The error-reduction rates showed a similar pattern in the infant-handling context, declining from 52% to 41.3%, respectively.

While the grunts uttered in three behavioural contexts could be statistically distinguished from others (foraging, infant handling, social interaction), this was not true for the fourth context (move), and the overall classification results were low across all four contexts (54% accuracy). The production specificity of baboon grunts was thus relatively poor. The analyses further indicated that the assessment of production specificity is sensitive to the number of contexts considered. For example, move grunts were rarely misclassified as infant grunts when only these two contexts were analysed, corroborating the findings of Owren, Seyfarth & Cheney (1997), but were frequently misclassified when foraging and social-interaction contexts were also included. These results clearly show that the true production specificity can only be assessed when all calls in all contexts are considered – something that is not always feasible in the field. Yet researchers should aim to include at least all of the contexts in which similar-sounding calls occur before assessing production specificity.

The issue of production specificity is not only relevant in determining whether certain calls are context-specific. A related issue is how reliably signal characteristics are tied to signaller quality, such as fighting ability or reproductive state. The theory of signal evolution provides a superb framework for understanding under which circumstances 'honest signalling' can evolve. Depending on the question of whether the interests of signaller and recipient overlap, the signalling behaviour has to bear a certain cost. Specifically, when interests diverge, signalling has to be costly, while cheap signalling can evolve when interests overlap (Maynard Smith & Harper, 2003; Searcy & Nowicki, 2005).

From the recipient's perspective, it is important to assess how reliable the association between signal features and sender quality is. For instance, how certain could a male baboon be that his rival's 'wahoo' calls accurately reflect his resource-holding potential (Fischer *et al.*, 2004)? And how accurately do female vocalisations indicate whether she is in her fertile period or not? We recently completed an analysis of the predictive value of changes in women's voices during their menstrual cycle. An earlier study had assessed changes in women's voices during two phases of the cycle: just prior to ovulation and before menstruation (Bryant & Haselton, 2009). The authors reported that women spoke with a higher-pitched voice prior to ovulation, when conception risk is highest. In our own study, we tracked the variation on a day-to-day basis throughout an entire cycle, for a set of 23 women. Although we were able to replicate the finding that women spoke with higher pitch just before ovulation, their fundamental frequency dropped substantially on the estimated day of ovulation, so that both the highest and lowest values were measured during the fertile phase. Moreover, women continued to speak with variable pitch throughout the cycle, suggesting that voice pitch or variability in speech patterns is not a good predictor of female fertility (Fischer *et al.*, 2011).

In sum, one crucial cognitive operation generating 'meaning' in listeners is inference. The processing of the signals themselves is constrained by species-specific design features of the perceptual apparatus, and typically, the recipient's behaviour is scaffolded by innate dispositions. Other than that, the statistical regularities in the world will constrain how reliably specific signals map onto different states, and this in turn will influence the certainty with which an animal is able to infer the meaning of a signal.

12.8 Referential signalling

What are the implications of these insights for the study of 'semantic' or 'referential' communication? I think we are left with two major research questions, and one well-supported conclusion – namely that the listener does all the work. The research questions concern, first, the selective pressures that favour (context-) specific calls, and, second, the evolutionary constraints that prevent a more flexible vocal communication (Fischer & Hammerschmidt, 2011). In terms of the selective pressures, systematic investigations of the role of predation pressure, habitat characteristics and social organisation are needed that take into account phylogenetic relationships. It seems likely that the existence of different predators with different hunting styles, which are connected with different response strategies, is the best predictor of the emergence of context-specific alarm calls (Macedonia & Evans, 1993). To clarify this issue, broad comparative analyses embedded in an evolutionary and ecological framework are needed.

In terms of the recipients' behaviour, I see no fundamental difference in the processing of context-specific calls, individually distinctive calls, or calls that vary with resource-holding potential or reproductive state. Differential responses to different call types are widespread in the animal kingdom, and

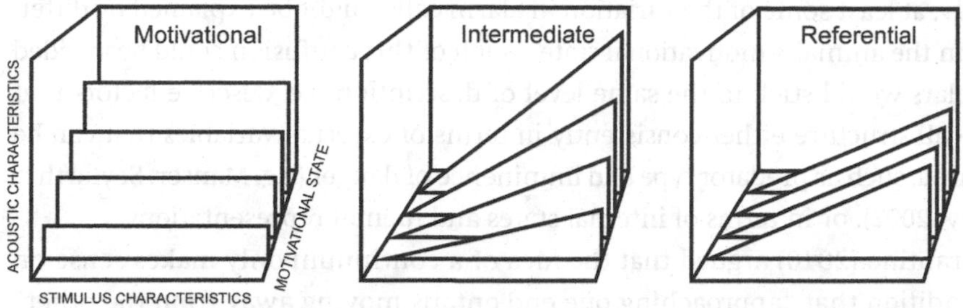

Figure 12.5 Motivational to Referential continuum. Marler and colleagues assumed two major axes that affect acoustic variation: the motivational state and the characteristics of the stimulus that elicits the calling. At the extremes would be calls that are fully 'motivational' (left) or fully 'referential' (right). The authors suggested that most vocalisations fall somewhere between the two extremes (middle). There are two problems with this conceptualisation: first, the axes are at two different levels of description (external versus internal); second, the model does not incorporate the possibility of independent variation along the two axes. Thus, certain call types could be given in response to a broad range of stimuli in situations of low urgency, while other variants could be given only in very specific contexts of high response urgency. Redrawn from Figure 4.1 in Marler *et al.* (1992) with permission from Cambridge University Press.

include not only functionally referential food and alarm calls, but also heterospecific calls, including verbal commands given by an animal trainer. The most impressive examples regarding 'call comprehension' can be found in dogs, whose ability to map a word onto an object ranges up to several hundred objects (Kaminski, Call & Fischer, 2004; Pilley & Reid, 2011).

Whether or not animal communication should be conceived as emotional, referential or both appears to be an issue of continuing debate, some of which may stem from an inconsistent and/or imprecise use of the terminology. In their classic paper, Marler *et al.* (1992) depicted a scheme to capture the fact that signals may be referential, motivational or both (Figure 12.5), a view taken up by Seyfarth and Cheney (2003b) who argued that calls can be both 'semantic' and 'emotional'. The problem with the idea of a continuum is that it lures scholars to confuse the two different levels of analysis, namely the production of signals, on the one hand, and the information that can be retrieved, on the other (see Scarantino, 2010). 'Motivational' changes refer to the internal state of the signaller, while (functional) reference is diagnosed when context-specific calls elicit specific responses. Importantly, motivational changes can also fulfil the criterion of production specificity and have thus the potential to elicit specific responses (Slocombe & Zuberbühler, 2005). Accordingly, calls that are purely motivational on the production end could still be functionally referential.

Possibly, at least some of the variation in alarm calls might be explained by differences in the animal's motivational state. Much of this confusion could be avoided if scholars would stick to the same level of description, i.e. describe factors that affect call structure either consistently in terms of external variables that can be measured, such as predator type and imminence of danger (e.g. Manser, Seyfarth & Cheney, 2002), or in terms of internal states and mental representations.

Scarantino (2010) argued that the idea of a continuum only makes sense on the condition that "approaching one end entails moving away from the other" (Scarantino, 2010, p. E3). I do not believe that this poses a problem, as long as one assumes the existence of two axes along which sounds may vary independently. As mentioned before, acoustic analyses suggested that calls can be mapped along an axis of aversion-to-hedonism and an axis encoding intensity (Fichtel *et al.*, 2001; Scheiner *et al.*, 2002), supporting the view that two or more dimensions are needed to explain acoustic variation. In other words, calls may be well correlated with the context (predator type) and imminence of danger (Fischer *et al.*, 1995; Manser, 2001).

Taking these facts together, I side with Rendall and colleagues (2009), who have aired some frustration about terminological sloppiness and hyperbole. On the other hand, I do not think that 'affect conditioning' (Owren & Rendall, 1997) is sufficient to explain the complexity of (primate) vocal communication. Specifically, it underestimates the cognitive components and decision-making processes that are involved in generating responses.

To conclude, the search for the origins of speech has proven to be an extremely fruitful research programme at many levels (Fitch, 2010). Somewhat disappointingly, after three decades of intensive research, we have to accept that non-human primate vocal communication bears little resemblance to human speech (Tomasello, 2008). At the same time, we have learned a great deal about the way monkeys and apes communicate. Instead of beating the 'speech' drum much longer, I suggest moving towards a more ecologically grounded research programme that addresses functional aspects and the selective pressures that shape communication. At the same time, I agree with Cheney and Seyfarth (1990) with regard to the power of vocalisations as a window into the animal's mind, and I believe that acoustic analyses and playback experiments will continue to be the most potent tools to identify the information content of primate vocalisations, and to elucidate what the calls mean to conspecific listeners.

Acknowledgements

I thank Ulrich Stegmann for inviting me to contribute to this volume and for his valuable comments on an earlier draft of the manuscript. I am grateful to Brandon Wheeler and Robert Seyfarth for discussion and valuable comments on the manuscript. Ludwig Ehrenreich kindly helped with the preparation of the figures.

References

Bauers, K. A. (1991). 'Coo' vocalizations in stumptailed macaques: a controlled functional analysis. *Behaviour*, **119**, 143–160.

Bryant, G. A. & Haselton, M. G. (2009). Vocal cues of ovulation in human females. *Biology Letters*, **5**, 12–15.

Cheney, D. L. & Seyfarth, R. M. (1990). *How Monkeys See the World.* Chicago, IL: University of Chicago Press.

Cheney, D. L., Seyfarth, R. M. & Silk, J. B. (1995). The role of grunts in reconciling opponents and facilitating interactions among adult female baboons. *Animal Behaviour*, **50**, 249–257.

Crockford, C., Wittig, R. M., Seyfarth, R. M. & Cheney, D. (2007). Baboons track the transient social relationships of others. *Animal Behaviour*, **73**, 885–890.

Dall, S. R. X., Giraldeau, L.-A., Olsson, O., McNamara, J. M. & Stephens, D. W. (2005). Information and its use by animals in evolutionary ecology. *Trends in Ecology and Evolution*, **20**, 187–193.

Dawkins, R. & Krebs, J. R. (1978). Animal signals: information or manipulation? In J. R. Krebs & N. B. Davies, eds., *Behavioural Ecology: An Evolutionary Approach.* Oxford: Blackwell Scientific Publications, pp. 282–309.

Dennett, D. C. (1971). Intentional systems. *Journal of Philosophy*, **68**, 68–87.

Fichtel, C. & Kappeler, P. M. (2002). Anti-predator behavior of group-living malagasy primates: mixed evidence for a referential alarm call system. *Behavioral Ecology and Sociobiology*, **51**, 262–275.

Fichtel, C., Hammerschmidt, K. & Jürgens, U. (2001). On the vocal expression of emotion. A multi-parametric analysis of different states of aversion in the squirrel monkey. *Behaviour*, **138**, 97–116.

Fischer, J. (1998). Barbary macaques categorize shrill barks into two call types. *Animal Behaviour*, **55**, 799–807.

Fischer, J. (2006). Categorical perception. In K. Brown, ed., *Encyclopedia of Language and Linguistics*, 2nd edn, Vol. 2. Oxford: Elsevier, pp. 248–251.

Fischer, J. (2008). Transmission of acquired information in non-human primates. In J. H. Byrne, ed., *Learning and Memory: A Comprehensive Reference.* Oxford: Elsevier, pp. 299–313.

Fischer, J. (2010). Nothing to talk about? On the linguistic abilities of non-human primates (and some other animal species). In U. Frey, C. Störmer & K. Willführ, eds., *Homo Novus – A Human Without Illusions.* New York: Springer, pp. 35–48.

Fischer, J. (2011). Where is the information in animal communication? In R. Menzel & J. Fischer, eds., *Animal Thinking: Contemporary Issues in Comparative Cognition.* Cambridge, MA: MIT Press, pp. 151–161.

Fischer, J. & Hammerschmidt, K. (2001). Functional referents and acoustic similarity revisited: the case of Barbary macaque alarm calls. *Animal Cognition*, **4**, 29–35.

Fischer, J. & Hammerschmidt, K. (2011). Ultrasonic vocalizations in mouse models for speech and socio-cognitive disorders: insights into the evolution of vocal communication. *Genes, Brain and Behavior*, **10**, 17–27.

Fischer, J., Hammerschmidt, K. & Todt, D. (1995). Factors affecting acoustic variation in Barbary macaque (*Macaca sylvanus*) disturbance calls. *Ethology*, **101**, 51–66.

Fischer, J., Hammerschmidt, K., Cheney, D. L. & Seyfarth, R. M. (2001a). Acoustic features of female chacma baboon barks. *Ethology*, **107**, 33–54.

Fischer, J., Kitchen, D. M., Seyfarth, R. M. & Cheney, D. L. (2004). Baboon loud calls advertise male quality: acoustic features and their relation to rank, age, and exhaustion. *Behavioral Ecology and Sociobiology*, **56**, 140–148.

Fischer, J., Metz, M., Cheney, D. L. & Seyfarth, R. M. (2001b). Baboon responses to graded bark variants. *Animal Behaviour*, **61**, 925–931.

Fischer, J., Semple, S., Fickenscher, G. *et al.* (2011). Do women's voices provide cues of the likelihood of ovulation? The importance of sampling regime. *PLoS ONE*, **6**, e24490.

Fitch, W. T. (2010). *The Evolution of Language*. Cambridge: Cambridge University Press.

Fitch, W. T. & Hauser, M. D. (1995). Vocal production in non-human primates – acoustics, physiology, and functional constraints on honest advertisement. *American Journal of Primatology*, **37**, 191–219.

Fitch, W. T., Neubauer, J. & Herzel, H. (2002). Calls out of chaos: the adaptive significance of nonlinear phenomena in mammalian vocal production. *Animal Behaviour*, **63**, 407–418.

Hammerschmidt, K. & Fischer, J. (1998). The vocal repertoire of Barbary macaques: a quantitative analysis of a graded signal system. *Ethology*, **104**, 203–216.

Hammerschmidt, K. & Fischer, J. (2008). Constraints in primate vocal production. In U. Griebel & K. Oller, eds., *The Evolution of Communicative Creativity: From Fixed Signals to Contextual Flexibility*. Cambridge. MA: MIT Press, pp. 93–119.

Hammerschmidt, K. & Todt, D. (1995). Individual differences in vocalizations of young Barbary macaques (*Macaca sylvanus*): a multi-parametric analysis to identify critical cues in acoustic signalling. *Behaviour*, **132**, 381–399.

Hesler, N. & Fischer, J. (2007). Gestural communication in Barbary macaques (*Macaca sylvanus*): an overview. In M. Tomasello & J. Call, eds., *The Gestural Communication of Apes and Monkeys*. New Jersey: Lawrence Erlbaum Associates, pp. 159–195.

Jablonka, E. & Lamb, M. J. (2005). *Evolution in Four Dimensions*. Cambridge, MA: MIT Press.

Kaminski, J., Call, J. & Fischer, J. (2004). Word learning in a domestic dog: evidence for 'fast mapping'. *Science*, **304**, 1682–1683.

Koch, C. (1999). *Biophysics of Computation: Information Processing in Single Neurons*. New York: Oxford University Press.

Krebs, J. R. & Dawkins, R. (1984). Animal signals: mind-reading and manipulation. In J. R. Krebs & N. B. Davies, eds., *Behavioural Ecology: An Evolutionary Approach*. Oxford: Blackwell, pp. 380–402.

Macedonia, J. M. & Evans, C. S. (1993). Variation among mammalian alarm call systems and the problem of meaning in animal signals. *Ethology*, **93**, 177–197.

Manser, M. B. (2001). The acoustic structure of suricates' alarm calls varies with predator type and the level of response urgency. *Proceedings of the Royal Society of London Series B: Biological Sciences*, **268**, 2315–2324.

Manser, M. B., Seyfarth, R. M. & Cheney, D. L. (2002). Suricate alarm calls signal predator class and urgency. *Trends in Cognitive Sciences*, **6**, 55–57.

Marler, P., Evans, C. S. & Hauser, M. D. (1992). Animal signals: motivational, referential, or both? In H. Papoušek, U. Jürgens & M. Papoušek, eds., *Nonverbal Vocal Communication*. Cambridge: Cambridge University Press, pp. 66–86.

Maynard Smith, J. & Harper, D. (2003). *Animal Signals*. Oxford: Oxford University Press.

Meise, K., Keller, C., Cowlishaw, G. & Fischer, J. (2011). Sources of acoustic variation: implications for production specificity and call categorization in chacma baboon (*Papio ursinus*) grunts. *Journal of the Acoustical Society of America*, **129**, 1631–1641.

Owren, M. J. & Bernacki, R. H. (1998). Applying linear predictive coding (LPC) to the frequency analysis of animal acoustic signals. In S. L. Hopp & C. S. Evans, eds., *Recent Advances in the Study of Animal Communication*. New York: Springer, pp. 129–162.

Owren, M. J. & Rendall, D. (1997). An affect-conditioning model of non-human primate vocal signaling. In D. H. Owings, M. D. Beecher & N. S. Thompson, eds., *Communication. Perspectives in Ethology*, Vol. 12. New York: Plenum Press, pp. 299–346.

Owren, M. J. & Rendall, D. (2001). Sound on the rebound: bringing form and function back to the forefront in understanding non-human primate vocal signaling. *Evolutionary Anthropology*, **10**, 58–71.

Owren, M. J., Seyfarth, R. M. & Cheney, D. L. (1997). The acoustic features of vowel-like grunt calls in chacma baboons (*Papio cyncephalus ursinus*): implications for production processes and functions. *Journal of the Acoustical Society of America*, **101**, 2951–2963.

Palombit, R. A., Seyfarth, R. M. & Cheney, D. L. (1997). The adaptive value of 'friendships' to female baboons: experimental and observational evidence. *Animal Behaviour*, **54**, 599–614.

Pfefferle, D., Heistermann, M., Pirow, R., Hodges, J. K. & Fischer, J. (2011). Estrogen and progestogen correlates of the structure of female copulation calls in semi free-ranging Barbary macaques (*Macaca sylvanus*). *International Journal of Primatology*, **32**, 992–1006.

Pilley, J. W. & Reid, A. K. (2011). Border collie comprehends object names as verbal referents. *Behavioural Processes*, **86**, 184–195.

Rendall, D., Owren, M. J. & Ryan, M. J. (2009). What do animal signals mean? *Animal Behaviour*, **78**, 233–240.

Rendall, D., Seyfarth, R. M., Cheney, D. L. & Owren, M. J. (1999). The meaning and function of grunt variants in baboons. *Animal Behaviour*, **57**, 583–592.

Ruxton, G. D. & Schaefer, H. M. (2011). Resolving current disagreements and ambiguities in the terminology of animal communication. *Journal of Evolutionary Biology*, doi:10.1111/j.1420-9101.2011.02386.x.

Scarantino, A. (2010). Animal communication between information and influence. *Animal Behaviour*, **79**, E1–E5.

Scheiner, E., Hammerschmidt, K., Jürgens, U. & Zwirner, P. (2002). Acoustic analyses of developmental changes and emotional expression in the preverbal vocalizations of infants. *Journal of Voice*, **16**, 509–529.

Scott-Phillips, T. C. (2008). Defining biological communication. *Journal of Evolutionary Biology*, **21**, 387–395.

Searcy, W. A. & Nowicki, S. (2005). *The Evolution of Animal Communication*. Princeton, NJ and Oxford: Princeton University Press.

Seyfarth, R. M. & Cheney, D. L. (2003a). Signalers and receivers in animal communication. *Annual Review of Psychology*, **54**, 145–173.

Seyfarth, R. M. & Cheney, D. L. (2003b). Meaning and emotion in animal vocalizations. *Annals of the New York Academy of Sciences*, **1000**, 32–55.

Seyfarth, R. M., Cheney, D. L., Bergman, T. *et al.* (2010). The central importance of information in studies of animal communication. *Animal Behaviour*, **80**, 3–8.

Seyfarth, R. M., Cheney, D. L. & Marler, P. (1980). Monkey responses to three different alarm calls: evidence of predator classification and semantic communication. *Science*, **210**, 801–803.

Shannon, C. E. & Weaver, W. (1949). *The Mathematical Theory of Communication*. Urbana, IL; University of Illinois Press.

Skyrms, B. (2010). *Signals. Evolution, Learning and Information*. Oxford: Oxford University Press.

Slocombe, K. E. & Zuberbühler, K. (2005). Agonistic screams in wild chimpanzees (*Pan troglodytes schweinfurthii*) vary as a function of social role. *Journal of Comparative Psychology*, **119**, 67–77.

Smith, W. J. (1977). *The Behavior of Communicating: An Ethological Approach*. Cambridge, MA: Harvard University Press.

Teufel, C., Fletcher, P. C. & Davis, G. (2010). Seeing other minds: attributed mental states influence perception. *Trends in Cognitive Sciences*, **14**, 376–382.

Tomasello, M. (2008). *Origins of Human Communication*. Cambridge, MA: MIT Press.

Wagner, R. H. & Danchin, É. (2010). A taxonomy of biological information. *Oikos*, **119**, 203–209.

Wheeler, B. C., Searcy, W. A., Christiansen, M. H. *et al.* (2011). Communication. In R. Menzel & J. Fischer, eds., *Animal Thinking: Contemporary Issues in Comparative Cognition*, Cambridge, MA: MIT Press pp. 187–205.

Zuberbühler, K. (2000). Referential labelling in diana monkeys. *Animal Behaviour*, **59**, 917–927.

Zuberbühler, K. (2006). Language evolution: the origin of meaning in primates. *Current Biology*, **16**, R123–R125.

Commentary

Fischer argues that "in the very strict sense, animal communication does not consist of information transmission, and animal signals do not contain information". Strictly speaking, "information is generated by the recipient". I disagree. Information is generated by the signal because of its capacity to allow a recipient to make a prediction. Capacities are what philosophers call dispositional properties, namely properties things have by virtue of their potentialities (e.g. fragility, solubility). But as we would say that a glass vase is (strictly speaking) fragile by virtue of its potential for breaking in suitable circumstances, so we should say that a signal is (strictly speaking) informative by virtue of its potential for informing a recipient in suitable circumstances. See my commentary to Rendall and Owren for further discussion.

Andrea Scarantino

Response

Scarantino makes an interesting point, but the problem with the proposed view is that it fails to specify who determines whether or not a signal is informative or has predictive value. Whether or not a signal reduces the uncertainty of the recipient also depends on his or her prior knowledge state. Therefore, I would prefer to link the determination of the informative value to a given recipient. In principle, this could be the observer of the communicative act (such as the philosopher analysing the incident). The point I want to make here is that the assessment of the value of information always needs to be tied to a specific vantage point, and from an evolutionary point of view, it makes much sense to use one part of the communicative dyad – the recipient – and be explicit about it.

Julia Fischer

13

Information and uncertainty in meerkats and monkeys

COLIN ALLEN

13.1 Introduction

The papers published in 1980 by Robert Seyfarth, Dorothy Cheney and Peter Marler on the alarm calls of vervet monkeys were instant classics. In a short paper in *Science* (Seyfarth *et al.*, 1980a) and the more detailed companion piece in *Animal Behaviour* (Seyfarth *et al.*, 1980b), they described experiments that Seyfarth and Cheney had conducted in Kenya's Amboseli National Park. They played pre-recorded vervet monkey vocalisations from loudspeakers hidden in bushes, to test the reactions of the monkeys who were within earshot. They used the different "alarm calls" that are commonly produced when vervet monkeys detect predatory eagles, leopards and snakes, and observed the vervets responding in predator-appropriate ways to the three kinds of calls. With Marler, their postdoctoral advisor who had initially suggested the experiments, they argued that these differential responses to the alarm calls showed that monkeys hearing these calls obtain specific information about the type of predator, not just the emotional or arousal state of the signaller. They claimed that these calls are thus an example of 'referential communication' in a non-human primate.

The vervet alarm calls have achieved iconic status, even among those philosophers who know little about the experimental details or scientific context in which the experiments were developed. Among biologists, the research has spawned a veritable industry that employs playback methods to investigate 'referential communication' in a variety of different species: primates, meerkats, prairie dogs, domesticated chickens and so on. The use of the playbacks in such experiments is now itself the subject of serious study within history and

Animal Communication Theory: Information and Influence, ed. Ulrich Stegmann. Published by Cambridge University Press.

philosophy of science (Radick, 2007). If there is one example of a successful research programme involving scientists who accept the label of 'cognitive ethologist' for themselves, it is the investigation of referential communication.

From an evolutionary point of view, the systems of alarm calls and responses found in various species can sometimes be understood in terms of kin selection. Individuals living together in groups often comprise a network of genetically related individuals, and insofar as the predator-appropriate responses of receivers decrease the mortality of related individuals hearing the calls, this increases inclusive fitness of the signallers even if they incur a potential cost by attracting the attention of predators to themselves. From a cognitive point of view, many ethologists have been inclined to say that such calls inform other group members about the presence of predators. However, and as other chapters in this volume discuss, this framing of animal communication in terms of information has proven controversial.

The most vociferous criticisms are to be found in a series of papers by Michael Owren, Drew Rendall and colleagues (e.g. Rendall & Owren, 2002; Rendall, Owren & Ryan, 2009; Owren, Rendall & Ryan, 2010). They argue that the notion of 'information' as used by ethologists imports metaphors from human language that are not scientifically grounded in the facts about animal communication. They assert that it is a mistake to try to understand more primitive forms of animal communication using features derived from more recently evolved human language. As an alternative, they suggest that a more fruitful approach would be to focus on the ways in which physical characteristics of signals, such as pitch, duration and intensity, activate emotion-related or motivational systems in receivers. Their view is summarised in the title of Owren, Rendall and Ryan's 2010 paper, "Redefining animal signaling: influence versus information in communication", urging ethologists to focus on the *influence* that signallers have on receivers (they prefer 'perceivers') rather than *information* conveyed from one to the other.

Seyfarth, Cheney and four co-authors have responded to this challenge with a paper titled 'The central importance of information in studies of animal communication' (Seyfarth *et al.*, 2010), in which they accuse their opponents of attacking a straw man. However, their response fails to deal with one of the main complaints raised by Owren *et al.* (2010), namely that the notion that animal signals convey or contain 'information' is not appropriately connected by the cognitive ethologists to the quantitative measure of information developed by Shannon and based in probability theory. Seyfarth *et al.* (2010) include a very brief section, consisting of exactly one paragraph, in which they refer to Shannon (1948) and Wiener (1961) to ground their use of the term 'information' as 'reduction of uncertainty'. They mention 'reduction of uncertainty' only once more – in the immediately following paragraph that heads the next section – while continuing to use the term 'information' throughout the rest of the paper without any further reference to probabilities. It is precisely this kind of pro forma mention of Shannon's definition that leads the critics to complain about failure to properly tie the notion of information in animal communication to Shannon's probabilistic theory of communication. As Adams and Beighley (Ch. 17 of this volume) put it, "The complaint is that people cite Shannon and Weaver (1949) and then move on without explanation."

There is both a practical point and a definitional point here. On the practical side, even though quantitative analyses of the information in animal communication have sometimes been attempted – the first effort in this direction being an analysis of honeybee communication by Haldane and Spurway (1954) – the assumptions about receiver perception and signal measurement that are required for absolute quantities to be calculated may be hard to verify (e.g. Beecher, 1989). On the definitional side, is the question of how (indeed, whether) to connect the probabilistic notion of 'reduction of uncertainty' to the notion of specific informational content. Owren *et al.* quote Weaver (from Shannon & Weaver, 1949, p. 99) to support their claim that "meaning and significance are quite different from Shannon information" (Owren *et al.*, 2010, p. 761). They also cite Dretske (1981) as supporting "the originators' admonition to separate information from meaning" and they go on to assert that Shannon's concept of information is "incommensurate" with the approach adopted by animal communication researchers. Philosophers familiar with Dretske's (1981) book may be somewhat puzzled by this. Distinctions do not imply incommensurability. Although Dretske does not equate semantic content to information, a major effort of the book is nevertheless to explicate content in information-theoretic terms. My main goal in this chapter, however, is not to set the record straight about Dretske's account of intentional content (but see Allen, 1995 for a comparative review of philosophical accounts, including Dretske's).

In this chapter, I argue that *information* versus *influence* presents a false dichotomy for the study of animal communication. The information eliminativists' argument that ethology would be better off without a notion of information is based on inordinate concern for what Owren *et al.* (2010, p. 766) describe as the "over-complicated accounts of perceiver processing" that they associate with the informational view of animal communication. The allegedly less complicated 'influence' view of communication may only seem less complicated when certain complexities of animal communication are wilfully ignored. Shannon (1956) cautioned against jumping on "the bandwagon" of information theory whose basic results, he wrote, were "aimed in a very specific direction . . . that is not necessarily relevant to such fields as psychology, economics, and other social sciences" (p. 3). Nevertheless, he went on to say that he personally believed that "many of the concepts of information theory would prove useful in these other fields" – but he insisted that the utility of what is essentially a deductive, mathematical theory would need to be established experimentally. After surveying the debate in more detail, I discuss two experiments illustrating the utility of Shannon's approach.

13.2 Information overload?

The pair of papers contributing to the debate among the ethologists in 2010 represent something of an in-house dispute among the academic progeny of Peter Marler. Many of the major protagonists (Robert Seyfarth, Dorothy Cheney, Marc Hauser, Chris Evans, Klaus Zuberbühler, Julia Fischer, Drew Rendall, Michael Owren etc.) were directly advised by Marler or by one of his advisees. Others in this debate, such as Don Owings, were colleagues of Marler at the University of California, Davis, or otherwise connected to the UC Davis department. Michael Owren was Cheney and Seyfarth's first postdoctoral advisee, working at UC Davis, and Drew Rendall, who did his PhD at UC Davis also later became their postdoctoral advisee.

Although Shannon's account of information played a role in Marler's thinking about animal communication, it is by no means the sole starting point. The debate in which Marler was engaged can be framed as follows (I owe the following list to my student Robert Rose; see also Radick, 2007):

(1) Haldane and Spurway's (1954) information-theoretic analysis of the honeybee waggle dance as carrying 5 bits of information of which 2.5 bits on average are picked up by the honeybee audience.
(2) The rejection by Lorenz and Tinbergen (and Haldane) of a 'mentalistic' or 'semantic' reading of claims about information, instead seeing such signals as 'triggers' of automatic responses. (See also Adams and Beighley, Ch. 17 of this volume, for a similar characterisation of the role of 'information' in analysing animal communication.)
(3) Marler's reading of Peircean semiotic theory (see Peirce, 1935), and descendants thereof, specifically Ogden and Richards (1923), Morris (1946) and Cherry (1957), according to which the triadic relationship among *object*, *sign* and *interpretant* is irreducible to binary relationships. Marler combines this with Morris' operationalised notion of 'interpretant' in terms of behavioural dispositions in the receiver.

Marler also accepts the semioticians' identification of the referent of a communicative act as the object in this triadic relationship.

(4) Marler's following of Ogden and Richards in taking the relationships linking signs and objects to be 'imputed' – meaning that these relations are mediated by psychological agents.

(5) The rejection by Marler (1961), following Morris (1946), of a dichotomous view of animal communication as either emotional or referential – a distinction that has its roots in Darwin (Radick, 2007). Why not both?

(6) Marler's rejection, following Cherry (1957), of a clean distinction between 'semantics' or the study of 'meaning' of signs and 'pragmatics' or "the significance of signals to the communicants" (Marler, 1961, p. 229), at least for the purposes of studying animal communication.

Although Marler read widely in the semiotics literature, little of this shows through in the papers that established the research programme at the heart of the current dispute. However, I believe that the notion of *imputed* significance is key to seeing our way through the current thicket of ideas about information in animal communication. Of course, the idea that perceivers 'impute significance' to signals suggests the kind of cognitive sophistication that makes Owren *et al.* nervous about metaphors drawn from human language understanding. I will use some recent research on meerkats in which I had a hand to try to illustrate how cognitive capacities can be related to animal communication and studied rigorously without assuming a linguistic conception of information.

Before introducing the meerkats, let me try to be a bit more specific about the standard linguistic conception of information. (I owe much of the following paragraph to conversations with Michael Ramscar, and to his paper "Information: a theory of human communication", in preparation.) The standard model of language takes meaning to be directly encoded in words and sentences, and thus extractable by a knowledgeable hearer or reader. A knowledgeable receiver knows the lexicon which associates words with meanings (or concepts) and, if the language is a sophisticated one, the rules for assembling larger meaningful utterances from the lexical items. The dominant metaphor becomes one of message passing – a fixed message is packaged by a speaker into a predetermined code that is extracted by a competent listener. In contrast to the orthodox view, even though certain aspects of this code may be conventionalised, it is better (and more consistent with Shannon) to think of these messages as something that competent receivers must *reconstruct*. The process is closer to probabilistic reasoning than semantic lookup. I will describe the application of these ideas to a study of meerkat communication below.

13.3 Meerkat individuals

Meerkats are a kind of mongoose endemic to southern Africa. They live in colonies of up to 50 individuals dominated by a dominant pair, and they produce a number of distinctive vocalisations that are functionally related to different social situations and predator threats. Meerkat vocalisations are also distinguishable at the individual level, but meerkat researchers had found themselves rather stumped when it came to testing whether the meerkats themselves were capable of recognising individuals by vocal cues alone. It was hard to find any naturally occurring situations in which the identity of the signaller mattered to the meerkats, except those involving the dominant animal. A study found that subordinate animals can distinguish the calls of the dominant female from those of other females based on sound alone (Reber, 2010). However, because there is exactly one dominant female in each group it could not be determined whether this discrimination indicated only category-level recognition (dominant versus subordinate) or more fine-grained individual recognition. No difference in social response to subordinate females could be discerned.

Years ago, I had helped brainstorm the design of Dorothy Cheney and Robert Seyfarth's habituation experiments with vervet monkeys, in which they repeatedly played the calls of a single individual, habituating the others to that call, and then tested with other calls from the same individual and different individuals. They found that habituation did not transfer between alarm calls, but that habituation did transfer between acoustically distinct social contact calls from the targeted individual, suggesting meaning-based categorisation of signaller reliability (Cheney & Seyfarth, 1988). In the present context, I am willing to treat the claim that vervets categorise calls by meaning as controversial. However, because the transferred habituation was limited to calls from the same individual, it should be uncontroversial that this can only be explained if the monkeys are sensitive to individually distinctive elements of the calls.

Such experiments are difficult to carry out. Cheney and Seyfarth had been very careful to play a call from the hidden speakers only when the monkey whose call was being played back was out of sight of the others. The habituation phase is especially difficult because multiple exposures are needed but appropriate opportunities are spread over days and weeks. Nevertheless, an attempt was made by Schibler and Manser to carry out a version of Cheney and Seyfarth's 1988 unreliable signaller experiment on the meerkats. However, the meerkats showed no transfer of habituation, leading the researchers to title their paper, "The irrelevance of individual discrimination in meerkat alarm calls" (Schibler & Manser, 2007). Schibler and Manser noted that individual discrimination might occur in some contexts, but that it was not important for the meerkats to respond differently in the specific context of this experiment.

At a meeting in Berlin in July 2010, I suggested a different approach to meerkat researchers Marta Manser and her postdoc Simon Townsend. The approach was based on violation of expectation that did not explicitly require prior habituation. The thought was this: if meerkats are able to identify individuals by their vocalisations alone and are sensitive to the direction from which a call is heard, then they ought to find it surprising if they receive evidence of a nearly instantaneous shift of location of a single individual. So, if it were possible to locate two speakers on opposite sides of a focal subject and play, in rapid succession, social contact calls from the same individual, at a time interval that was too short for the caller to have changed location, then an attentive listener ought to show some sign that this was unusual. Meerkats have a 'close' call which Manser had hypothesised to play a function in maintaining group cohesion (Manser, 1998) and that had been shown by Townsend, Hollen and Manser (2010) to be individually distinctive by acoustic analysis. The 'close' call seemed, therefore, to be a good candidate to use in this experiment. Although we did not know exactly what meerkats would do in the situation where they heard separately recorded 'close' calls from the same individual (AA′ pattern), we reasoned that a different reaction to the AA′ pattern versus calls from two different individuals coming from different sides (AB pattern) would show that the animals were tracking individual identity by vocal calls alone. To short-circuit an even longer story, this is indeed what Townsend found when he ran the experiment at the Kalahari Meerkat Project study site. (Yes, Meerkat Manor!) Meerkats hearing the AA′ pattern with approximately 4 s separation between calls became more vigilant and were more likely to look in the direction of the second loudspeaker than those hearing the AB pattern. In the published description of this experiment we argued that it showed within-category discrimination amongst the subordinate individuals who are tracked spatially (Townsend, Allen & Manser, 2011).

It would be more succinct to say that meerkats obtain information about identity and location from the 'close' calls of group members, but because the issue of information is contested by Owren, Rendall and Ryan (Rendall *et al.*, 2009; Owren *et al.*, 2010) it is necessary in the present context to justify speaking that way. But why introduce the notion of information at all when we did not use the term in the written report? The short answer is that the language we did use, of tracking identities and locations of individuals through time, concerns information available to the hearer rather than immediate behavioural influence exerted by the caller on the perceiver. The long answer follows.

13.4 What meerkats impute

In our paper we argued that the experimental results "suggest that meerkats do indeed have a concept of conspecifics as 'individuals' recognised perceptually" (Townsend *et al.*, 2011). Our circumspection about this claim derives from a lack of a cognitive model or mechanism to explain the meerkats' spontaneous tracking of the location of nearby individuals from moment to moment. Nor do we have any evidence pertaining to whether meerkats can integrate individual identity cues from different modalities such as sight, hearing and smell, or track individuals over the long term. The attribution of individual concepts serves as a placeholder pending further investigation of the processes and mechanisms. In the context of the present volume, nothing depends on the claim that the meerkats have individual concepts. Nevertheless, I would argue that the issues that lead some to be skeptical of animal concepts are analogous to those in the controversy about information in animal communication.

One way to make the connection is via the critique offered by Chater and Heyes (1994) of the notion of 'concept' in animal cognition. Similar to the complaint by Owren *et al.* that the notion of information as deployed by ethologists imports metaphors from human language, Chater and Heyes' argument is that the notion of concept is not well defined outside the context of language users. I will not rehearse the full responses to their argument here, but in my view (elaborated in Allen, 1999; see also Newen & Bartels, 2007) the best justification for concept attribution involves the sensitivity of the animals to epistemic failure, i.e. noticing and learning from their own errors of categorisation when an expectation is violated. When categorisation seems to be going smoothly and there are no errors, the notion of a concept may seem superfluous because one can simply regard the categoriser's response as directly driven by properties of immediate stimuli. But when things go wrong and expectations are violated, sophisticated configural learners – concept users – simultaneously update their responses not just to features of the stimulus directly involved in the event but to various related features that were absent during the violation of expectation. Contra Chater and Heyes, the use of the word 'concept' is meaningfully attributed even when the categorising animals do not have explicit labels (words) for their categories. When cognitive agents learn from their prediction errors about specific instances, they reconfigure the relational structure among the features relevant to the entire category, even features absent from the instance generating the error. The cognitive structures that are constructed and reorganised by discriminative learners are the concepts. And while the best discriminative learning models are associationist in flavour, this is not your grandfather's behaviourism (Smith, 2000; also, M. Ramscar, in preparation).

The idea of multiple adjustments within a category is implicit at the core of the 'unreliable signaller' experiment of Cheney and Seyfarth (1988). The habituated group members did not just come to ignore the one individual's signal that was played repeatedly during the habituation phase of the experiment (a 'wrr'). They also came to ignore another kind of acoustically distinct call from the same individual played in the test phase (the 'chutter'). This cannot be explained without attributing some cognitive structure to the monkeys to connect wrrs to chutters. They both belong to the category of social contact calls. The change of significance of the chutters is 'imputed' insofar as nothing intrinsic to the signs themselves (the wrrs and chutters are acoustically distinct) or to the sign–object relationship suffices to explain the pattern of results without bringing the 'interpretant' – and hence the receiver's cognitive architecture – into it.

Now, it might be argued, from a behaviourist point of view, that stimulus contexts are what wrrs and chutters have in common. Both kinds of social signal tend to occur in similar contexts, allowing the animal to learn their association. Putting this in semiotic terms (but abandoning the semioticians' insistence on the irreducible ternary nature of communication), one might say that because wrrs and chutters both connect to situations involving social contact with other groups, the binary relationship between sign and contexts involving social contact (the object of communication) is sufficient to explain the receiver's transfer of habituation between the two calls. This will not do, however. Different alarm calls all connect to situations involving contact with predators, yet the monkeys did not transfer habituation between the alarm calls that were used in the experiment. Perhaps, though, predators and the corresponding alarm calls tend to occur in noticeably different contexts (bushy areas for snakes, more open spaces for eagles, for example). Even so, the monkeys would need to have learned to discriminate social contact among the contexts for alarm calls, while they learned to ignore the same contextual features surrounding calls. It is only against the background of this difference – a fact about the acquired cognitive structure of the receivers – that we can understand why the transfer of habituation occurs in some cases and not in others.

The fact that the monkeys group some sign–object relationships together but discriminate others is a fact that necessarily involves their role in imputing significance to the calls, not merely to externally given sign–object relationships. The role of their cognitive architecture goes beyond perception of the physical characteristics of the signal such as pitch and volume (the aspects of receiver psychology that Owren, Rendall and Ryan emphasise by insisting on using 'perceiver' in place of 'receiver'). It requires our attention, as theorists, to the informational properties of the signals. Of course, the calls *influence* receivers too. Receivers could hardly be informed without being influenced. But the nature of that influence fits Shannon's conception. When monkeys cease responding to an individual's chutters, it is not because the objective relationship between chutters and the environment has changed. The relationship of that individual's chutters to social contact with another group is exactly the same at the end of the experiment as it was at the beginning. Only the informational entropy of the individual's wrrs has been objectively changed (by changing the probabilistic relationship between the wrrs and social contact with another group). Nevertheless, the receivers' expectations about chutters have changed, which is an imputed change in significance.

The violation of expectation in our meerkat experiment forces similar considerations. In normal interactions, 'close calls' influence perceivers' overt behaviour rather minimally. But the very same call can have a different influence based not on anything intrinsic to the call, or to the signal–object relationship per se, but depending on an imputed significance given what information the meerkat has about the prior location of the caller. By attending to prediction errors, the meerkats learn to better predict, and in this sense understand, the world around them (cf. M. Ramscar, in preparation).

How does this connect back to Shannon? A Haldane-style calculation of the average bit rate of any single call might be possible, in principle if not in full practicality. If we start with the assumptions that in any given situation a meerkat initially has no information about the location of a fellow group member, that all relative directions are equiprobable, and that the physics of sound production and sound wave propagation provides much greater potential for identifying the source than meerkats can discriminate, then the average amount of locational information conveyed by these calls depends on the directional and distance resolution of the perceiver (how many radial sectors can be distinguished and what kind of range discrimination exists) and the amount of individual information depends on how many individuals can be discriminated. In any given situation, the amount of information actually extracted by the receiver depends on her prior information state. So, given two 'close' calls from the same individual in the same location, the second might provide only a small amount of new information to the receiver, which is related to reducing any uncertainty that comes from the signaller's having moved location since the first call.

Only some very rough, back-of-the-envelope calculations are possible here. We could make an assumption about the average amount of information conveyed by a 'close' call by assuming something about the radial discriminability of the signals (say 32 equal-sized sectors within the 360° range, which gives 5 bits), the range discrimination (assume just two range bands, 'very close' and 'close', for 1 bit) and the individual discrimination capabilities (say a maximal group size of 64 individuals, for another 6 bits). We could then estimate the reduction of uncertainty provided by a second call, based on the typical movement patterns of meerkats. This corresponds to the entropy (uncertainty) of a joint event (x, y) which Shannon (1948, p. 22) defined as the sum of the entropy of x and the *conditional entropy* of y given x, i.e. the uncertainty of y when x is known. If meerkats never moved, the second call would be entirely redundant – its conditional entropy would be 0. If meerkats typically move within 10 seconds with a 50% probability, then another call 10 seconds later by the same individual from the same location conveys one bit of information etc. However, these back-of-the-envelope calculations depend on many assumptions about meerkat psychophysics, patterns of movement etc, for which ethologists do not have supporting evidence (see also Beecher, 1989) although they might be able to collect them. Some of those assumptions might be better investigated in the laboratory than the field, but the fact that they have not been investigated does not undermine the utility of talking about communicative information despite our present inability to assign an exact entropy value for the communication.

To say that meerkats obtain information about the location of individuals from their 'close' calls is not to say that these vocalisations have phonologically distinct elements for different locations. They are 'articulated' for location of utterance (in the sense of Millikan, 1984) only in the sense that their location is a significant aspect of the sign. Human language allows us to say things that articulate range and direction relative to another person by varying not just the location of utterance but also the form of the acoustic signal, such as "On your left!" versus "On your right!" Production of such statements is a cognitively complex task because successful allocentric references to the other person's left or right require the signaller to predict how the receiver will interpret 'left' versus 'right', in some sense adopting the receiver's point of view. Given the desire to communicate position rapidly, when the situation permits, people are much more likely to say "Here!" or "Hey!" and rely on the receiver's ability to discriminate who said it and from where. In principle, any vocalisation whatever would do, even if its conventionalised meaning is unrelated ("I hear the gooseberries are doing well this year...") or opposite ("I'm not here") to the location and identity information extracted by the receiver. However, because they require superfluous processing, such fanciful examples would be inefficient as signals whose primary function is to maintain social cohesion smoothly. Alternatively, a sound that is lacking in conventional meaning but still conventionalised ("hey!") is a quite effective tool for communicating location to a receiver. The physics of vocalising supplies the information needed for individual identification and the physics of sound travel provides direction to the source, while the receiver takes care of decoding the message. Informational and physical aspects of signals co-exist.

This notion of information does not fit the conception of meaning provided by the standard message-passing conception of language. Recalling Marler's (1961) claim that the significance of signals to the communicants – what he calls 'pragmatics' – should be our focus, I argue that it is the right conception of information for the study of animal communication (and perhaps a good alternative to the message-passing model for human language, too, but there is no space to defend that here; cf. M. Ramscar, in preparation). Some aspects of animal communication are conventionalised, albeit not to the same degree that human language is. Insofar as there are social mechanisms within a group of communicators that serve to stabilise the communicative functions of specific signals, the significance of these calls will be partly conventionalised, although contexts will allow for a lot of variation in the information that receivers impute. Even the absence of such mechanisms – which are not involved in maintaining the relationship of vocal quality to identity unless imitators are dissuaded by social means – the influence of such signals on receivers is highly dependent on what information receivers already have.

So long as the meerkats' 'close' calls follow the normal, smooth pattern of meerkat movements and interactions, the influence that signallers have on receivers is rather subtle. But when a call is perceived from an unexpected location, the influence is much greater. The difference that otherwise identical calls have on an audience requires us to take account of the role of receivers in imputing significance to them. The meerkat who hears a call from a completely unexpected direction is surprised. In a psychological sense, its uncertainty appears to have increased as it looks in the direction of the second call as if searching for confirming evidence. But if the function of the call is to communicate location, and communication involves reduction of uncertainty, how is this possible? The meerkat's surprise seems unlikely to be explained simply in terms of the change in subjective probability attached to the other's location because the initial call produces a comparable change without engendering surprise. Nor does Shannon's measure allow negative entropy, i.e. increase of uncertainty. We should be mindful of possible mathematical alternatives to Shannon's account (see Vigo, 2011, for a mathematical account of categorical information that does allow negative information). Nevertheless, it is possible to make sense of the meerkat's psychological uncertainty as a case of *mis*communication that provides information about the signaller and the code.

In Shannon's engineering context, there is an idealised communication system in which sender and receiver share a fixed code and the task of the ideal receiver is to use the signal to reconstruct the message encoded by the signaller, i.e. to select one message from a predetermined set of possible messages (Shannon, 1948, p. 5). Miscommunication in this kind of idealised system consists solely in the receiver's selecting the wrong message. However, in the real world of communication between cognitively complex agents, including meerkats, the code is not uniquely determined in advance. Each signal can be considered as potentially encoding not one message but a range of possible messages, serving multiple possible purposes. Successful communication systems are shaped by social and natural selection pressures that enable signallers and receivers to converge, more or less, on signals that serve their biological purposes. But such convergence generally happens not because one precise message comes to be associated with each signal. Rather, the process requires continuous adjustments of signallers' and receivers' expectations against the background of a dynamic set of experiences. The predominant role of individual experience in interpreting signals is, I believe, why Marler emphasised pragmatics ("the significance of signals to the communicants") over semantics (a fixed relationship of signs to meanings) in the study of animal communication. When a signal violates expectations, it could be because a low-probability event occurred, because the signal was misperceived or because the communication system itself is not what was assumed. In this way, violated expectations provide evidence of real-world miscommunication. Such violations may provide information about the larger system of signals and messages that receivers must learn about. The surprised meerkat may have received a signal that normally would reduce uncertainty about the present location of the signaller, and so we may talk about the content of the message in this relatively context-free way. But as an interpretant, the meerkat has received information about the whole system of communication in which it is embedded. This information is not, however, encoded in the signal it received, and thus we do not have to say that it was communicated. Nevertheless, the cognitive animal can use information about the unlikeliness of the message it imputed to learn something about the reliability of the signaller and of the communicative system itself, and thus it looks around to learn more.

13.5 Conclusions

Messages have meaning, according to Shannon, by which he meant that "they refer to or are correlated according to some system with certain physical or conceptual entities" (1948, p. 3). But, he explained, such meanings are not relevant to the engineering problem of designing efficient communication channels. Shannon (1956) urged caution about extending the engineer's concept to biology and psychology, but he was also optimistic that the theory would prove useful. I believe that neither side of the recent dispute has fully absorbed Shannon's lessons.

The reference to information in animal communication is not bound to metaphors drawn from human language. The Marlerians are right that the information eliminativists attack a straw man, although I am sympathetic to some elements of their critique. More can and should be done to connect the mathematics of information to claims about animal communication, but mathematical modelling is not an absolute requirement for progress to be made. There are general benefits to mathematical models, namely more precise predictions, and Shannon's seminal theory is a natural starting point. But there may be other ways of building mathematical models of information that would be even more useful for cognitive science (Vigo, 2011). Nevertheless, it is worth re-emphasising that Shannon's theory has held centre stage for many solid reasons, and given its seminal status, the theory is a natural starting point.

There is information available from communicative signals. The communicative systems of animals do not have the full structure of human language (see also McAninch, Goodrich & Allen, 2009). Nonetheless, the signals are appropriately described in terms of meaning or significance. That significance derives from an objective relationship between signal and source, but requires an organism to interpret it. One and the same signal has different significance to different receivers, or to the same receiver at different times. Owren *et al.* claim that ethologists should be cautious about using the metaphors of 'transmission', 'container' and 'conduit' (Owren *et al.*, 2010, p. 760) because they prefer to focus on the ways in which signals influence the emotions and behaviours of perceivers rather than presupposing a message literally being conveyed from signaller to receiver. I also urge caution about these metaphors, but for a different reason: they tend to reinforce the idea of fixed messages being passed between communicants through well-defined channels. The system is a lot more malleable than that, and communicators have various strategies for adjusting to violations of their expectations. Understanding these adjustments requires attention to the epistemically significant learning capacities of animals – they are not just influenced, but they actively seek additional information when expectations are violated. Here, information models have strong leverage over mere influence models because they connect to learning theory in deep ways (M. Ramscar, in preparation).

The information eliminativists urge attention to affective-emotional processes in understanding animal communication rather than information processing, but following Marler, I believe this to be a false dichotomy (again, see McAninch *et al.*, 2009). Emotions are part of the information-processing system, not separate from it (Damasio, 1995). A meerkat that is surprised on hearing a 'close' call from an unexpected direction becomes aroused and alert, actively acquiring more information. Differential responses to repeated calls in the meerkats are not due to the intrinsically arousing properties of 'close' calls. The effect of a second call from the same individual within a few seconds and coming from the opposite direction is explained in terms of the informational state of the meerkat in relation to both calls. Contra Owren *et al.*, so long as we have to take into account the receiver's informational state to make sense of its reaction to the signal then we cannot regard the meerkat as solely driven by a fixed relationship between physical properties of the signal and an emotional/affective response. Smooth communication fails when expectations are violated. But expectancies exist only in those organisms which impute significance to the signals they receive.

Acknowledgements

I am grateful to Marta Manser, Michael Ramscar, Robert Rose, Ulrich Stegmann and Simon Townsend, as well as two unnamed referees for helpful comments on earlier drafts. Drew Rendall also helpfully connected some of the dots among Marler's academic descendants.

References

Allen, C. (1995). Intentionality: natural and artificial. In J. A. Meyer & H. L. Roitblat, eds., *Comparative Approaches to Cognitive Science*. Cambridge, MA: MIT Press, pp. 93–110.

Allen, C. (1999). Animal concepts revisited: the use of self-monitoring as an empirical approach. *Erkenntnis*, **51**, 33–40.

Beecher, M. D. (1989). Signalling systems for individual recognition: an information theory approach. *Animal Behavior*, **38**, 248–261.

Chater, N. & Heyes, C. (1994). Animal concepts: content and discontent. *Mind and Language*, **9**, 209–246.

Cheney, D. L. & Seyfarth, R. M (1988). Assessment of meaning and detection of unreliable signals by vervet monkeys. *Animal Behaviour*, **36**, 477–486.

Cherry, C. (1957). *On Human Communication: A Review, a Survey, and a Criticism*. Cambridge, MA: MIT Press.

Damasio, A. (1995). *Descartes' Error: Emotion, Reasoning, and the Human Brain*. New York: Harper Perennial.

Dretske, F. I. (1981). *Knowledge and the Flow of Information*. Cambridge, MA: MIT Press.

Haldane, J. B. S. & Spurway, H. (1954). A statistical analysis of communication in '*Apis Mellifera*' and a comparison with communication in other animals. *Insectes Sociaux*, **1**, 247–284.

Manser, M. B. (1998). The evolution of auditory communication in suricates (*Suricata suricatta*). PhD thesis, University of Cambridge.

Marler, P. (1961). The logical analysis of animal communication. *Journal of Theoretical Biology*, **1**, 295–317.

McAninch, A., Goodrich, G. & Allen, C. (2009). Animal communication and neo-expressivism. In R. W. Lurz, ed., *Philosophy of Animal Minds: New Essays on Animal Thought and Consciousness*. Cambridge: Cambridge University Press, pp. 128–144.

Millikan, R. G. (1984). *Language, Thought, and Other Biological Categories*. Cambridge, MA: MIT Press.

Morris, C. (1946). *Signs, Language and Behavior*. New York: Prentice Hall.

Newen, A. & Bartels, A. (2007). Animal minds and the possession of concepts. *Philosophical Psychology*, **20**, 283–308.

Ogden, C. & Richards, I. (1923/1946). *The Meaning of Meaning*, 8th edn. New York: Harcourt, Brace and World.

Owren, M. J., Rendall, D. & Ryan, M. J. (2010). Redefining animal signaling: influence versus information in communication. *Biology and Philosophy*, **25**, 755–780.

Peirce, C. S. (1935). *Collected Papers*. Cambridge, MA: Harvard University Press.

Radick, G. (2007). *The Simian Tongue: The Long Debate on Animal Language*. Chicago, IL: University of Chicago Press.

Reber, S. A. (2010). Discrimination of close calls is related to conflict situations in female meerkats. MSc thesis, University of Zurich, Switzerland.

Rendall, D. & Owren, M. J. (2002). Animal vocal communication: say what? In M. Bekoff, C. Allen & G. M. Burghardt, eds., *The Cognitive Animal: Empirical and Theoretical Perspectives on Animal Cognition*. Cambridge, MA: MIT Press, pp. 307–314.

Rendall, D., Owren, M. J. & Ryan, M. J. (2009). What do animal signals mean? *Animal Behaviour*, **78**, 233–240.

Schibler, F. & Manser, M. B. (2007). The irrelevance of individual discrimination in meerkat alarm calls. *Animal Behaviour*, **74**, 1259–1268.

Seyfarth, R. M., Cheney, D. L., Bergman, T. *et al.* (2010). The central importance of information in studies of animal communication. *Animal Behaviour*, **80**, 3–8.

Seyfarth, R. M., Cheney, D. L. & Marler, P. (1980a). Monkey responses to three different alarm calls: evidence for predator classification and semantic communication. *Science*, **210**, 801–803.

Seyfarth, R. M., Cheney, D. L. & Marler, P. (1980b). Vervet monkey alarm calls: semantic communication in a free-ranging primate. *Animal Behaviour*, **28**, 1070–1094.

Shannon, C. E. (1948). A mathematical theory of communication. *Bell Systems Technical Journal*, **27**, 379–423, 623–656.

Shannon, C. E. (1956). The bandwagon. *IEEE Transactions Information Theory*, **2**.

Shannon, C. E. & Weaver W. (1949). *A Mathematical Model of Communication*. Urbana, IL: University of Illinois Press.

Smith, L. B. (2000). Avoiding association when it's behaviorism you really hate. In R. Golinkoff & K. Hirsh-Pasek, eds., *Breaking the Word Learning Barrier*. Oxford: Oxford University Press, pp. 169–174.

Townsend, S. W., Allen, C. & Manser, M. B. (2011). A simple test of vocal individual recognition in wild meerkats. *Biology Letters*, epub doi: 10.1098/rsbl.2011.0844.

Townsend, S. W., Hollen, L. I. & Manser, M. B. (2010). Meerkat close calls encode group-specific signatures but receivers fail to discriminate. *Animal Behaviour*, **80**, 133–138.

Vigo, R. (2011). Representational Information. *Information Sciences*, **181**, 4847–4859.

Wiener, N. (1961). *Cybernetics; or Control and Communication in the Animal and the Machine*. Cambridge, MA: MIT Press.

14

The neural representation of vocalisation perception

KATE L. CHRISTISON-LAGAY AND YALE E. COHEN

14.1 Introduction

The idea that the brain may have regions that are specialised for different tasks can be traced back to the pseudoscience of phrenology (Castro-Caldas & Grafman, 2000). Phrenologists believed that various bumps and enlargements on the skull reflected enlarged areas of the brain underneath, and that they could therefore interpret the peculiarities of one's skull to determine one's personality and intellectual capacities. Although this pseudoscience luckily fell out of favour, one aspect of it did not: the idea that certain functions were localised to specific regions of the brain. This supposition of phrenology is now a tenet of how we currently understand the brain: specific brain functions are mediated by specific circuits. More specifically, there are regions of the brain that handle the processing of sensory stimuli; regions that are involved in coordinating movements; areas implicated as central to memory and decision-making. We also now understand that these areas seem be subdivided, such that small regions may be highly specialised for specific types of stimuli or tasks.

This specialisation appears to be what happens in the case of the neural processing of vocalisation perception and production. To hear and subsequently perceive sounds, we and other animals need a functioning auditory cortex. However, Wernicke (1874) and Broca (1861) showed that humans who had experienced insult to two particular portions of the brain – portions that were not primary auditory cortex – had trouble in language production and language processing. Broca's area in the inferior frontal gyrus and Wernicke's area in the posterior superior temporal gyrus have both been implicated in the

Animal Communication Theory: Information and Influence, ed. Ulrich Stegmann. Published by Cambridge University Press.

comprehension of human language and vocalisations. Although the specific role of Broca's area has been revised over the years to reflect its involvement in comprehension and cognitive control of linguistic tasks rather than in language production (Novick, Trueswell & Thompson-Schill, 2005), these early case studies provided a knowledge base that has been expanded upon over the intervening years with other case studies and later psychological and neuroscientific experiments. In humans, it has been found that not only is language processing localised to specific regions within the brain, but that it is also, to a great extent, lateralised to the left hemisphere of the brain (Broca, 1865; Bethmann *et al.*, 2007).

Early work focused largely on humans, perhaps because it is self-evident that human language is a valid and informative form of communication. But what about animals? Certainly, animals make vocalisations. Can these vocalisations be considered communication in the same way that human language can be? The answer is not entirely clear. Tomasello (2008) argues that in order for vocalisations to be considered communicative in the way that human language is communicative, the vocalisations must be intentionally informative. Not all sounds that an animal might make can be considered intentionally informative, even if they are information-rich. For example, a sneeze can be information-rich: perhaps the sneezer is sick, or there is something sneeze-inducing in the area. Listeners would be able to glean this information from the sneeze. However, the sneezer did not intend to sneeze, nor did he intend to communicate the information carried in the sneeze, and therefore, the sneeze should not be considered a form of communication. It is arguable that although primates can identify the identity, sex, group identity and size of an individual based upon vocalisations (Rendall, Rodman & Emond, 1996; Fitch, 1997; Rendall, Owren & Rodman, 1998; Gouzoules & Gouzoules, 2000; Miller, Dibble & Hauser, 2001; Weiss, Garibaldi & Hauser, 2001), and can discriminate between different exemplars of the same call and categorise calls (Seyfarth, Cheney & Marler, 1980; Fischer, 1998; Fitch & Fritz, 2006), none of this information is, in fact, intentionally communicated. Therefore, although the vocalisations are certainly information-rich, perhaps they should not be considered a form of communication.

Seyfarth and Cheney (2010) suggest, however, that while humans may be unique within the animal kingdom with regards to the extent of our ability to create new words, use syntax, understand that a speaker/vocaliser is intentionally vocalising and understand precisely what that vocalisation means, it does seem that some species of animals may be able to communicate via vocalisation in a manner not entirely dissimilar to our own. Specifically, it is arguable that some animals have referential vocalisations, intentionally vocalise and are capable of combining vocalisations using a simple syntax. Many non-human primates have different categories of vocalisations (i.e. different types of calls) that are acoustically different and may be used differentially in different situations. For example, vervets make different alarm calls based upon the type of predator present (Seyfarth *et al.*, 1980). These calls can be understood by conspecifics and even by individuals from other species. These calls elicit avoidance behaviours in listeners and prompt them to hide – clearly, the vocalisations are information-rich. One might assume that the call was intentionally made to warn others. But such a conclusion is, in this case, only supposition. The case for intentionality is made stronger when looking at chimpanzee vocalisations elicited by food. Chimpanzees vocalise in the presence of food, and therefore draw others to the food source. However, they are less likely to vocalise if there is not much food present or if the food is rare and favoured (Hauser & Wrangham, 1987; Hauser *et al.*, 1993). This withholding of vocalisation when it would not be beneficial to the animal suggests that the vocalisation in other contexts is an intentional form of communication; or, at the very least, that the chimpanzee can and does control whether or not he vocalises. It has also been found that in some species, different types of calls may be strung together to modify their meanings (Arnold & Zuberbuhler, 2006), which suggests that the animals are using a simple syntax to modify vocalisation meanings.

14.2 Vocalisation production

Although vocalisation behaviour is relatively well studied, there is a notable dearth of studies on the neurobiology of vocalisation production. This dearth of neurobiological studies is especially glaring in the case of non-human primates. Although there have been microstimulation studies of the anterior cingulate cortex, the periaqueductal grey and the reticular formation – all of which, when stimulated, lead animals to produce natural-sounding vocalisations (Jürgens, 2009) – these studies do not cast light on the neural code underlying differentiated and nuanced vocalisation production. Furthermore, because these studies evoke the vocalisations through stimulation, they cannot address whether a vocalisation is intentional, and thus cannot study the neural code underlying vocalisation production intentionality. The few neuroscientific studies that have used single-cell recordings to address vocalisation production have examined the response of neurons in the auditory cortex while an animal vocalises. These studies have found that during self-initiated vocalisations, the activity of most of the observed neurons in the auditory cortex is suppressed, while a small subset of the neurons shows greater activation during vocalisation (Eliades & Wang, 2003, 2005, 2008). Furthermore, the response of auditory cortex neurons during vocalisation seems to be context-dependent: the neurons of a common marmoset that are active during antiphonal calling do not have similar activity when the same vocalisation (*phee*) is produced in a non-antiphonal context (Miller & Wang, 2009). However, at present, few other studies have examined vocalisation production at the neural level, and none to our knowledge have been able to address whether there is a difference in the neural representation of vocalisations believed to be intentional and those that are not.

14.3 Processing of vocalisations

Because of the lack of studies on the neuroscience behind vocalisation production, our discussion for the rest of the chapter will be limited to the processing of vocalisations by conspecific animals. We have already established that there is the possibility that some animals can communicate via vocalisations in a manner not dissimilar to humans. If that is indeed the case, do these animals' brains process communication in a manner similar to humans as well? Even before considering direct evidence that communication signal processing in animals is privileged (i.e. that vocalisations are processed differently from other sounds), several facts are highly suggestive that it is. First, if the perception of communication signals and language is a specialised, privileged process in humans, it stands to reason that our degree of specialisation must have evolved from something. Furthermore, primates can extract many of the same features from vocalisations that humans can. This similarity suggests that perhaps animals may extract these features from conspecific communication calls in a manner similar to the way that humans process spoken language. Because of these facts, and because humans are known to have brain regions that are specialised for communication, it is perhaps natural to look for similar specialisation in our close phylogenetic cousins, the non-human primates.

Primates are certainly not the only animals who vocalise, nor are they the only ones believed to have informative, referential vocalisations: to name a few, chickens, chickadees and meerkats are believed to make referential vocalisations (Evans & Evans, 1999; Templeton, Greene & Davis, 2005; Hollén & Manser, 2007). Nor are primates the only model systems whose communication signals have been studied: there has been extensive study of the motor circuits, learning and auditory feedback involved in bird song (Hausberger & Cousillas, 1995; Leonardo & Fee, 2005; Mooney, 2009). However, because the bird song literature is full of topics far outside the purview of this chapter, and because that literature does not add substantively to the question of how information contained within a vocalisation is processed, we will dedicate the rest of our discussion to the perception of conspecific vocalisations in primates.

Before we begin to explore the topic of neural representations of vocalisation, we must acknowledge some of the current limits and limitations of neuroscience.

When we say that neurons are 'selective' for a certain type of vocalisation, we cannot (at present) say exactly which features of vocalisations those neurons select; nor can we say that the brain understands, for example, that exactly four action potentials in this region mean X, whereas six action potentials mean Y. Neural activity is highly variable, and subject to the influence of uncountable other neurons as well as other chemical and electrical events. Additionally, when an imaging study shows more activity in one area over another, we cannot say what exactly that activity is – it could be the action of inhibitory or excitatory neurons, increased metabolism of nearby support cells, or any number of other reasons that blood flow might increase to an area of the brain. We also cannot say definitively that a given neuron or region is selective for just one (or even a few) types of vocalisations or sounds: we cannot possibly test the response to every conceivable auditory stimulus. Therefore, when we discuss selectivity, we can only say that a neuron is selective for a given sound (or sounds) as compared with the rest of the assemblage of sounds tested. When we discuss neural responses to a given vocalisation, we refer to the distribution of responses over multiple presentations of the stimulus.

In addition to limitations on interpreting data, the methods needed to acquire neural data from animals places experimental restrictions on data collection. During data acquisition, the animals are not in natural or even naturalistic environments; they must be trained to be still and complete tasks; the sounds that they hear are often played through speakers instead of occurring 'naturally'; and the sounds are often presented without the gestures and expressions that would accompany them in natural contexts. Thus, there are limitations on the types of experiments that currently can be conducted. Furthermore, differences in training may alter the neural representation of a vocalisation when presented in a certain context. Therefore, because of limitations on data collection, analysis and experimental design, and because the study of the neural representation of communication is still in early stages, the field is conservative in its conclusions.

14.3.1 *Processing in the auditory cortex*

There are several more-or-less complementary models of the auditory processing pathways. The first holds that auditory processing is broken into two streams: the 'what' ventral pathway and the 'where' dorsal pathway (Kaas & Hackett, 1999; Romanski *et al.*, 1999). The 'what' pathway is thought to be used to process the content of the auditory signal, including identifying what kind of sound it is, what it means and the identity of the source. The purpose of the 'where' pathway should be self-evident. The second model is largely the same, except that instead of 'what' and 'where' pathways, there are 'perception' and 'action' pathways (Griffiths, 2008; Rauschecker & Scott, 2009). The 'perception' pathway is largely the same as the 'what' pathway: it is responsible for the conscious perception of a sound's identity. The 'action' pathway allows appropriate motor actions to be executed in response to sounds even in the absence of conscious perception of that sound (Griffiths, 2008). The third model holds that there are multiple, parallel pathways involved in auditory processing: one for auditory objects (perceived sounds and speech), a pathway that is nearly identical to the 'what' or 'perception' pathway; one for spatial information, which is largely the 'where' pathway; and one (or several) for other auditory functions (Rauschecker & Scott, 2009). Although the main pathways are similar to the 'what'/'where' dual stream model, this model differs in its inclusion of feed-forward and feedback mechanisms at nearly every level of processing (Rauschecker & Scott, 2009). Those who favour this conceptual model claim that these feed-forward and feedback mechanisms explain how self-initiated vocalisations are compared and their production updated (Rauschecker & Scott, 2009). In our discussion of the identification and perception of vocalisations, the 'what' pathway – whose purpose remains fairly consistent across models – is the more salient pathway to discuss. However, in order to avoid confusion between the different names for the pathway in different models, we will refer to the pathway responsible for the processing and perception of a sound's identity as the 'auditory object' pathway. From the primary auditory cortex (the core), the 'auditory object' pathway proceeds through the anterior portions of the secondary and higher-order auditory cortices (belt and parabelt regions, respectively) in the temporal lobe before proceeding to the prefrontal cortex (Romanski *et al.*, 1999; see Figure 14.1). Because this pathway is sensitive to the type of sound presented, it is a natural path to examine for the neural correlates of vocalisation perception. Owing to the complexities of identifying the exact region of auditory cortex being reported on in various studies, here we will refer to the primary auditory cortex as 'core regions', and to secondary and higher-order auditory cortices as 'non-core regions'.

Studies of the selective processing of vocalisations at the cortical start of the 'auditory object' pathway have yielded mixed findings. It is clear that core regions are necessary to process these sounds: without the core regions, animals are functionally deaf. Moreover, even when accounting for their degree of deafness, the processing of conspecific vocalisations is disturbed (Heffner & Heffner, 1984, 1986, 1989). However, it is unclear whether there are neurons (or indeed, populations of neurons) that are selective for conspecific vocalisations. Findings from Wollberg and Newman (1972), Winter and Funkenstein (1973), Manley and Muller-Preuss (1978), Wang *et al.* (1995) and Wang and Kadia (2001) suggest that there may be some neurons, or populations of neurons, that

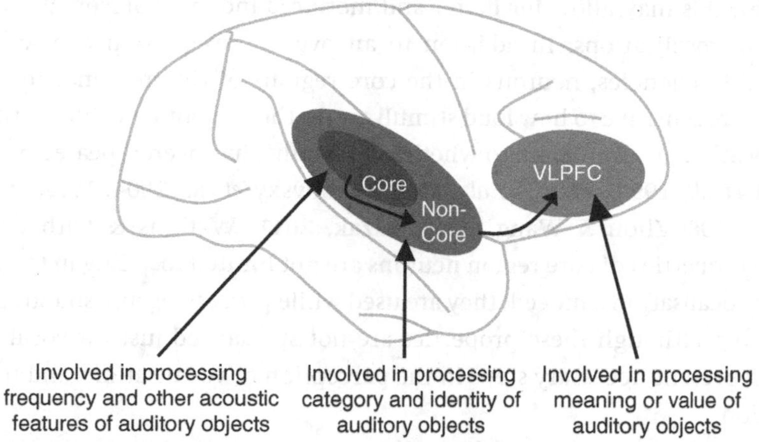

Figure 14.1 The 'auditory object' pathway of auditory processing with putative processing steps. **Core:** primary auditory cortex; **non-core:** secondary and higher-order auditory cortices; **VLPFC:** ventrolateral prefrontal cortex.

The 'auditory object' pathway of auditory processing is responsible for the conscious perception of a sound's identity, including the type of sound, its meaning and the identity of its source. From the core regions of the auditory cortex, the 'auditory object' pathway proceeds ventrally and anteriorly through the non-core regions of the auditory cortex to the VLPFC. The core is believed to be responsible for processing the frequency and other acoustic features and representations relating to auditory objects, including vocalisations; non-core regions are believed to be involved in the processing of the category and identity of auditory objects (here, vocalisation category and vocaliser's identity); and the VLPFC is believed to be involved in processing the meaning and value of auditory objects (here, the meaning of vocalisations).

are more sensitive to conspecific vocalisations than to other sounds, but there is no strong evidence to suggest that there are 'call detectors' in core regions of the model systems used. There is, however, evidence that core regions of the auditory cortex may have an over-representation of frequencies that are characteristic of the conspecific vocalisations of a given species (Epple, 1968; Aitkin *et al.*, 1986; Owren *et al.*, 1988; Wang, 2000). The interpretation of this fact should be approached cautiously, as the frequency ranges associated with conspecific vocalisations and the range of best hearing may be a type of chicken-or-egg situation: it is possible that the frequency range best represented for a given species is so evolved in order to best represent conspecific vocalisations, but it is also possible that conspecific vocalisations have evolved to be centred in the best frequency range for a given species. Whichever the case may be, because conspecific vocalisations do exploit the best-represented frequencies for a given species, this may allow for better and more redundant representation of conspecific vocalisations. In addition to an over-representation of vocalisation-related frequencies, neurons in the core regions of the mammalian auditory cortex are sensitive to how loud stimuli are, to the temporal profile of stimuli, to the location of stimuli and to whether a stimulus has been repeated or is novel (Javitt *et al.*, 1994; Wang *et al.*, 1995; Ulanovsky *et al.*, 2004; Werner-Reiss & Groh, 2008; Zhou & Wang, 2010; Razak, 2011; Watkins & Barbour, 2011). These properties of core region neurons are not limited to aiding in the processing of vocalisations; indeed, they are used while processing any sound stimulus. However, although these properties are not specialised just for vocalisations, they represent necessary steps in the perception of vocalisations and thus bear mention.

Although core regions of the auditory cortex may not be particularly specialised to process vocalisations, there is evidence to suggest that non-core regions of the auditory cortex and prefrontal cortical areas are more selective. Rauschecker and Tian (2000) and Tian *et al.* (2001) found that in non-core regions, there are neurons that are relatively selective for conspecific vocalisations. Specifically, they found neurons in the anterior lateral belt of an anaesthetised rhesus macaque that responded selectively to different types of calls (different vocalisation categories). The recorded cells showed a range of selectivity to different vocalisations. However, most were not selective to just one call, but rather showed robust activity in response to three to five types of vocalisation. Notably, the vocalisations that activated a given neuron were not necessarily those that were the vocalisations with bandwidths most similar to each other. This suggests that it is not merely the frequency components of the vocalisations that are activating the neuron. Non-core regions of the auditory cortex have also been shown by positron emission tomography (PET) to be active in response to conspecific vocalisations (Poremba *et al.*, 2004). Specifically, the anterior regions of the left temporal cortex showed more metabolic activity in response to conspecific vocalisations than other regions of the auditory cortex. Recent studies also showed that within non-core regions that are responsive to vocalisations, there are clusters of neurons that are highly selective specifically for conspecific vocalisations, and that, furthermore, neurons within these clusters are highly selective as to which conspecific vocalisations they respond to (Petkov *et al.*, 2008; Perrodin *et al.*, 2011). Some neurons in this area were found to be selective for the category of vocalisation. Tsunada, Lee and Cohen (2011) showed that neurons in the superior temporal gyrus, a non-core region, have categorical activity in response to complex auditory stimuli. Although this study used human phonemes and not conspecific vocalisations, the findings further corroborate the idea that non-core regions are responsive to complex stimuli, and that the responses of neurons in these regions are not based solely on the acoustics of a sound. Taken together, these findings suggest that while the non-core regions of the auditory cortex are likely to be part of the network that processes vocalisations, these regions are not the end of vocalisation processing.

The findings discussed above suggest that non-core regions of the auditory cortex may be involved in encoding the category of vocalisation. But vocalisation category is not the only information carried in a vocalisation. Portions of the 'auditory object' pathway have been found to be selective not to the type or category of the vocalisation, but rather to the identity of the vocaliser. Using a functional magnetic resonance imaging (fMRI) adaptation paradigm, Petkov *et al.* (2008) found an area within non-core regions of the auditory cortex that responded more to the voice of an individual conspecific vocaliser than it did to specific types of vocalisation or other environmental sounds. This suggests that the processing of communication signals may be split into different sub-processes: there may be regions in the 'auditory object' pathway that are specialised for processing the type of vocalisation and others for processing the identity of the vocaliser. These results have also been shown on the single-neuron level: within clusters of vocalisation-selective neurons, single neurons have been shown to be selective for a vocaliser's identity (Perrodin *et al.*, 2011).

14.4.2 *Prefrontal processing*

As discussed above, the processing of vocalisations does not seem to be completed in the auditory cortex. After processing in the non-core regions of the auditory cortex, information in the 'auditory object' processing pathway proceeds to the ventrolateral prefrontal cortex. Romanski and Goldman-Rakic (2002) and Romanski, Averbeck and Diltz (2005) found that neurons in the ventrolateral prefrontal cortex responded to a number of sounds, including human and monkey vocalisations. They found that most neurons responded to several vocalisations, although some responded either to just one or non-selectively to the auditory stimuli presented. However, they also found that the auditory stimuli to which the neurons were selective were not necessarily similar in meaning, but may have shared acoustic characteristics. While this is in keeping with Romanski *et al.*'s (2005) view that the ventrolateral prefrontal cortex has a role in assessing acoustic features, Gifford *et al.* (2005) found that neurons in the ventrolateral prefrontal cortex responded similarly to food calls that had similar meanings, even though those calls were acoustically distinct. Further supporting this, Russ, Orr and Cohen (2008) and Lee *et al.* (2009) suggest that activity in ventrolateral prefrontal cortex neurons correlates best not with the auditory stimuli, but with a monkey's behavioural choices about those stimuli. It should be noted that the Romanski and Goldman-Rakic (2002) and

Romanski *et al.* (2005) papers differ in many ways from the Russ *et al.* (2008) and Lee *et al.* (2009) papers, including the stimuli and paradigms used: Russ *et al.* (2008) and Lee *et al.* (2009) used manipulations of human phonemes, but also used a paradigm that required the animals to pay attention to the specific auditory stimuli. Therefore, it is possible that the differences in findings between these papers arise because of the requirements of the specific experiment, or it may be that there are subsets of neurons within the ventrolateral prefrontal cortex that perform different roles. Differences in the specifics of findings aside, these studies all suggest that neurons in the ventrolateral prefrontal cortex do seem to process conspecific vocalisations, and do so in a fairly specific manner.

Therefore, it seems that the 'auditory object' pathway does indeed process vocal communication signals in primates. However, a notable feature of human language perception is that it is largely lateralised to the left hemisphere; and many of the above-discussed studies do not explicitly examine the existence or extent of lateralised processing. So a question remains: is vocalisation processing in primates similarly lateralised?

14.4.3 *Lateralisation*

Many early studies in the neural correlates of communication perception in monkeys were conducted in experiments that paralleled early human studies. In these experiments, primarily two techniques were used: various portions of the core and non-core regions of the auditory cortex were ablated or otherwise lesioned; and dichotic listening paradigms in which sounds are presented to only one ear (and thus, the sound is presumably processed largely by the auditory cortex contralateral to sound presentation).

A study by Beecher *et al.* (1979) trained Japanese macaques and three other species of monkeys to recognise two categories of Japanese macaque vocalisations (both were types of *coo*): by category or by pitch (as either high- or low-pitched; both categories of vocalisation had both high- and low-pitched exemplars). Using a dichotic listening paradigm, and comparing the performance across species, tasks and ears, Beecher *et al.* found that the Japanese macaques learned the task more quickly when the vocalisations were sorted by vocalisation category than when sorted by pitch; that macaques showed a right ear (left hemisphere) advantage when the task was based upon vocalisation class instead of pitch; and finally, that the control species showed no ear advantage and were faster to learn the pitch-sorted identification task than they were to learn the category-sorted task. These results are supported by a similar experiment by Petersen *et al.* (1984). In both cases, it is notable that it was only the Japanese macaques that showed a right ear/left hemisphere advantage, which suggests that the processing of communication calls may be specific to conspecific vocalisations, and not the vocalisations of other species even when those species are closely related.

Results from Hauser, Agnetta and Perez (1998) and Ghazanfar, Smith-Rohrberg and Hauser (2001) support the idea that lateralisation of processing may be specific to conspecific vocalisations. In these studies, vocalisations were presented to rhesus macaques. When the vocalisations were not manipulated, there was a right ear preference for most vocalisations, whereas when the vocalisations were altered so that they were faster, slower (Hauser *et al.*, 1998) or reversed (Ghazanfar *et al.*, 2001), this right ear advantage was eliminated. This suggests that there is lateralisation of the processing of many natural vocalisations.

Lesions studies also support the idea of lateralisation in the processing of conspecific vocalisations. In a series of experiments, Heffner and Heffner (1984, 1986, 1989) found that Japanese macaques with ablations of the left auditory cortex, and those with ablations limited to left non-core regions, were unable to discriminate between vocalisation categories. Moreover, the deficit was not merely due to cortical deafness: control experiments showed that hearing monkeys could identify conspecific vocalisations, even if those vocalisations were distorted in a way that mimicked hearing loss. Because hearing loss alone does not account for the degree of decrement in the identification of conspecific vocalisations that was observed in the lesioned animals, this suggests that the identification of vocalisations does not rely merely upon 'normal' hearing, but seems to require both specialised and lateralised processing.

These studies suggest that the processing of conspecific vocalisations is left-lateralised. There is, however, some evidence to suggest that not all conspecific vocalisation processing follows this rule. Hauser *et al.* (1998) noted that while most vocalisations elicited a right-ear, left-hemisphere listening bias, the copulation scream elicited a left-ear, right-hemisphere listening bias. Right lateralisation of vocalisation processing has also been found in chimpanzees using PET (Taglialatela *et al.*, 2009), and in macaques using fMRI (Joly *et al.*, 2011). However, in chimpanzees, the right lateralisation was limited to posterior portions of the temporal lobe, which are not within the traditional 'auditory object' pathway. Also, the right lateralisation for macaques was limited to core regions: the greatest activity in non-core regions of the auditory cortex in response to vocalisations was observed on the left, not the right, side of the brain. This suggests that the lateralisation of the processing of communication signals may be more complicated than originally believed. This more complicated story is substantiated by corroborating studies in humans, which suggest that different aspects of vocal communication signals may affect the lateralisation of processing (Zatorre & Belin, 2001; Belin, Zatorre & Ahad, 2002; Zatorre, Belin & Penhune, 2002; Boemio *et al.*, 2005).

14.5 Conclusions

In summary, the processing of conspecific vocalisations seems to follow the 'auditory object' processing pathway, and there may be further specialisations of that pathway that are specific to conspecific vocalisations. Furthermore, there may be lateralisation of at least certain aspects of conspecific vocalisation processing. However, the neurobiological study of animal communication is still in its nascent phases. Many questions remain, and the field is ripe with possibilities for future studies.

A broader range of vocalisations, and potentially a broader range of model organisms, need to be used to expand upon results discussed in this chapter. For example, single neuron recordings and imaging studies comparing the neural response to vocalisations that have yielded left-lateralised results in the past should be compared with those that have been suggested to be right-lateralised (for example a grunt versus a copulation scream). Furthermore, a study looking at the neural response to calls with specific meanings, such as the vervet's predator alarm calls, could yield important findings regarding the neural correlates of the meaning of vocalisations.

It should also not be ignored that communication does not consist merely of acoustic signals. Even if the study of communication were to be limited to communicative vocalisations, those vocalisations have both denotative and connotative elements. For example, if a vervet were to make the 'eagle' alarm call, this would denote that an eagle had been spotted. However, there is an affective component to the call – the call connotes a present danger. It is possible that while the 'auditory object' pathway may process the acoustics of a sound, further processing may take place elsewhere to process both denotative and connotative meanings of vocalisations. Kuraoka and Nakamura (2007) found that neurons in the amygdala are selective for certain types of emotional content in conspecific vocalisations, and Gil-da-Costa *et al.* (2004) also found activity in limbic structures while primates listen to conspecific vocalisations. Therefore, it is possible that the emotion valence of vocalisations may, in part, be processed and encoded in the limbic system.

Several papers observe that vocalisations produced in states of high emotional arousal, such as screams, seem to elicit a startle reflex in animals, and they suggest that perhaps these vocalisations are processed subcortically (Owren & Rendall, 2001; Rendall, 2009). Certainly, auditory startle reflexes are mediated by subcortical regions (Brown *et al.*, 1991), and auditory content is processed in the brainstem (Griffiths *et al.*, 2001). No systematic study of the processing of conspecific vocalisations of primates in early auditory nuclei has been undertaken, so the degree of processing that occurs subcortically is unknown. However, neurons in the mouse inferior colliculus (an early auditory nucleus) have been shown to respond selectively to certain vocalisations, even when the vocalisation's sound energy falls outside that preferred by the neuron (Portfors, Roberts & Jonson, 2009). This suggests that perhaps vocalisations are privileged even at the subcortical level. Considerably more study is needed to explore the mechanisms and extent of any such processing.

If one does not limit the study of communication to acoustic processing, even more experimental possibilities present themselves. While Tomasello (2008) argues that the intentionality of primate vocalisations may be questionable, there are certainly meaningful, intentional gestures and expressions used by primates. A systematic study of the neural correlates of the perception of motor components of communication signals could yield interesting findings about a form of primate communication that is perhaps more nuanced than non-human primate vocalisations.

Furthermore, it should be acknowledged that the perception of vocalisations does not exist in a vacuum, and thus, the context in which a vocalisation is produced and perceived is likely to contribute to the neural representation of the event. Context-dependent activity has already been shown in the case of marmoset's antiphonal calling (Miller & Wang, 2009). Another contextual variable is whether a listening primate both sees and hears a conspecific vocaliser. It has been shown that primates can match facial expression with vocalisation (Massaro, 1998; Ghazanfar & Logothetis, 2003; Izumi & Kojima, 2004); furthermore, there is integration of information about facial expression even in areas that are traditionally considered to be unimodal, auditory responsive areas (Ghazanfar *et al.*, 2005). Similarly, Gil-da-Costa *et al.* (2004) showed that when an animal listens to conspecific vocalisations, activity is elicited in higher-order visual areas, as well as in limbic and paralimbic regions. This supports the idea that the processing of communication signals is far more complicated than merely processing acoustic signals, which is, in and of itself, non-trivial. Instead, the processing of communication signals evokes activity related to memory, affect and multimodal sensory representations. Therefore, in order to glean a full understanding of the neural correlates of communication perception, there need to be studies to examine the multimodal and affective components of perception at every step in the 'auditory object' pathway, at the level of the limbic system and into the frontal and prefrontal cortices.

References

Aitkin, L. M., Merzenich, M. M., Irvine, D. R. F., Clarey, J. C. & Nelson, J. E. (1986). Frequency representation in auditory-cortex of the common marmoset (*Callithrix jacchus jacchus*). *Journal of Comparative Neurology*, **252**, 175–185.

Arnold, K. & Zuberbuhler, K. (2006). The alarm-calling system of adult male putty-nosed monkeys, *Cercopithecus nictitans martini*. *Animal Behaviour*, **72**, 643–653.

Beecher, M. D., Petersen, M. R., Zoloth, S. R., Moody, D. B. & Stebbins, W. C. (1979). Perception of conspecific vocalizations by Japanese macaques – evidence for selective attention and neural lateralization. *Brain Behavior and Evolution*, **16**, 443–460.

Belin, P., Zatorre, R. J. & Ahad, P. (2002). Human temporal-lobe response to vocal sounds. *Cognitive Brain Research*, **13**, 17–26.

Bethmann, A., Tempelmann, C., De Bleser, R., Scheich, H. & Brechmann, A. (2007). Determining language laterality by fMRI and dichotic listening. *Brain Research*, **1133**, 145–157.

Boemio, A., Fromm, S., Braun, A. & Poeppel, D. (2005). Hierarchical and asymmetric temporal sensitivity in human auditory cortices. *Nature Neuroscience*, **8**, 389–395.

Broca, P. (1861). Remarques sur le siège de la faculté de langage articulé, suivis d'une observation d'aphemie (perte de la parole). *Bulletins de la Societe Anatomique*, **6**, 330–357.

Broca, P. (1865). Sur le siège de la faculté du langage articulé. *Bulletins de la Societe d'Anthropologie*, **6**, 377–399.

Brown, P., Rothwell, J. C., Thompson, P. D. *et al.* (1991). New observations on the normal auditory startle reflex in man. *Brain*, **114**, 1891–1902.

Castro-Caldas, A. & Grafman, J. (2000). Those were the (phrenological) days. *The Neuroscientist*, **6**, 297–302.

Eliades, S. J. & Wang, X. (2003). Sensory-motor interaction in the primate auditory cortex during self-initiated vocalizations. *Journal of Neurophysiology*, **89**, 2194–2207.

Eliades, S. J. & Wang, X. (2005). Dynamics of auditory–vocal interaction in monkey auditory cortex. *Cerebral Cortex*, **15**, 1510–1523.

Eliades, S. J. & Wang, X. (2008). Neural substrates of vocalization feedback monitoring in primate auditory cortex. *Nature*, **453**, 1102–1106.

Epple, G. (1968). Comparative studies on vocalization in marmoset monkeys (*Hapalidae*). *Folia Primatologica*, **8**, 1–40.

Evans, C. S. & Evans, L. (1999). Chicken food calls are functionally referential. *Animal Behaviour*, **58**, 307–319.

Fischer, J. (1998). Barbary macaques categorize shrill barks into two call types. *Animal Behaviour*, **55**, 799–807.

Fitch, W. T. (1997). Vocal tract length and formant frequency dispersion correlate with body size in rhesus macaques. *Journal of the Acoustical Society of America*, **102**, 1213–1222.

Fitch, W. T. & Fritz, J. B. (2006). Rhesus macaques spontaneously perceive formants in conspecific vocalizations. *Journal of the Acoustical Society of America*, **120**, 2132–2141.

Ghazanfar, A. A. & Logothetis, N. K. (2003). Neuroperception: facial expressions linked to monkey calls. *Nature*, **423**, 937–938.

Ghazanfar, A. A., Maier, J. X., Hoffman, K. L. & Logothetis, N. K. (2005). Multisensory integration of dynamic faces and voices in rhesus monkey auditory cortex. *Journal of Neuroscience*, **25**, 5004–5012.

Ghazanfar, A. A., Smith-Rohrberg, D. & Hauser, M. D. (2001). The role of temporal cues in rhesus monkey vocal recognition: orienting asymmetries to reversed calls. *Brain Behavior and Evolution*, **58**, 163–172.

Gifford, G. W., MacLean, K. A., Hauser, M. D. & Cohen, Y. E. (2005). The neurophysiology of functionally meaningful categories: macaque ventrolateral prefrontal cortex plays a critical role in spontaneous categorization of species-specific vocalizations. *Journal of Cognitive Neuroscience*, **17**, 1471–1482.

Gil-da-Costa, R., Braun, A., Lopes, M. *et al.* (2004). Toward an evolutionary perspective on conceptual representation: species-specific calls activate visual and affective processing systems in the macaque. *Proceedings of the National Academy of Sciences USA*, **101**, 17516–17521.

Gouzoules, H. & Gouzoules, S. (2000). Agonistic screams differ among four species of macaques: the significance of motivation-structural rules. *Animal Behaviour*, **59**, 501–512.

Griffiths, T. D. (2008). Sensory systems: auditory action streams? *Current Biology*, **18**, R387–R388.

Griffiths, T. D., Uppenkamp, S., Johnsrude, I., Josephs, O. & Patterson, R. D. (2001). Encoding of the temporal regularity of sound in the human brainstem. *Nature Neuroscience*, **4**, 633–637.

Hausberger, M. & Cousillas, H. (1995). Categorization in birdsong: from behavioural to neuronal responses. *Behavioural Processes*, **35**, 83–91.

Hauser, M. D. & Wrangham, R. W. (1987). Manipulation of food calls in captive chimpanzees – a preliminary-report. *Folia Primatologica*, **48**, 207–210.

Hauser, M. D., Agnetta, B. & Perez, C. (1998). Orienting asymmetries in rhesus monkeys: the effect of time-domain changes on acoustic perception. *Animal Behaviour*, **56**, 41–47.

Hauser, M. D., Teixidor, P., Field, L. & Flaherty, R. (1993). Food-elicited calls in chimpanzees – effects of food quantity and divisibility. *Animal Behaviour*, **45**, 817–819.

Heffner, H. E. & Heffner, R. S. (1984). Temporal-lobe lesions and perception of species-specific vocalizations by macaques. *Science*, **226**, 75–76.

Heffner, H. E. & Heffner, R. S. (1986). Effect of unilateral and bilateral auditory cortex lesions on the discrimination of vocalizations by Japanese macaques. *Journal of Neurophysiology*, **56**, 683–701.

Heffner, H. E. & Heffner, R. S. (1989). Cortical deafness cannot account for the inability of Japanese macaques to discriminate species-specific vocalizations. *Brain and Language*, **36**, 275–285.

Hollén, L. I. & Manser, M. B. (2007). Motivation before meaning: motivational information encoded in meerkat alarm calls develops earlier than referential information. *American Naturalist*, **169**, 758–767.

Izumi, A. & Kojima, S. (2004). Matching vocalizations to vocalizing faces in a chimpanzee (*Pan troglodytes*). *Animal Cognition*, **7**, 179–184.

Javitt, D. C., Steinschneider, M., Schroeder, C. E., Vaughan Jr, H. G. & Arezzo, J. C. (1994). Detection of stimulus deviance within primate primary auditory cortex: intracortical mechanisms of mismatch negativity (MMN) generation. *Brain Research*, **667**, 192–200.

Joly, O., Ramus, F., Pressnitzer, D., Vanduffel, W. & Orban, G. A. (2011). Interhemispheric differences in auditory processing revealed by fMRI in awake rhesus monkeys. *Cerebral Cortex*, **22**, 838–853.

Jürgens, U. (2009). The neural control of vocalization in mammals: a review. *Journal of Voice*, **23**, 1–10.

Kaas, J. H. & Hackett, T. A. (1999). 'What' and 'where' processing in auditory cortex. *Nature Neuroscience*, **2**, 1045–1047.

Kuraoka, K. & Nakamura, K. (2007). Responses of single neurons in monkey amygdala to facial and vocal emotions. *Journal of Neurophysiology*, **97**, 1379–1387.

Lee, J. H., Russ, B. E., Orr, L. E. & Cohen, Y. (2009). Prefrontal activity predicts monkeys' decisions during an auditory category task. *Frontiers in Integrative Neuroscience*, **3**, doi: 10.3389/neuro.07.016.2009.

Leonardo, A. & Fee, M. S. (2005). Ensemble coding of vocal control in birdsong. *Journal of Neuroscience*, **25**, 652–661.

Manley, J. A. & Muller-Preuss, P. (1978). Response variability of auditory-cortex cells in the squirrel monkey to constant acoustic stimuli. *Experimental Brain Research*, **32**, 171–180.

Massaro, D. W. (1998). *Perceiving Talking Faces: From Speech Perception to a Behavioral Principle*. Cambridge, MA: MIT Press.

Miller, C. T. & Wang, X. (2009). Behavior-dependent modulation of primate prefrontal cortex neurons during natural behavior. Paper presented at the Society for Neuroscience.

Miller, C. T., Dibble, E. & Hauser, M. D. (2001). Amodal completion of acoustic signals by a non-human primate. *Nature Neuroscience*, **4**, 783–784.

Mooney, R. (2009). Neural mechanisms for learned birdsong. *Learning and Memory*, **16**, 655–669.

Novick, J., Trueswell, J. & Thompson-Schill, S. (2005). Cognitive control and parsing: reexamining the role of Broca's area in sentence comprehension. *Cognitive, Affective and Behavioral Neuroscience*, **5**, 263–281.

Owren, M. J. & Rendall, D. (2001). Sound on the rebound: bringing form and function back to the forefront in understanding non-human primate vocal signaling. *Evolutionary Anthropology: Issues, News, and Reviews*, **10**, 58–71.

Owren, M. J., Hopp, S. L., Sinnott, J. M. & Petersen, M. R. (1988). Absolute auditory-thresholds in three Old World monkey species (*Cercopithecus aethiops, Cercopithecus neglectus, Macaca fuscata*) and humans (*Homo sapiens*). *Journal of Comparative Psychology*, **102**, 99–107.

Perrodin, C., Kayser, C., Logothetis, N. K. & Petkov, C. I. (2011). Voice cells in the primate temporal lobe. *Current Biology*, **21**, 1408–1415.

Petersen, M. R., Zoloth, S. R., Beecher, M. D. *et al.* (1984). Neural lateralization of vocalizations by Japanese macaques – communicative significance is more important than acoustic structure. *Behavioral Neuroscience*, **98**, 779–790.

Petkov, C. I., Kayser, C., Steudel, T. *et al.* (2008). A voice region in the monkey brain. *Nature Neuroscience*, **11**, 367–374.

Poremba, A., Malloy, M., Saunders, R. C. *et al.* (2004). Species-specific calls evoke asymmetric activity in the monkey's temporal poles. *Nature*, **427**, 448–451.

Portfors, C. V., Roberts, P. D. & Jonson, K. (2009). Over-representation of species-specific vocalizations in the awake mouse inferior colliculus. *Neuroscience*, **162**, 486–500.

Rauschecker, J. P. & Scott, S. K. (2009). Maps and streams in the auditory cortex: non-human primates illuminate human speech processing. *Nature Neuroscience*, **12**, 718–724.

Rauschecker, J. P. & Tian, B. (2000). Mechanisms and streams for processing of 'what' and 'where' in auditory cortex. *Proceedings of the National Academy of Sciences USA*, **97**, 11800–11806.

Razak, K. A. (2011). Systematic representation of sound locations in the primary auditory cortex. *Journal of Neuroscience*, **31**, 13848–13859.

Rendall, D. (2009). Asymmetries in the individual distinctiveness and maternal recognition of infant contact calls and distress screams in baboons. *Journal of the Acoustical Society of America*, **125**, 1792.

Rendall, D., Owren, M. J. & Rodman, P. S. (1998). The role of vocal tract filtering in identity cueing in rhesus monkey (*Macaca mulatta*) vocalizations. *Journal of the Acoustical Society of America*, **103**, 602–614.

Rendall, D., Rodman, P. S. & Emond, R. E. (1996). Vocal recognition of individuals and kin in free-ranging rhesus monkeys. *Animal Behaviour*, **51**, 1007–1015.

Romanski, L. M. & Goldman-Rakic, P. S. (2002). An auditory domain in primate prefrontal cortex. *Nature Neuroscience*, **5**, 15–16.

Romanski, L. M., Averbeck, B. B. & Diltz, M. (2005). Neural representation of vocalizations in the primate ventrolateral prefrontal cortex. *Journal of Neurophysiology*, **93**, 734–747.

Romanski, L. M., Tian, B., Fritz, J. *et al.* (1999). Dual streams of auditory afferents target multiple domains in the primate prefrontal cortex. *Nature Neuroscience*, **2**, 1131–1136.

Russ, B. E., Orr, L. E. & Cohen, Y. E. (2008). Prefrontal neurons predict choices during an auditory same–different task. *Current Biology*, **18**, 1483–1488.

Seyfarth, R. M. & Cheney, D. L. (2010). Primate vocal communication. In M. L. Platt & A. A. Ghanzanfar, eds., *Primate Neuroethology*. New York: Oxford University Press, pp. 84–96.

Seyfarth, R. M., Cheney, D. L. & Marler, P. (1980). Monkey responses to three different alarm calls – evidence of predator classification and semantic communication. *Science*, **210**, 801–803.

Taglialatela, J. P., Russell, J. L., Schaeffer, J. A. & Hopkins, W. D. (2009). Visualizing vocal perception in the chimpanzee brain. *Cerebral Cortex*, **19**, 1151–1157.

Templeton, C. N., Greene, E. & Davis, K. (2005). Allometry of alarm calls: black-capped chickadees encode information about predator size. *Science*, **308**, 1934–1937.

Tian, B., Reser, D., Durham, A., Kustov, A. & Rauschecker, J. P. (2001). Functional specialization in rhesus monkey auditory cortex. *Science*, **292**, 290–293.

Tomasello, M. (2008). *Origins of Human Communication*. Cambridge, MA: MIT Press.

Tsunada, J., Lee, J. H. & Cohen, Y. E. (2011). Representation of speech categories in the primate auditory cortex. *Journal of Neurophysiology*, **105**, 2634–2646.

Ulanovsky, N., Las, L., Farkas, D. & Nelken, I. (2004). Multiple time scales of adaptation in auditory cortex neurons. *Journal of Neuroscience*, **24**, 10440–10453.

Wang, X., Merzenich, M. M., Beitel, R. & Schreiner, C. E. (1995). Representation of a species-specific vocalization in the primary auditory cortex of the common marmoset: temporal and spectral characteristics. *Journal of Neurophysiology*, **74**, 2685–2706.

Wang, X. Q. (2000). On cortical coding of vocal communication sounds in primates. *Proceedings of the National Academy of Sciences USA*, **97**, 11843–11849.

Wang, X. Q. & Kadia, S. C. (2001). Differential representation of species-specific primate vocalizations in the auditory cortices of marmoset and cat. *Journal of Neurophysiology*, **86**, 2616–2620.

Watkins, P. V. & Barbour, D. L. (2011). Level-tuned neurons in primary auditory cortex adapt differently to loud versus soft sounds. *Cerebral Cortex*, **21**, 178–190.

Weiss, D. J., Garibaldi, B. T. & Hauser, M. D. (2001). The production and perception of long calls by cotton-top tamarins (*Saguinus oedipus*): acoustic analyses and playback experiments. *Journal of Comparative Psychology*, **115**, 258–271.

Werner-Reiss, U. & Groh, J. M. (2008). A rate code for sound azimuth in monkey auditory cortex: implications for human neuroimaging studies. *Journal of Neuroscience*, **28**, 3747–3758.

Wernicke, C. (1874). *Der Aphasische Symptomencomplex: Eine Psychologische Studie auf Anatomischer Basis*. Breslau: Max Cohn & Weigert.

Winter, P. & Funkenstein, H. (1973). Effect of species-specific vocalization on discharge of auditory cortical-cells in awake squirrel-monkey (*Saimiri sciureus*). *Experimental Brain Research*, **18**, 489–504.

Wollberg, Z. & Newman, J. D. (1972). Auditory cortex of squirrel-monkey – response patterns of single cells to species-specific vocalizations. *Science*, **175**, 212–214.

Zatorre, R. J. & Belin, P. (2001). Spectral and temporal processing in human auditory cortex. *Cerebral Cortex*, **11**, 946–953.

Zatorre, R. J., Belin, P. & Penhune, V. B. (2002). Structure and function of auditory cortex: music and speech. *Trends in Cognitive Sciences*, **6**, 37–46.

Zhou, Y. & Wang, X. Q. (2010). Cortical processing of dynamic sound envelope transitions. *Journal of Neuroscience*, **30**, 16741–16754.

PART IV ANIMAL SIGNALS IN EVOLUTIONARY PERSPECTIVE

15

The value of information in signals and cues

MICHAEL LACHMANN

In this chapter I will discuss some uses of information measures in animal behaviour and genetics. Instead of delving into the question of when, whether and how a signalling system evolves, I will examine a simpler definition of information transfer and mutual information from statistical mechanics and the theory of communication. This circumvents, but does not solve, the question of whether or not signalling systems exist in biology. However, in my opinion, understanding the evolution of information use and transfer in biology is an important step in understanding the evolution of signals and cues.

In describing the many possible ways in which animals can interact, manipulate or maybe transmit information, the field of animal signalling borrowed many different concepts, which sadly still do not even begin to cover all the different possible types of biological 'signals', their origin and stability. Two of these concepts are 'signals' and 'cues'. Maynard Smith and Harper (2003) define a signal as "any act or structure that alters the behavior of other organisms, which evolved because of that effect, and which is effective because the receiver's response has also evolved". They also add: "It follows that the signal must carry information – about the external world – that is of interest to the receiver."

A cue, on the other hand, is defined as "a feature of the world, animate or inanimate, which can be used by an animal to guide future actions" (Maynard Smith & Harper, 2003, after Hasson, 1994).

Thus both signal and cue carry information about the world. When an organism evolves to respond to a cue its fitness can only increase, since a

Animal Communication Theory: Information and Influence, ed. Ulrich Stegmann. Published by Cambridge University Press.

strategy of ignoring the cue must have been less fit. The same is not true for a signalling system or when interacting with other organisms. Once signaller and receiver evolve to signal and respond, their interaction can change so that both might lose (Hirschleifer, 1971; Box 15.1).

Box 15.1 Is information always beneficial?

When an organism has a cue, i.e. a feature of the environment that it can respond to, it usually also has the option to ignore it. If a strategy of responding to the cue invades, it means that

$$\text{Fitness(responding to cue)} > \text{Fitness(ignoring cue)}$$

which of course means that there is a fitness gain from responding to the cue.

When we deal with an interaction between two or more actors, there is not always a gain. Imagine two female, F1 and F2, competing over the mating possibilities with two males. Assume that one of the males has higher quality than the other, though it is not necessarily known which, and that F1 had first choice. F2 can then decide whether to mate with the same male as F1, or with the other male. Let us assume that the fitness gain from mating alone with the high-quality male is 5, and with the low-quality male 1. Assume that two females mating with the same high-quality male get a fitness of 2 each, and both mating with the low-quality male get a fitness of 0 each.

If no female has information about male quality, the second female does best in choosing the other male. Half the time she would then mate with the high-quality male, and half of the time with the low-quality male, for an average fitness of $(5 + 1)/2 = 3$. Mating with the same male as F1 would give her a fitness of 2 or 0, both lower than 3.

What happens if F1 has information about male quality? In this case F1 would choose the high-quality male. If F2 now took the other male, she would always get the low-quality male, and an average fitness of 0. Therefore, she should prefer to choose the same male as F1, for a fitness of 2. In this case, F1 would also get a fitness of 2 – lower than her original average fitness of 3, without information.

Notice that for F1 the strategy of ignoring the information and flipping a coin in her choice of male is not stable: in that case F2 would choose the other male, and F1 would be tempted to switch to the strategy of choosing the high-quality male, and gain a fitness of 5 instead of 3. Thus in this case gaining additional information has reduced F1's average fitness at equilibrium.

In the following I will introduce the notion of mutual information, and explain its simple connection to the notion of fitness or relative growth rate. I will then present some of the uses of information measures in genetics. This chapter is not aimed as a review of the uses of information measures in biology (see instead, for example, Adami, 2004; Dall *et al.*, 2005; Dall Schmidt & Van Gils, 2010 and other articles in the same issue of *Oikos*; Sherwin, 2010). Instead, I want to explain why such measures have their value in theoretical biology and in particular in the theory of animal communication.

15.1 Entropy and mutual information

Uncertainty is closely related or identical to the concept of 'entropy' in various fields. In physics, two different but closely related definitions of entropy are used. The first, introduced by Clausius (1867), is based on macroscopic measures of the system, such as temperature, pressure and volume. Clausius defines the change in entropy as the integral of dQ/T, the heatflow divided by the temperature, and writes

> I propose to call the magnitude *S* the entropy of the body, from the Greek word *τροπή*, transformation. I have intentionally formed the word entropy so as to be as similar as possible to the word energy; for the two magnitudes to be denoted by these words are so nearly allied their physical meanings, that a certain similarity in designation appears to be desirable. (Clausius, 1867, p. 357).

The other, based in statistical mechanics, is a measure of the number of possible states a system could be in given its macroscopic properties. To describe a glass of water fully is impossible – we would need to know the position and velocity of more than 10^{24} atoms, and we cannot even measure the position or wavefunction of a single atom precisely. Instead we know some macroscopic properties of the water – volume, temperature, weight etc. We do not know a system's complete description, and yet, when someone tells us the temperature of the water, we gain information. Entropy in statistical mechanics is a measure for the 'number'[1] of possible states a system could be in given its macroscopic properties, or more precisely the log of the number of states. The importance of this measure in physics comes mainly from what is known as 'Liouville's theorem', which states that for isolated physical systems, two distinct states of the system cannot converge. So if we have a system that could be in one of

[1] For simplicity I talk in this chapter about number of states, instead of talking about the volume of an ensemble in phase space.

1000 possible states, and let it evolve for three hours, we will still be looking at 1000 different possible states. Thus, for example, if we start with all 1000 possible states associated with the current macroscopic properties of the system, then at any time in the future we must still be looking at 1000 different possible states. This means that the system cannot reach a condition where its macroscopic properties are associated with only 500 possible states. It must have macroscopic properties associated with *at least* 1000 possible states. This is one possible explanation why entropy, the number of possible states of the system given its macroscopic properties, cannot decrease – this is the second law of thermodynamics.

In the theory of communication, entropy is also a name for uncertainty, e.g. the number of possible states a signal could be associated with. Claude Shannon developed a measure for the uncertainty, and found it to be very similar to Boltzmann's derivation of entropy. Tribus and McIrvine (1971, p. 180) cite Shannon as saying:

> My greatest concern was what to call it. I thought of calling it 'information', but the word was overly used, so I decided to call it 'uncertainty'. When I discussed it with John von Neumann, he had a better idea. Von Neumann told me, "You should call it entropy, for two reasons. In the first place your uncertainty function has been used in statistical mechanics under that name, so it already has a name. In the second place, and more important, no one knows what entropy really is, so in a debate you will always have the advantage."

Entropy measures are also seeing an increased use in statistics, mainly in Bayesian and likelihood analysis. Jaynes' (1957a, 1957b) maximum entropy principle suggests a way to choose a prior distribution for Bayesian analysis: one that maximises our uncertainty but is consistent with what we know.

The use of a measure related to entropy makes sense when we are interested in a count or a quantification of the number of states of a system, and especially when one is interested in the change in the number of states. Here we should distinguish two ways to calculate the difference in uncertainty.

The first is called 'mutual information'. Mutual information tells us how much knowing one thing helps us in knowing something else – for example, how much knowing the season tells us about the temperature. The second way of calculating a difference in uncertainty, which does not seem to have a name, but is used often, is to calculate the difference in entropy after a *particular* change in our knowledge has occurred. We might, for example, hear that the forecast is for rain tomorrow, and as a result of hearing that particular message "rain tomorrow" our uncertainty changes. So in the first way of calculating the difference in uncertainty we ask how much our uncertainty changes on average when we hear the weather report, in the second way we ask how much it changed after we heard a specific weather report, namely that it will rain.

Of these two, mutual information is the one that is more intuitive to understand. As we would expect from gaining information, this measure is never below zero – being given information should not increase our uncertainty. Thus, knowing the month reduces our uncertainty about the temperature. The second measure described above *can* be negative – imagine living in a place where it is sunny most of the time, say Palo Alto, California, and hearing a weather report saying that tomorrow there is a 50% chance of rain. Without this information, there was a 99% chance of sunshine, 1% chance of rain – the average weather. But the particular report gave rain a 50% chance, so now we are much less certain whether to take an umbrella with us or not.

To state this again: on average, listening to a weather report whose precision we know cannot increase our uncertainty, averaging over all possible reports and their probability. But a certain report for a certain day can increase our uncertainty.

If we write $H(X)$ for the entropy, or uncertainty associated with not knowing X (for example not knowing if it will rain), $H(X|Y)$ for the uncertainty in X given that we know the state of Y (Y could, for example, be the weather report) and $H(X|Y = s)$ for the uncertainty of X when Y is in a certain state s, then the mutual information between X and Y, written as $I(X;Y)$, can be written as

$$I(X;Y) = \sum_{\text{all states } s \text{ of } Y} p(s)\,[H(X) - H(X\,|\,Y = s)] \tag{15.1}$$

where $p(s)$ stands for the probability that Y is in state s (for more explanation see Box 15.2). We see the connection between the mutual information and the difference in entropy conditioning on a single state – the first is an average of the second. Mutual information is the weighted average, over all states of Y, of the difference in entropy conditional on each single state. Mutual information has some very convenient properties. Thus $I(X;Y) = I(Y;X)$: how much the month tells us about the temperature is equal to how much the temperature tells us about the month. Mutual information is also independent of recoding the variables. So, if instead of measuring temperature in Celsius we measure it in Fahrenheit, or maybe we look at the log of the temperature, the

Box 15.2 Mutual information

Mutual information tells us how much our uncertainty about one thing is reduced when we are told about another. In the figure, we are looking at two variables X and Y. Not all values of X and Y are possible. The white square outlines the possible values of X and Y, and I assume that all rectangles are equally likely. Thus Y can take a value of 4 when X is 5, 6, 7 or 8, but not when X is 1, 2, 3 or 4.

The down-pointing arrow shows what happens if we are interested in X, and ignore Y, or have no information about Y. For example, X can be 1 when Y is 1 or 2. In this case we don't know Y, but the chance for $X = 1$ is equal to the sum of these two rectangles, or 1/8. So, when Y is not known X can take 8 different values, all equally likely, and therefore the missing information is $H(X) = \log(8) = 3$ bits. If we know Y, we know something about X. Thus, when we know that $Y = 4$, X can only be one of 5, 6, 7 or 8. For any value of Y, X can take on 4 values, so once we know Y, we have $H(X|Y) = \log(4) = 2$ bits of information missing. The difference in the missing information when we don't know Y and when we know Y is the difference between these two values, so $I(X;Y) = H(X) - H(X|Y) = 3 - 2 = 1$. Knowing Y gives us 1 bit of information about X; it halves the number of possible states of X from 8 to 4.

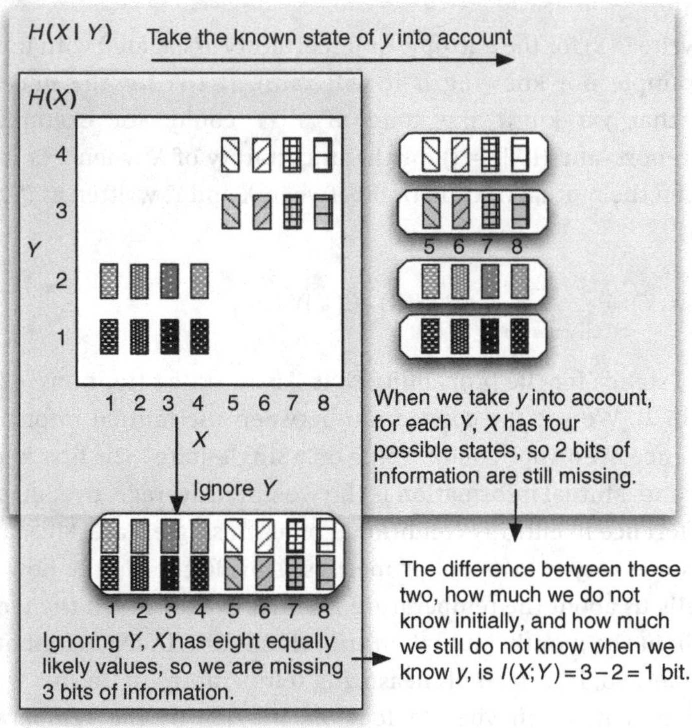

Figure 15.2

mutual information stays the same. The same is not true, for example, for the closely related concept of statistical correlation, which does change if we remap our variables. Box 15.3 explains why this is the case. It is also true that whenever there is a statistical correlation between two variables, they carry mutual information about one another. The converse is not true – it could be that two variables have mutual information and yet have a correlation of zero.

Box 15.3 Effect of rescaling a variable on mutual information and on correlation

Most variables we measure have no natural scale. One researcher might look at the weight of the organism in kilograms and another in pounds, or maybe in log scale, when comparing many different orders of magnitude. Such changes have an effect on correlation measures of variables, but not on the mutual information between them. Let us take X and Y from Box 15.1, and rescale Y so that the possible values are 1, 2, 8 or 9. Rescale X so that the possible values are 1, 2, 3, 4 or 15, 16, 17, 18. We can now complete the same calculation we did in Box 15.1: when ignoring Y, X still has 8 possible equally likely values, and for every value of Y there are 4 possible values of X. Nothing has changed from Box 15.1: we still gain $3 - 2 = 1$ bit of information about X when we know Y, so $I(X;Y) = 1$. It is easy to understand why rescaling Y and X will never have an effect – in calculating the mutual information we are interested in the probabilities of the different values, and not in where they sit.

Correlation changes when we rescale the values. Graphical representations of the correlation coefficient are not easy to understand (see "Thirteen ways to look at the correlation coefficient" by Rodgers & Nicewander, 1988.) One interpretation of the correlation draws a rough ellipse around the sample points, and compares the height of the ellipse in the Y direction to its width in the middle (see grey arrows below). The smaller the width of the ellipse in the middle relative to its height, the larger the correlation. When we rescale the variables we will transform this ellipse, and the correlation will change. In the example I gave above, the correlation between X and Y increases.

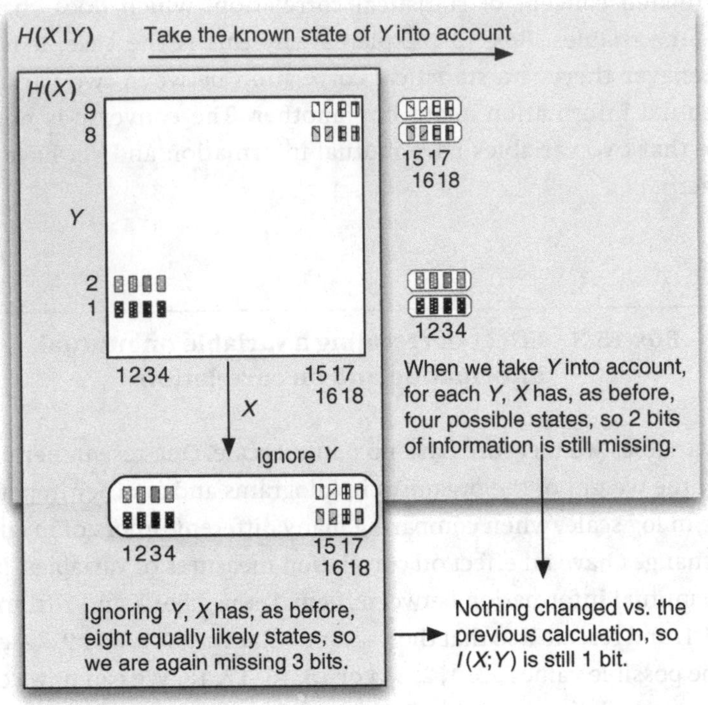

Figure 15.3A

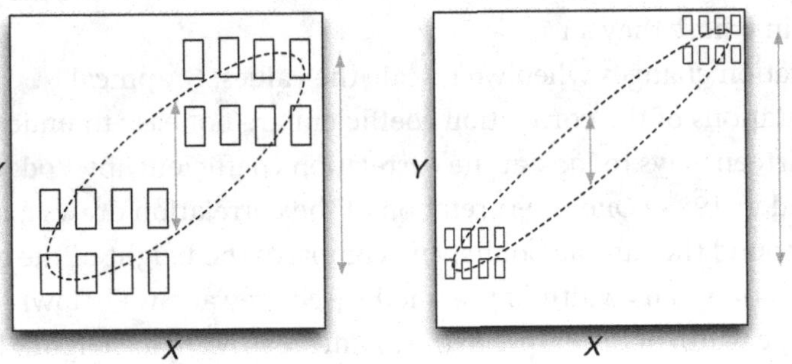

Figure 15.3B

15.2 The information value of cues and signals

In the following, I will examine the information content of a cue or signal given to an organism. Following arguments used in previous papers (Bergstrom & Lachmann, 2004; Donaldson-Matasci, Bergstrom & Lachmann, 2010), I will argue that even in cases where we are interested in the fitness of organisms, information theoretic measures will be related to fitness gain of lineages. I will look at two measures of the information content. The first is the mutual information between the cue and some aspect of the organism's environment. The second looks at the effect of the signal or cue on the organism's fitness. I begin with the latter.

Consider the difference between the optimal fitness without the cue, and the optimal fitness with the cue. Let us write $F(X)$ for the optimal fitness possible when the state of X is not known to the organism, and $F(X|c)$ for the optimal fitness when X is not known, but a cue c is received – i.e. the fitness conditional on X. We can then look at the "value of information" (Stephens, 1989).

$$\text{Fitness gain} = \sum_{\text{all cues } c} p(s)[F(X) - F(X|c)] \qquad (15.2)$$

The similarity of this equation to the definition of mutual information in Equation 15.1 is apparent, except that here we measure fitness, and above bits. Is there any connection between these two?

In information theory we look at the frequency of events, for example how often the word 'me' is used in the English language versus the word 'encyclopaedia', or how often the bit 0 is stored in a file versus the bit 1. Using these frequencies we can then find an optimal coding – how long should the word that stands for 'me' be versus the word that stands for an encyclopaedia. What is not taken into account is the meaning of the signals. Thus, we calculate the information capacity of a channel, without taking into account whether it serves as a police dispatch, or a television channel for late-night infomercials. Let us look at a simple example: we could use information theory to reduce the number of key presses one needs to use on average to dial a number, making often-used numbers shorter. Imagine that our dial pad had just two keys with the digits 1 and 2 on them, and we want to be able to quickly dial three contacts, Aaron, Ben and Claudia, but we call Aaron twice as often as each of the other two. In this case it would be optimal to assign Aaron the number '1', and assign Ben and Claudia the numbers '21' and '22'. With this assignment, half the time we would have to dial just one digit (when dialling Aaron we would dial '1'), and half the time we would have to dial two digits (when reaching one of the other two we would dial '21' or '22'). Our average dial length would be 1.5 digits, which is optimal in this case. But usually the assignment of telephone numbers also takes into account other considerations: the reason that emergency numbers are short and easy to remember is that they are important, and not that they are dialled more often (though they probably are). In the above example, if an expecting couple was assigning the numbers, and Ben was their contact in the maternity ward, the couple might use the shorter number '1' for Ben, even though they do not need to reach him very often – because when they do need to reach him it is urgent. We see that in many real-world examples, one needs to take into account not only frequency, but also meaning.

One can ask a similar question in biology. Why would a measure of the mutual information between a cue and the environment be at all relevant to understanding an organism, if it is not specified what this cue is about? Why would the information content of a cue carrying two bits of information about the location of an ant be important if we do not know whether it is perceived by a beetle or by a lion? In a world that cares about survival and reproduction, is the information content of a cue as measured in bits relevant?

The surprising result is that entropy-based measures are also relevant to such cases. In economics it turns out that the information in a signal about stocks is closely related to how much faster your money will double when using the information (Kelly, 1956; Cover & Thomas, 1991). What we and others have shown (Cohen, 1966; Bergstrom & Lachmann, 2004; Kussell & Leibler, 2005; Donaldson-Matasci *et al.*, 2010) is that a similar result also holds in biology: under certain conditions, the Shannon information of an environmental cue is exactly the fitness benefit one could gain from heeding it. Heeding a cue giving one bit of information will then allow a two-fold increase in fitness, without specifying what this cue is about, or the fitness consequences of the different strategies available to the organism! In the following I will try to explain this somewhat unintuitive result.

When dealing with the evolution of strategies of organisms, we are interested in which strategy will out-survive its competitors. The simple case examined is an organism living in a variable environment. We assume it reacts to a cue reducing its uncertainty about the environment, and we want to ask how relevant is the information content of the cue about the environment as measured by Shannon's information measure, i.e. the mutual information between the environment and the cue.

It turns out that for evolutionary questions one needs to specify not only whether an environment is variable, but also how the uncertainty is distributed between individuals in the population (Donaldson-Matasci, Lachmann & Bergstrom, 2008; Rivoire & Leibler, 2011). At the one extreme are environments that are shared by all individuals in the population, for example whether it was a cold or warm winter. At the other extreme are variable environments that are different for every individual in the population, for example whether a predator is hiding close by. Between these extremes are environments whose variability is partly shared, or ones whose variability is only shared between some individuals – for example all those living in a certain location. For simplicity, I assume that the variability is shared between all individuals in the current generation, and that if an individual is adapted to the wrong environment, it dies. Here I also assume that each generation is exactly one year long.

A central concept in information theory is the idea of 'typical sequences' (Shannon & Weaver, 1948; McMillan, 1953; Cover & Thomas, 1991). Imagine an environment that has 'cold years' with probability 70% and 'warm years' with probability 30%: then for long enough sequences of years we will see with high probability a sequence that has around 70% cold years and 30% warm years. See Box 15.4 for more explanation on typical sequences.

A hypothetical organism with no information about the environment has little choice but to either have a fixed genetically defined phenotype, or have its phenotype randomly determined by a 'roll of dice' – the juvenile develops into an adult adapted to cold years with probability q, and adapted to warm years with probability $(1 - q)$. The genes will determine only the chance q, but not the phenotype of each offspring. Thus, each organism will have a fraction q of offspring adapted to cold and $1 - q$ adapted for warmth, and each of those again will have a fraction q of its offspring adapted to cold and $1 - q$ to warmth and so on. In Box 15.5 I explain why, in this case, it is optimal for the organism to have a genotype so that q is equal to p. The optimal strategy thus involves bet-hedging. Without information, a lineage has to divide its bets equally between all possible typical environments *and match gthe proportion of phenotypes to the proportion of corresponding environments.* When having the wrong phenotype does not result in

Box 15.4 Typical sequences

If we look at a sequence of independent events, each of which has a chance p of occurring, then for long enough sequences we will mostly see sequences that have a ratio of around p to $1 - p$ of the two event types. Thus, if we throw a coin with even chances for heads and tails, most of the time we will see a sequence that has around 50% heads and 50% tails.

In the figure we see the four possible outcomes of two coin tosses (with heads and tails represented by black and white), all equally likely. A ratio of 0.5 occurs most often, but not by a huge margin. With four tosses, we will have 6/16 possibilities with 50% heads and 50% tails. Now 14/16 = 87% of the possibilities are between 25% and 75%.

With a large enough sequence, almost all sequences we observe will have that ratio; they will all be approximately equally likely. In N events, Np times an event with chance p happens, and $N(1 - p)$ times one with chance $(1 - p)$, so the chance for each sequence is $p^{Np}(1 - p)^{N\,(1 - p)}$, which can be written as $2^{N\,[p \log p\, +\, (1 - p) \log(1 - p)]}$. In general there will be 2^{NH} typical sequences all equally likely, with H the entropy of each event.

Typical sequences have a central importance in understanding information theory. Thus, if we wish to compress the outcomes of N coin tosses, we can just number the events that are likely to occur from 1 to 2^{NH}. Since other events almost never occur, it does not matter how we encode those. This means that to encode N tosses we will only need NH bits. In a similar way we can calculate how many different messages the English language can transmit. If we assume that words occur at certain frequencies, independent of each other, then we will mainly be observing typical sequences of words, and we know how many of those there are: 2^{NH}. Words, of course, do not occur independently of each other, so we can expand our treatment to pairs of words, sentences and paragraphs. (This example is very similar to those used in Shannon's original paper.)

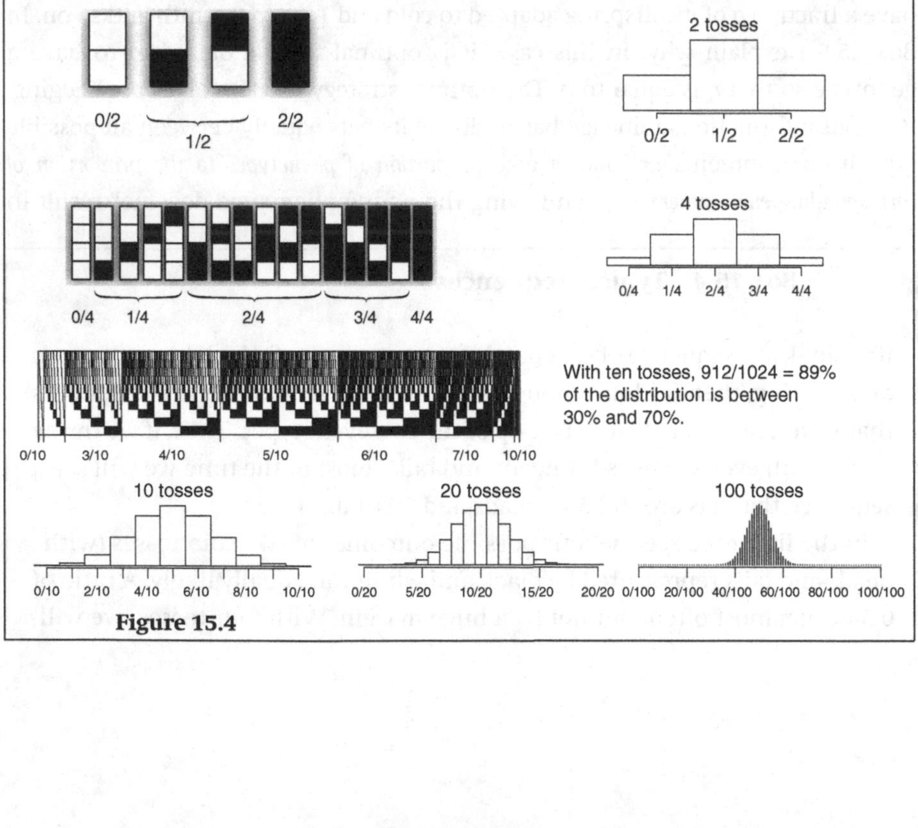

Figure 15.4

death, just in lower fitness, the optimal strategy can still be one with bet-hedging, but finding the optimal strategy is a bit more complicated. In this case there will be some frequencies of warm and cold years for which there will be no bet-hedging – instead the individuals will always develop the same phenotype. Other, intermediate, frequencies will still have bet-hedging as the optimal strategy.

Real organisms will, of course, always have some information about the relevant state of the environment. Below I discuss the optimal strategy in those cases, which will, for minuscule amounts of information, be very close to that without any information.

How will additional information about the environmental state help the lineage? As mentioned above, information is a measure of the (fold) reduction in uncertainty. (I will use the word 'fold' in this chapter for the amount multiplied or divided by. A four-fold reduction thus means that we divide the number of possible states by four, and I will talk about the 'fold reduction' to speak about an unspecified amount of reduction.) If there are 100 equally likely states, and we get one bit of information about them, we can see our updated uncertainty as 50 equally likely states; two bits of information will leave us with 25 states and so on. Thus, if a lineage has to divide its resources equally between 100 possible outcomes because it is relying on bet-hedging, and it gains one bit of information, it will need to divide its resources only between 50 possible outcomes, and thus have twice as many surviving lineages. Therefore, if along the tree of future possibilities a lineage gains every generation one bit of information it means that it can exactly double its fitness – the growth rate is multiplied by two. The fitness gain of x bits of information is in these cases exactly a 2^x-fold gain in fitness. Quite an amazing result: without knowing what the system in question is, lions or bacteria, without knowing the exact conditions or fitness effects and how many different environments the organism experiences, we can say that one bit of information given to the organism can gain it a two-fold increase in fitness.

How can one bit of information about an important or unimportant part of the individual's life lead to the same fitness benefit? The trick is that one bit of information equals one bit of fitness increase only for the case where the organism bet-hedges on the outcomes before and after the information is provided. If the optimal strategy before having information is to bet-hedge on the outcomes, and after information is received the optimal strategy is still to bet-hedge (with modified probabilities since additional information modified the probabilities of the different outcomes), then the value of information is equal to the mutual information. When the information is about a feature of the organism's environment that is of little consequence, the optimal strategy will not be to bet-hedge, and the value of the information in terms of fitness will be less than the information content. This pre-selects on the type of information

Box 15.5 Typical sequences in the environment and in a lineage

In our example, an organism survives only if its phenotype (fill pattern shown in the circle) matches the environment in the generation (fill pattern shown in the background rectangles). If the environment is white with probability p and striped with probability $(1 - p)$, a typical sequence of environments will have almost exactly that ratio of white to striped states. For a future lineage of an organism to survive (all lineages originating from circle on left), its phenotypes must match the environmental phenotypes exactly.

If in every generation a fraction q of the offspring are white and a fraction $(1 - q)$ striped, then a typical sequence of phenotypes along a lineage will have almost exactly that fraction of white versus striped phenotypes. For the phenotype to match the environment every generation, q has to be equal to p (see, for example, along the marked surviving lineage).

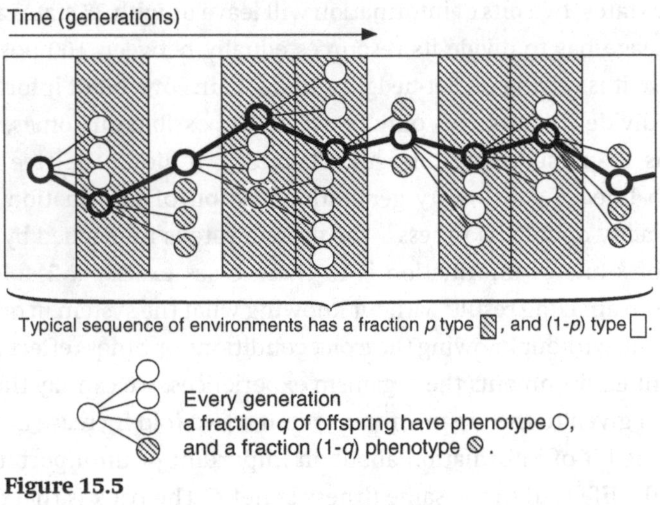

Time (generations)
Typical sequence of environments has a fraction p type ▨, and (1-p) type □.
Every generation
a fraction q of offspring have phenotype ○,
and a fraction (1-q) phenotype ◍.

Figure 15.5

that our claim applies to. When we give a lion information about the location of an ant, then because the location of the ant is not important enough for the lion, it will not have bet-hedged on the location of the ant. It might, for example, have bet-hedged on the location of antelopes, so information about antelopes will fulfil our criterion. A beetle will not bet-hedge on the location of antelopes, but might do so on the location of ants. Thus bet-hedging is an equalising criterion. Only when we provide a certain amount of information about a system to organisms that bet-hedge on the state of the system can we get exactly the same fitness effects as the information content. Since the organism will not bet-hedge on unimportant aspects of its environment, these cases are excluded from our result.

The connection between information and fitness comes from counting. Shannon's information measure is about a fold reduction of possible states. When we ask about compression of a file, we have to count how many possible equally likely states there are. When we talk about the difference in entropy between a cup of tea at 100 or 25 °C, we ask about the difference in the number of possible states between these two temperatures. Fitness can also be seen as a measure of the number of possible future lineages, and since we again look at a measure of equally likely possibilities, information and entropy can be applied.

It is interesting to note that Wagner (2007) used quite a different approach to reach very similar results. He looked at the fitness effects of the sensing of a limiting nutrient's abundance, using a model for the metabolic network. In the model, he again arrived at the result of a connection between information content and fitness.

15.3 Information and genomes

Many bacteria live in a constant arms-race of producing toxins, anti-toxins and other countermeasures. Some of the countermeasures to antibiotic toxins, such as tetracycline produced by actinobacteria, involve arrested or slowed growth – obviously a phenotype with a big cost. In these cases, an environmental cue about the presence of a toxin could be 'lineage-saving'. Often, however, the action of the toxin could be so quick that the cells die before they can respond to it. Bacteria might also be using bet-hedging, producing a subpopulation of individuals that grow more slowly, to save their lineages from unexpected exposure to toxins. Kussel and Leibler (2005) looked at the efficiency of response to a cue versus a bet-hedging strategy, and found the conditions under which one or the other gives a faster average growth rate. They noticed the connection between information and fitness effect. We can do a quick analysis based on the tools described above. When the bacteria have no information about the environment, not even the phenotypic/genotypic state of their parents, their fitness will be reduced by at least $H(\text{Env})$ relative to ones that know the exact state of the environment. If there are cues available about the environment, their fitness can increase by up to $I(\text{cue; Env})$ – the mutual information between the cue and the environment (the 'relevant' environment, i.e. the environmental states over which bet-hedging is used). But the bacteria can use an alternate method – evolutionary switching between states. We can then see the state of the genome with respect to arrested growth as a 'cue' to the state of the environment. The increase in fitness from using this strategy will be I(Genome; Env) or less – the mutual information between the genome and the environment. What creates a correlation between the genome and the environment is selection, and the fact that recent environmental states, those during which selection acted, contain information about the current environment.

Kimura (1961) tried to calculate the rate at which natural selection inserts information into the genome:

> If those individuals which are to be eliminated by natural selection in the process of progressive evolution were kept alive and allowed to reproduce at the same rate as the favored individuals, the population number would become, after t generations, e^{-Lt}. This means that natural selection allows an incident to occur with probability one, which, without selection, could occur only with a probability of e^{-Lt} … and therefore information gained per generation is $L/\log(2)$ bits.

Here L refers to the 'load', a measure saying how many lineages are lost to the population because not all individuals have the same fitness as the best in the population (Kimura used the notation L_e for this). The load L is defined so that if in a generation half the lineages are lost through their low fitness then $\exp(L)= 2$, so that $L = \log(2)$. Kimura then balanced the above measure with the rate at which deleterious mutations destroy information per generation, to estimate the total number of bits gained since the Cambrian explosion – around 10^8 bits. Recently, Adami (2004) re-examined such an approach to estimate the selection that acts on a sequence. Sites that are neutral are under no evolutionary constraints, and thus are free to take any possible sequence. Over enough evolutionary time we should see every one of them. Missing sequences hint at selection, for example if at a certain site we only see a 'G' across many species. As before, we can measure the fold reduction in the number of sequences (again, I use the word 'fold' to stand for the amount by which we divide the number of sequences). The exact reduction is sometimes hard to calculate, because the number of species is so much smaller than the number of possible sequences. As a proxy, we can look base by base, ignoring interactions between bases. As above, the additivity of mutual information would allow us to add the measure for each base to get the overall amount of conservation of the site. Adami also showed how one can find interacting sites in an RNA molecule by looking at their mutual information.

An interesting related use of entropy introduced to biology is for counting possible states of the genome fulfilling some condition. We can measure the specificity of a binding motif by counting the number of possible sequences that bind to a certain molecule relative to the number of all possible sequences of the genome in a region of the same size. Thus the method introduced by Schneider and Stephens (1990) represents each base with a height proportional to the information content of the position, i.e. a height related to how constrained the motif in that position is. If the motif can have only one possible base, say an 'A', then we reduce the number of possibilities from 4 to 1, i.e. a four-fold reduction. This four-fold reduction is represented by its log in base 2, so we say that the position specifies two bits of information about the possible binding motif, and its height is proportional to 2. If a position is not constrained at all, and can have any of the four bases, there is no reduction. Then that position specifies zero bits of information, and the height of that position is zero. Because of the additive properties of information, one can add the heights of all bases in the motif to get its overall specificity – two motifs with similar total height put the same amount of constraint on the sequence for binding. (This method of representation, only looking at single positions, ignores correlations between different bases.) We can also use a similar representation to specify motifs of amino acids in proteins.

Notice that the measure used here is not mutual information, but instead the reduction in uncertainty only for the regions that bind to the motif. The expression for mutual information between the binding of a molecule and the sequence of the genome will involve at least two possible outcomes of the binding state, e.g. either the molecule binds or it does not bind in the region, and then we will have a second term involving the reduction in uncertainty when we know the molecule does not bind in a region. Or it could be that we had a certain chance to be told that the molecule binds in the region in case it does, so the two possible events would be that we are told and we are not told that the molecule binds in the region. The measure introduced by Schneider and Stephens only includes the difference in binding regions. However, since the effect on non-binding regions is so slight, the second term has an insignificant contribution to the mutual information.

15.4 Conclusion

I have tried to highlight some of the uses of quantitative measures of information and entropy in cues and communication between organisms. Many biologists, including myself, hope that at some point entropy measures could take as central a role in the theory of evolution as they do in physics and information theory. But for now these promises are unfulfilled – few would argue that a course in information theory should be in the standard biology curriculum. On the other hand, small local uses of entropy are appearing, such as describing the specificity of a binding motif. In the narrow sense described in this chapter, it is easy to agree that there is mutual information between a certain cue in the environment or signal given by another organism and the relevant environmental state of an organism. One might also look at the information in the genome in the same way – mutual information between the genome and the environment. The sense in which the term 'information' is then used is similar to its use in statistical mechanics and the theory of communication. Beyond these static measures, if we try to analyse the behaviour of organisms providing cues to one another, the mathematical analysis becomes much harder. One needs to then take into account factors such as manipulation or the stability of the signalling system to mutations and strategy changes by the participants. Other important factors would be how the detection of the cue originates, or how the detection of a signal or the emission of a signal originates in evolution. All these, however, are mathematical or modelling questions, more easily addressed than the question of whether or not the organism really sent a 'signal' or was just manipulating the receiver.

References

Adami, C. (2004). Information theory in molecular biology. *Physics of Life Reviews*, **1**, 3–22.

Bergstrom, C. & Lachmann, M. (2004). Shannon information and biological fitness. *Proceedings of the Information Theory Workshop, 2004. IEEE*, pp. 50–54.

Clausius, R. (1867). *The Mechanical Theory of Heat: With its Applications to the Steam-engine and to the Physical Properties of Bodies*. London: John Van Voorst.

Cohen, D. (1966). Optimizing reproduction in a randomly varying environment, *Journal of Theoretical Biology*, **12**, 119–129.

Cover, T. & Thomas, J. (1991). *Elements of Information Theory*. New York: Wiley.

Dall, S. R., Giraldeau, L.-A., Olsson, O., McNamara, J. M. & Stephens, D. W. (2005). Information and its use by animals in evolutionary ecology. *Trends in Ecology and Evolution*, **20**, 187–193.

Dall, S. R. X., Schmidt, K. A. & Van Gils, J. A. (2010). Biological information in an ecological context. *Oikos*, **119**, 201–202.

Donaldson-Matasci, M., Bergstrom, C. T. & Lachmann, M. (2010). The fitness value of information. *Oikos*, **119**, 219–230.

Donaldson-Matasci, M., Lachmann, M. & Bergstrom, C. T. (2008). Phenotypic diversity as an adaptation to environmental uncertainty. *Evolutionary Ecology Research*, **10**, 493–515.

Hasson, O. (1994). Cheating signals. *Journal of Theoretical Biology* **167**, 223–238.

Hirschleifer, J. (1971). The private and social value of information and the reward to inventive activity. *American Economic Review*, **61**, 561–574.

Jaynes, E. T. (1957a). Information theory and statistical mechanics. *Physical Review*, **106**, 620–630.

Jaynes, E. T. (1957b). Information theory and statistical mechanics. II. *Physical Review*, **108**, 171–190.

Kelly Jr, J. (1956). A new interpretation of information rate. *Bell System Technical Journal*, **35**, 917–926.

Kimura, M. (1961). Natural selection as the process of accumulating genetic information in adaptive evolution. *Genetics Research*, **2**, 127–140.

Kussell, E. & Leibler, S. (2005). Phenotypic diversity, population growth, and information in fluctuating environments. *Science*, **309**, 2075–2078.

Maynard Smith, J. & Harper, D. (2003). *Animal Signals*. New York: Oxford University Press.

McMillan, B. (1953). The basic theorems of information theory. *Annals of Mathematical Statistics*, **24**, 196.

Rivoire, O. & Leibler, S. (2011). The value of information for populations in varying environments. *Journal of Statistical Physics*, **142**, 1124–1166.

Rodgers, J. L. & Nicewander, W. A. (1988). Thirteen ways to look at the correlation coefficient. *American Statistician*, **42**, 59–66.

Schneider, T. D. & Stephens, R. M. (1990). Sequence logos: a new way to display consensus sequences. *Nucleic Acids Research*, **18**, 6097–6100.

Shannon, C. (1948). The mathematical theory of communication. *Bell System Technical Journal*, **27**, 379–423.

Sherwin, W. B. (2010). Entropy and information approaches to genetic diversity and its expression: genomic geography. *Entropy*, **12**, 1765–1798.

Stephens, D. (1989). Variance and the value of information. *American Naturalist*, **134**, 128–140.

Tribus, M. & McIrvine, E. (1971). Energy and information. *Scientific American*, **225**, 179–188.

Wagner, A. (2007). From bit to it: how a complex metabolic network transforms information into living matter. *BMC Systems Biology*, **1**, 33.

16

Information and influence in sender–receiver models, with applications to animal behaviour

PETER GODFREY-SMITH

16.1 Introduction

Debates about animal communication often mirror philosophical debates about communication and meaning in human affairs, especially debates about language.[1] In both contexts there is suspicion in one camp about familiar ways of describing signs in terms of 'representation' and the 'carrying of information'. In some discussions people say that to treat animal communication in this way is 'anthropomorphic'. But plenty of philosophers would say that these concepts are the wrong ones to apply in the *human* case, as they are part of a discredited picture of human cognitive activity, one that sees us as passively mirroring the world. There is a diverse anti-representationalist tradition in philosophy of language and philosophy of mind.[2]

All options are possible here: an information-based approach might be good in the human case and bad in the animal case. It might be bad in both, or good in both. In an article in the *New York Times* in 2011, Simon Blackburn admiringly notes that biologists studying animal signals have moved beyond a simple representationalist view, and he hopes that philosophers of language will follow their lead. An information-based view might even be bad in the human case and

[1] Thanks to Jack Bradbury, Carl Bergstrom, Rosa Cao and Nick Shea for helpful comments and correspondence. I benefited also from many other chapters in this volume, which I was able to use as a result of Ulrich Stegmann's patience and my colleagues' greater punctuality, for both of which I am grateful.

[2] See Rorty (1982) for a gathering of those threads.

Animal Communication Theory: Information and Influence, ed. Ulrich Stegmann. Published by Cambridge University Press.

good in the animal case, because the complexities of human language use have overwhelmed a simpler information-carrying role that still exists in animal signalling.

In the animal case, a shift in thinking about communication was linked to a shift in thinking about cooperation. Early work on animal communication was done within a framework that took cooperation and group-level adaptation as common.[3] Some influential criticism of information-based views of signalling, developing from the 1970s, has been associated with a less cooperative view of animal behaviour. Dawkins and Krebs (1978) argued that animal communication is a process in which signallers manipulate receivers, rather than informing them. A signaller uses another animal as a tool for producing behaviours that help the signaller, regardless of whether the receiver is better off. Given this, it is probably a good idea to "abandon the concept of information altogether" (Dawkins & Krebs, 1978, p. 309) when describing animal signalling. Their own later work moderated this view (Krebs & Dawkins, 1984), admitting some role for information and recognising the role of the receiver as a 'mind-reader'. Some subsequent work opposed to an informational approach has emphasised that a view based on 'manipulation' or 'influence' need not be a view according to which receivers are doing badly (Ryan, Ch.9 of this volume).

Is a concept of information useful in understanding animal communication at all? If so, is it useful only in understanding cases where there is cooperation? Does the divide between approaches based on information and those based on influence merely reflect a difference in emphasis, without disagreement about underlying processes, or is there a substantive disagreement? If the latter is true, how might further modelling and data collection decide the issue? This chapter tries to make progress on all these questions, using a model of sender–receiver relationships that draws on several fields. I argue that within this model, information and influence are complementary – they come as a 'package deal'. With respect to the role of cooperation, explaining signalling requires a finer-grained framework than a standard dichotomy between cooperation and conflict, or even a 'scale' between them. There are many varieties of *partial common interest*, some of which can stabilise signalling and some of which cannot. In a nutshell, the stabilisation of sender–receiver systems ties information and influence together.

16.2 Senders and receivers

Suppose there is a *sender* doing something that can be perceived or tracked by another agent, a *receiver*, who acts in a way influenced by what the

[3] See Searcy and Nowicki (2005) for a discussion of this historical sequence.

sender does. Talk of 'sending' and 'receiving' here is understood minimally, and does not imply anything about information, meaning or cooperation.

Why are they behaving this way? The question can be asked on many time-scales. The two agents might be making rational moment-to-moment decisions, or inflexibly following behavioural programmes shaped by a history of natural selection. But suppose we know that *something* is maintaining this pair of behaviours. Then here is one possibility: the state of the world varies, and acts by the receiver have consequences for both sides. The sender can track the state of the world in a way the receiver cannot. Further, the sender and receiver have *common interest*; they have the same preference orderings over acts that the receiver might produce in each state. For each state they agree about which act is worst, which are better, through to the best. Then a combination of behaviours in which senders produce signals and receivers shape their behaviour with the signals can be a *Nash equilibrium*: no unilateral deviation from those behaviours would make either of them better off.[4] If there are enough signals available, perfect coordination can be achieved: in each state of the world a distinctive signal is sent by the sender and it enables the receiver to produce an act tuned to that state.

If a situation like this is found, and provided there is no act that is best in every state, the signals must *carry information*. This formulation has a metaphorical element. Is it really true that information is the sort of thing that can be carried, transferred or contained? Several critics of information-based views of communication, both in humans and in animals, have questioned this point (see Chapters 6, 8 and 18 by Rendall & Owren, Morton & Coss, and Scott-Phillips & Kirby, in this volume). The metaphor of containment is indeed probably unhelpful, but what I have in mind can be described in other ways: the state of the signal affects the probabilities of various states of the world. More exactly, the probabilities of states of the world conditional on the state of the signal differ from the states' unconditional probabilities. This is information in roughly Shannon's (1948) sense. Although this is a 'thin' sense of information, many questions arise about it. The use of a physical concept of probability is rightly controversial, and I take its availability for granted. There are also various ways of specifying and measuring the information in a signal. At this stage all that matters is an idea common to many views: in order for the receiver

[4] A combination of behaviours by two or more agents is in *weak* Nash equilibrium if no unilateral change by any of the agents would make them better off; the combination is a *strict* Nash equilibrium if every unilateral change would make the agent who made the change worse off. Whether the equilibrium here is strict depends on whether some relevant payoffs are tied.

to coordinate acts with conditions in the world, the signal's state must be associated with the state of the world, not independent of it.[5]

The model above is essentially David Lewis' 1969 model of conventional signalling. There is no explanation of how the equilibrium is reached, and Lewis assumed rational choice as the means by which behaviours are maintained. Brian Skyrms (1996, 2010) gave an evolutionary recasting of Lewis' model. "Preference" is replaced by fitness, and rational choice is replaced by a selection process in which present success affects the future frequency of a strategy in a population. Related models have been given in economics.[6] When there is common interest in the sense above, informative signalling can be maintained in a wide range of cases and with various selection mechanisms.

In this kind of signalling, information and influence are coupled together. The signal must be one that carries information about the state of the world, or there is no reason for the receiver to attend to it. The signal must also be one that influences the receiver's actions, or there is no reason for the sender to send it. *Whether the signals carry information about the world* is up to the sender. It is the sender's choice, the outcome of evolution affecting the sender's side, or perhaps a matter of constraint with respect to the properties of the sender. For whatever reason, the sender is producing signals that vary, and that do so non-randomly with respect to some condition in the world. *Whether the signals have influence* is up to the receiver. It is the receiver's choice, the outcome of evolution affecting the receiver's side, or a matter of constraint with respect to the properties of the receiver. The receiver is acting in a variable way, and non-randomly with respect to the state of the signal.

Perhaps the stabilisation of the behaviours in some case is *not* due to common interest. One side may be constrained in a way that enables the other to exploit it. It may be that the sender is doing something that is so well tuned to the receiver's physiology that it cannot be ignored. This kind of constraint is the basis for a view of animal signalling defended by Owren, Rendall and Ryan (2010). Even if a signal cannot be ignored, can't its effects be filtered by the receiver? Owren, Rendall and Ryan argue that senders tend to have the upper hand in a process of this kind. On the other side, the receiver might be tracking something that the sender cannot help but produce – a scent, or reflected light. Camouflage is an attempt not to signal, in this minimal sense of signalling. Another kind of constraint affecting receivers is illustrated by fireflies of one

[5] For discussion, see Dretske (1981), Skyrms (2010), Godfrey-Smith (2012) and Millikan's contribution to this volume.

[6] For a survey of relevant ideas in economics, see Farrell and Rabin (1996). Throughout this discussion unless otherwise noted, no special costs for signalling are assumed; this is a 'cheap talk' model in Farrell and Rabin's sense.

species that produce mating signals of another species to lure males in to be eaten (Lloyd, 1975, Stegmann, 2009). Given the importance of mating, a tendency to respond to potentially lethal invitations remains in place. These are all cases where one side, sender or receiver, is subject to a constraint that prevents it from responding optimally to the policies pursued by the other.

Setting aside constraints of this kind, let us contrast the wholly cooperative situation with another. Suppose there is complete conflict of interest. In each state of the world, sender and receiver have reversed preferences with respect to actions that might be produced by the receiver. Then any information in the signals will be used by the receiver to coordinate acts with the world in a way that suits them, and that is opposed to the sender's preferences. Similarly, any tendency in the receiver to be influenced by signals of the relevant kind will be exploited by the sender to induce acts that are opposed to the receiver's own interests. Any sensitivity on either side can be exploited by the other. So any equilibrium we see will be one where the sender's 'signals' say nothing useful and the receiver is not sensitive to them. At equilibrium, there is no information in any signs and no influence either.

This second case will be revisited below, but if the argument is accepted for now, some consequences follow. Information and influence go together in these cases. At equilibrium we have both or neither. When there is common interest, if information is present in a signal it will come to have influence by receiver adaptation, and if there is influence then the signals will acquire information by sender adaptation.[7] When there is conflict of interest, any influence will be degraded, and any information will be degraded, too.

This reasoning assumes a kind of symmetry with respect to the control that the processes of sender and receiver adaptation have over the situation. This is a strong assumption that may not be realistic in biological cases. When the assumption does not apply, the result can be ongoing exploitation of one side by another, of the kind discussed in the 'constraints' paragraph above. In my discussion here, though, I will assume that adaptation is unconstrained on both sides. My focus will be another part of the Lewis model that surely looks biologically contentious, the assumptions about common interest.

So far I have discussed extremes – what I referred to as "common interest" is really *complete* common interest, and what I called "conflict" is *complete* conflict of interest. In complete common interest, sender and receiver have the same preference ordering over actions in every state. In complete conflict of interest,

[7] Here I assume that both sides do want different acts to be performed across at least some states of the world. If the receiver has an act which is best in all states, it does not matter what the sender does and whether their interests are aligned.

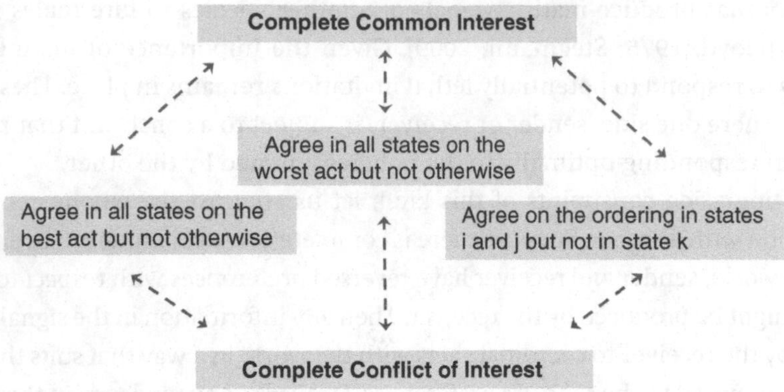

Figure 16.1 Relations between sender and receiver payoffs. The special cases of complete common interest and complete conflict of interest are linked by many paths that traverse different kinds of partial common interest.

sender and receiver have reversed preference ordering over actions in every state. Clearly there are many other cases – many kinds of *partial common interest*. Sender and receiver might agree on what is the best action in every state, but disagree otherwise. They might agree on what is worst, but disagree otherwise. If there are enough acts that are relevant, they might agree on best and worst, but flip some in the middle. They might agree entirely in some states but not in others. Complete common interest and complete conflict of interest are extremes, and there are many 'paths' between them, as illustrated in Figure 16.1.

This suggests a hypothesis: informative signalling (when all signals are equally costly to produce) is viable to the extent that there is common interest. In economics, a famous model due to Crawford and Sobel (1982) has this message. That model used a framework where common interest could be measured on a scale. This is not always true; agreeing on the worst-case outcome in every state does not show more, or less, common interest than agreeing on the ordering in most states but disagreeing in others. So it is really only a sketch of a hypothesis to say that informative signalling is viable 'to the extent' that there is common interest, but it may be a good sketch. The sketch can be filled out by looking for different ways in which partially informative signalling can be maintained through partial common interest.

16.3 Model cases with different relations between sender and receiver interests

This section will explore different kinds of common interest, using simple abstract cases. The cases all assume three equally probable states

(S1, S2, S3), three acts (A1, A2, A3) and three cost-less signals (m1, m2, m3). The sender perceives the state of world (perhaps its own condition), and can send any of three signals. The receiver perceives the signal and produces any of three actions. None of these steps is affected by 'noise' or mis-perception.

The three-state framework is a good way to look at different kinds of partial common interest, but systems with three states are complicated to analyse; even with complete common interest these systems show complex phenomena (Huttegger *et al.*, 2010). My analyses will be very simple. I will describe some equilibria – combinations of sender and receiver policies where each is the best response to the other – and give some dynamic arguments assuming adaptive responses made by one side to a previous move by the other. This is done without considering all equilibria or all possible invaders. In particular, no 'mixed strategies' are considered. The only rules considered map states to single messages, and messages to single acts. Where possible, the discussion will be neutral about how the sender and receiver roles are realised – for example, whether senders and receivers evolve in separate but interacting populations, or a single population contains individuals who take both roles in turn.

Case 1 (Table 16.1) is a case of complete common interest. If three messages are available (m1, m2 and m3), there are several ways of using the signals to achieve maximum payoff for both sides. For example, suppose senders send m1 in S1, m2 in S2, and m3 in S3, a policy which can be written as (S1 → m1, S2 → m2, S3 → m3). Suppose receivers do A1 in response to m1, A2 in response to m2, and A3 in response to m3, which is (m1 → A1, m2 → A2, m3 → A3). Lewis (1969) and Skyrms (2010) call this outcome a "signalling system" – a combination of policies in which maximum payoffs are achieved by both sides through the use of signals to achieve the best possible match between acts and states. Senders and receivers are then in a strict Nash equilibrium; if either side deviates unilaterally their payoff is reduced. There are six different ways of using the three available messages to achieve a signalling system.

Table 16.1 *Case 1: Complete common interest*

		States		
		S1	S2	S3
Acts	**A1**	3, 3	2, 2	0, 0
	A2	2, 2	3, 3	2, 2
	A3	0, 0	0, 0	3, 3

The entries in each cell specify sender payoff and receiver payoff, respectively, for each combination of receiver's act and state of the world.

Table 16.2 *Case 2: Agreement on the best act in all states*

		States		
		S1	S2	S3
Acts	**A1**	3, 3	2, 0	0, 2
	A2	2, 0	3, 3	2, 0
	A3	0, 2	0, 2	3, 3

As for Table 16.1, the entries in each cell specify sender payoff and receiver payoff, respectively, for each combination of receiver's act and state of the world.

When there is complete common interest, signalling systems can be found by various evolutionary processes. Evolutionary dynamics are complicated in a three-state case, with other equilibria present and the behaviour of the system depending on detailed assumptions about the process. All that matters here, though, is that complete common interest does allow signalling systems to evolve and remain stable.

What effect does moving to *partial* common interest have? First, we can note a shift away from complete common interest that does not make a difference to the stability of a signalling system. Suppose the two parties agree on what is the best action in all states, but not otherwise. This is case 2 (Table 16.2). Then the same sender's and receiver's rules that achieved a signalling system in case 1 can again be used to achieve a strict Nash equilibrium. Any deviation from such a system harms the deviator, although how much harm any given deviation brings will differ for sender and receiver. (For example, a move to A2 in S1 harms the receiver more than it harms the sender, but it does harm them both.) The changes to the payoff matrix from case 1 to 2 may affect how likely a system is to find this equilibrium, but once a signalling system has been found it is stable.

Next, suppose that sender and receiver agree about the worst act in each state, but do not agree otherwise. There are various ways this could happen, and one is shown as case 3 (Table 16.3). Another possibility is that the parties could agree entirely about what is good in two states, but disagree in the third – this is seen in case 4 (Table 16.4).

I will use the phrase *fully informative signalling* for cases where the sender maps states to signals in a one-to-one manner. In cases 3 and 4, fully informative signalling is not an equilibrium. However, in both cases there is an equilibrium in which some informative signalling goes on. In the terminology of Bergstrom and Lachmann (1998), there is a "partial pooling" equilibrium, in which the sender uses the same signal in two of the states, but sends a different signal in the third. In case 3, the following combination of policies is a weak Nash equilibrium: sender

Table 16.3 *Case 3: Agreement on the worst act in all states*

		States		
		S1	S2	S3
Acts	**A1**	0, 0	2, 3	2, 3
	A2	2, 3	0, 0	3, 2
	A3	3, 2	3, 2	0, 0

Table 16.4 *Case 4: Complete agreement in two states*

		States		
		S1	S2	S3
Acts	**A1**	3, 3	3, 0	0, 0
	A2	2, 2	2, 2	2, 2
	A3	0, 0	0, 3	3, 3

Cases of partial common interest that support informative signalling. As before, the entries in each cell specify sender payoff and receiver payoff, respectively.

does (S1 → m1, S2 → m2, S3 → m1); receiver does (m1 → A2, m2 → A1, m3 → A1). Case 4 has a similar equilibrium: sender does (S1 → m1, S2 → m1, S3 → m2); receiver does (m1 → A2, m2 → A3, m3 → A3).[8]

These are situations with different kinds of partial common interest (PCI), and both have partially informative signalling. As noted earlier, there are different ways of measuring the informational content of a signal, but several of them agree with something like this: if a signal reduces the possible states of the world from three to two, it carries less information than a signal that reduces the possible states from three to one. In case 3 (Table 16.3), m1 excludes the possibility of S2. It can be seen as having the informational content *S1 or S3*

[8] These examples are influenced by a case due to Skyrms (2010, p. 81). In Skyrms' case the two parties agree on the worst act in every state *and* agree entirely in one of the three states. The phenomena are separated here. The method used to find the equilibria in the text was to assume a starting point in which the sender uses a one-to-one mapping of states to messages, to note the receiver's 'best response' to this policy and to continue allowing each side to adapt in turn until an equilibrium was reached. Note that in both equilibria given here, the receiver has a policy for m3 even though this signal is never sent by the sender. These do matter because some receivers' rules for unseen signs open up adaptive possibilities for the sender.

obtains, whereas m2 has the informational content *S2 obtains*. Because m2 rules out more states, it has more informational content than m1.[9] So at equilibrium, there are *fewer* signals used in these cases and one of the signals carries *less* information than is seen in the equilibria described in cases 1 and 2.

Some general arguments can be given for cases where there are *n* states, *n* messages and *n* acts. Suppose fully informative signals are sent by the sender, there is disagreement on the best act for at least some states, neither sender nor receiver has a 'tie' for their top-scoring acts in any state, and the receiver does not have an act which is top-scoring for more than one state.[10] Then no matter what the receiver is doing, either sender payoffs or receiver payoffs (or both) are not maximal. If receiver payoff is not maximal, there is some change that takes the receiver to their maximum payoff. If, on the other hand, sender payoff is not maximal, then as long as the receiver maps some signal to each act, there is some way of changing the mapping of states to signals that induces the receiver to act in a way that delivers maximum payoff to the sender.

Things are not as simple if the receiver has an act that is optimal in more than one state. Then if the sender sends fully informative signals, the receiver can in some cases achieve maximum payoff by mapping two signals to a single act, and the sender cannot improve their outcome by changing their sending policy, although they can abandon fully informative signalling without penalty. Outside this special case, and the case of *agreement on the best*, partial common interest cannot, in the model used here, maintain fully informative signalling.

I said earlier that informative signalling cannot be maintained when there is complete conflict of interest. This claim has been expressed frequently, but there are some phenomena that can seem to be at odds with it. I will discuss two.

Bradbury and Vehrencamp (2000) present a model that embeds signalling within a general treatment of information use. A receiver is assumed to have various sources of information about a situation of uncertainty, and these establish a 'default' behaviour. The question the model asks is when attending to a given signal should override this default. And given the effects that the signal will have on the receiver's action, is it worth a sender *sending* the signal, or is the sender better off letting the receiver stick to their default behaviour? Bradbury and Vehrencamp discuss four relationships between sender and receiver interests, including what I call complete common interest, complete conflict, and two kinds of PCI. The surprising result is that it is possible for

[9] See Godfrey-Smith (2012) for more detail on some of these measures.

[10] The mention of 'ties' is included because there is a sense in which sender and receiver can 'disagree about the best' without there being an incentive to change, if one party gains equal and maximum payoffs from two acts in a given state, while the other gets maximum payoff from only one of those acts.

signalling to be beneficial to both sender and receiver in a situation of complete conflict of interest: "senders that completely disagree with receivers about appropriate receiver decisions may still benefit by providing moderately honest and accurate signals" (Bradbury and Vehrencamp, 2000, p. 259).

The result can be presented with their hypothetical example, which involves territorial behaviour in a mantis shrimp. The owner of a burrow is usually not moulting but occasionally is. When not moulting, a resident will win a contest with an intruder. When moulting, the resident will lose. Intruders have to decide whether to attack or pass by. The question for a resident is whether to threaten intruders, in a way that is a function of whether the resident is moulting. Suppose a resident does threaten in a way that conveys some information about its moult status; it is about twice as likely to threaten when not moulting as when moulting. Once it does this, in effect there are two signals, 'threaten' and 'meek'. It is easy to see that this signalling may be beneficial to the receiver, an intruder. The information about moult status may be sufficiently reliable for the intruder to adopt a policy of passing by if threatened, attacking if not. But this signalling may also be worthwhile to the sender, the resident, because it is not so reliable that intruders do not make mistakes – mistakes they would not make if there was no signalling. If an intruder attacks when the resident is not moulting, the intruder is badly injured and local competition is reduced for the resident. This is complete conflict of interest: in a non-moulting state, the resident is better off if the intruder attacks and the intruder is better if he does not. In a moulting state, the resident is better off if the intruder does not attack and the intruder is better if he does. The model uses some payoff assumptions that might be questioned, but suppose we grant the assumptions of the case.[11] It seems then to be a situation where informative signalling is viable despite complete conflict of interest.

With respect to the criteria used in this chapter, however, it is not such a case. The comparison that Bradbury and Vehrencamp address is this: is signalling of a given reliability better than not signalling at all, for both sender and receiver? This leaves open the question of whether signalling that passes this test will be stable against relevant invasions and modifications, a question their model is not intended to address. Suppose signalling of the kind described in the model is operating, so intruders attack if and only if they see the 'meek' behaviour from the resident. Then given that a non-moulting resident would prefer that intruders attack, non-moulting residents should modify their behaviour to threaten less, and let receivers attack more often. Given the receiver's present

[11] In Bradbury and Vehrencamp's scenario, the summed payoff to both sides is always higher if there is a fight than if there is not.

dispositions, the sender benefits from *never* threatening, in fact. Once they do this, signalling has collapsed and receivers will respond by no longer paying attention.[12] The Bradbury and Vehrencamp model describes necessary, but not sufficient, conditions for stable signal use.

There is a second possible challenge to the idea that signalling is not viable with complete conflict of interest. I said that in this situation the only equilibrium can be one where the sender pays no attention to the world and the receiver pays no attention to the sender. But this equilibrium might not be reached. Suppose we have a model like the ones above, with 3, 2, 0 payoffs possible in each state for each player, complete reversal of preferences in each state, and we start from a situation of fully informative signalling. Assume that each player changes their policy in turn, choosing a 'best response' to the present policy of the other player. In at least some cases this produces cycles where each player exploits and is exploited in turn. Each message is produced in a restricted set of states of the world, but the mapping is always changing.[13] It might be thought that this behaviour is an artifact of the simple framework used here, but Elliott Wagner (2011) has a model using a more sophisticated framework that yields a similar result in a situation of complete conflict of interest. His model generates chaotic change, where signals retain informational content at every stage.

In a sense, these are situations in which 'informative signalling is maintained'. At each moment in time, there is some restriction on the states of the world that can be predicted to obtain, based on the state of the signal. But the dynamic operating does not maintain a particular mapping between signals and states; the mapping is always changing, as the sender adapts to what the receiver has just become.

Situations like this also motivate a distinction between informational content and a concept of *functional* content (N. Shea, P. Godfrey-Smith & R. Cao, in preparation). Where informational content has to do merely with the way the state of the signal predicts the state of the world, one way to understand functional content is in terms of which states of the world (if any) figure in the explanation of the stabilisation of the sender and receiver policies with respect to that signal. In some cases functional content and informational content coincide, and in others they diverge. Many animal alarm calls prompted by

[12] In the framework of an 'evolutionarily stable strategy' (ESS) model, a population of shrimp who each use the sender and receiver strategies described by Bradbury and Vehrencamp (switching between roles according to their situation) could be invaded by a mutant which always gives the 'meek' display when sender, and follows the prevailing rule for receivers.

[13] The length of the cycle depends on the payoff details. There are also 'agree on the worst' cases, similar to my case 3, that can cycle in this way.

flying objects are very unreliable (Searcy & Nowicki, 2005, p. 66), being caused most often by non-dangerous birds and other things. When a high 'false alarm' rate is adaptive, the informational content of an alarm call may be *predator or harmless bird or. . .*, even though its functional content is *predator*. This distinction can also be used to describe cycles and chaos due to complete conflict of interest. In those cases signals have ever-shifting informational content, and no functional content at all.

16.4 Applications

In this section I will apply these ideas to some empirical cases. I do this cautiously, as applying idealised models to real-world systems is a scientific craft acquired by immersion in the details of such cases. A simple case with particular relevance, though, is signals by prey animals to predators. One example is 'stotting' by gazelles – stiff-legged vertical leaps, performed on seeing a predator and while moving away. The current consensus is that at least some of these displays are directed at the predators, rather than other members of the prey species, and a variety of animals use displays of this kind (Searcy & Nowicki, 2005; Bradbury & Vehrencamp, 2011).

Searcy and Nowicki describe these cases as follows: "If signaling is from prey to predator, then signaling is between individuals with interests that are diametrically opposed, rather than convergent" (2005, p. 53). Clearly predator and prey have opposing interests in many respects, but this is not a case of complete conflict. There are some states of the world in which their preferences for predator behaviour match, because some outcomes of an interaction are bad for both sides. A payoff matrix is given in Table 16.5: sender and receiver agree in one state of the world but not the other. If the prey animal is healthy and strong enough to escape, a chase is undesirable for both sides. If the prey is weak, a chase is good for predator and bad for prey.

A case like this is also discussed by Bradbury and Vehrencamp (2000), using the model described earlier. They show that if a signal is sufficiently reliable, both sides can do better with signal use than without it. This is another case with

Table 16.5 *Predator and prey*

		States	
		Strong	Weak
Acts	**Chase**	2, 2	0, 5
	No chase	3, 3	3, 3

a possibility of adaptive degrading of the signal's informativeness by the sender, however. Once receivers do not chase an individual that sends a certain signal, prey animals weak enough to be caught will benefit from sending this signal. Senders will degrade the information content of signals, and receivers will adapt by paying no attention to them. This suggests that given that such signals do persist, additional factors are needed to explain them (Fitzgibbon & Fanshawe, 1998). In the gazelle case, a likely extra factor is that weak animals can rarely manage an impressive stott. Stotting is a signal of vigour that is hard to fake.

Some other signals apparently directed at predators do not seem to have this feature. One is 'tail-flagging' by white-tailed deer (*Odocoileus virginianus*), in which the deer raises its tail to reveal white patches on its rump and the underside of the tail itself (Caro, 1995). Another is seen in some kinds of squid (e.g. *Sepioteuthis*), which display with colour changes and elaborate arrangements of arms when predatory fish approach (Moynihan & Rodaniche, 1982). These do not seem to be displays of vigour, like stotting, and may just be signals to the predator that they have been perceived.[14]

Evidence that these other signals actually deter predators is often weaker, but let us assume that they do. Why would the informativeness of these signals not degrade? Once an "I've seen you" display deters predation, why not maintain it all the time, whether you have seen a predator or not? Bradbury and Vehrencamp (2011, Ch. 14) note that some displays directed at predators emphasise that the prey is attending in exactly the right direction, which makes dishonesty difficult. Another factor may also become relevant. In the squid case, it is not that these displays would be difficult to fake, but they probably use energy and interfere with other behaviours. If predators are in fact rare, there may be no sense in disrupting other activities to perform the display when a predator has not been seen. The economics of the display, from this point of view, are no different from the economics of hiding, or running away. So at least to some degree, an "I've seen you" signal will naturally be reliable, as it will only be when a predator has been seen that the signal is worth producing. The signal is not hard to produce falsely but pointless to produce falsely. This argument relies on the assumption that the display does in fact disrupt other activities or use resources. In the case of squid displays this seems likely, but in the case of tail-flagging by deer it perhaps seems less so.

Bergstrom and Lachmann (2001) give a model in which yet another reason for the stability of predator-directed signals is suggested, which may also apply to

[14] Hanlon and Messenger (1996) note that in the case of squid, the display may have the function of startling the predator and disrupting the behavioural routines it employs in predation.

the squid case and perhaps to the deer. When an individual produces a signal directed at predators when none has been perceived, it risks alerting unseen predators to the individual's presence and location. These further explanations for the maintenance of honesty in the signal are complements, not alternatives, to the explanation in terms of partial common interest; it is partial common interest that makes the signals worth producing at all, and other factors that prevent the system being undermined by dishonest senders.

Another situation with partial common interest is mating signals. A standard picture of these cases is as follows (Chapter 3 of Searcy & Nowicki, 2005). In many though not all cases, males are the main signallers and females are receivers. This is because a female would like to mate if a male is of high quality but not otherwise, while males are less choosy. So males will advertise, and the females' problem is sorting the advertisements and choosing good males. This is a case of partial common interest, as both parties would prefer to mate if the male is high quality, and the problem of maintaining the informativeness of signals is also clear. If females respond to indicators of quality that can easily be faked, then they will be faked, and females will stop attending to them.

While accepting the assumptions of the standard picture for purposes of discussion, further factors can be noted. The range of relevant states of the world does not only include high- and low-quality states of the male. Male signals often achieve other reductions of uncertainty, by indicating that the sender is of appropriate species, age and sex, along in some cases with location. Neither side has an interest in attempting a mating with someone of the wrong species, age or sex: to that extent there is common interest. Against that background, there are states of the world where common interest breaks down, when a female discriminates between high- and low-quality males. This divergence motivates receivers to attend to displays of quality that are hard to fake, or too costly for low-quality senders to produce. So the overall story has a 'layered' structure. Common interest explains why signalling is done at all, and the particular form that signalling takes is due to selection by the receiver of signals whose information content is hard to degrade. If receivers in some cases did not have any way of enforcing use of a hard-to-fake indicator of quality, and had to deal with use of a simple cheap-talk signal of availability by senders, then we would have a PCI payoff matrix of the kind discussed earlier, where the two parties share preferences in two states of the world and diverge in one. Depending on the assumptions made about payoff relations and probabilities of states, receivers may accept the refusal of senders to distinguish low- and high-quality states, and use the less informative signals that result to guide their mating behaviour, or they might ignore the signals and use other cues.[15]

In sum: in sender–receiver systems, common interest maintains informative signalling by connecting information with influence. Without common interest, both information and influence should degrade, unless constraints of some kind prevent this, and this they may do; my discussion assumes unconstrained and comparable processes of adaptation on the sender and receiver sides. A contrast might be drawn between the human and animal cases. In animal signalling, where change is slow and often involves genetic evolution, much of what might compromise the application of these simple adaptationist models is constraint on adaptation. In the human case, the problem comes from our multifarious interests and capacities – from our flexibility. Returning to the model: common interest is not a yes-or-no matter, but is structured with two extreme cases (complete common interest and complete conflict) linked by many intermediates. One aim of this chapter is to supplement talk of 'cooperation and competition' with this finer-grained framework. Complete common interest may be rare in a between-organism context, but partial common interest is not, and various kinds of partial common interest support partially informative signalling, even in situations where talk is free.

References

Bergstrom, C. & Lachmann, M. (1998). Signaling among relatives. III. Talk is cheap. *Proceedings of the National Academy of Sciences USA*, **95**, 5100–5105.

Bergstrom, C. & Lachmann, M. (2001). Alarm calls as costly signals of antipredator vigilance: the watchful babbler game. *Animal Behaviour*,**61**, 535–543.

Blackburn, S. (2011). Of Hume and bondage. *New York Times*, 11 December.

Bradbury, J. & Vehrencamp, S. (2000). Economic models of animal communication. *Animal Behaviour*, **59**, 259–268.

Bradbury, J. & Vehrencamp, S. (2011). *Principles of Animal Communication*, 2nd edn. Sunderland, MA: Sinauer.

Caro, T. (1995). Pursuit deterence revisited. *Trends in Ecology and Evolution*, **10**, 500–503.

Crawford, V. P. & Sobel, J. (1982). Strategic information transmission. *Econometrica*, **50**, 1431–1451.

[15] For example, suppose the payoffs for sender and receiver, respectively, if a mating occurs are (5, 5) in the case of a high-quality male, (5, 0) if low-quality male and (1, 1) if the male is of the wrong species (this means no pregnancy, whereas pregnancy with a low-quality male is expensive), while the payoffs if no mating occurs are (2, 2) regardless of the state of the male. Then if the system starts with unique signals being sent in each state and the receiver making their best response, senders will 'pool' two states into one signal, obscuring the distinction between low- and high-quality males. If states are equiprobable then receivers should continue to respond to the signals.

Dawkins. R. & Krebs. J. (1978). Animal signals: information or manipulation? In J. Krebs & R. Davies, eds., *Behavioural Ecology, An Evolutionary Approach*. Oxford: Blackwell, pp. 282–309.

Dretske, F. (1981). *Knowledge and the Flow of Information*. Cambridge, MA: MIT Press.

Farrell, J. & M. Rabin (1996). Cheap talk. *Journal of Economic Perspectives*, **10**, 103–118.

Fitzgibbon, C. D. & Fanshawe, J. H. (1988). Stotting in Thomson's gazelles: an honest signal of condition. *Behavioral Ecology and Sociobiology*, **23**, 69–74.

Godfrey-Smith, P. (2012). *Review of Brian Skyrms' Signals (2010)*. *Mind*, in press.

Hanlon, R. & Messenger, J. (1996). *Cephalopod Behaviour*. Cambridge: Cambridge University Press.

Huttegger, S., Skyrms, B., Smead, R. & Zollman, K. (2010). Evolutionary dynamics of Lewis signaling games: signaling systems vs. partial pooling. *Synthese*, **172**, 177–191.

Krebs, J. & Dawkins, R. (1984). Animal signals: mind-reading and manipulation. In J. Krebs & R. Davies (eds.), *Behavioural Ecology: An Evolutionary Approach*, 2nd edn. Oxford: Blackwell, pp. 380–402.

Lewis, D. K. (1969). *Convention*. Cambridge, MA: Harvard University Press.

Lloyd, J. E. (1975). Aggressive mimicry in *Photuris* fireflies: signal repertoires by femmes fatales. *Science*, **187**, 452–453.

Moynihan, M. & Rodaniche, A. (1982). The behaviour and natural history of the Caribbean reef squid *Sepioteuthis sepioidea* with a consideration of social, signal and defensive patterns for difficult and dangerous environments. *Advances in Ethology*, **125**, 1–150.

Owren, M., Rendall, D. & Ryan, M. (2010). Redefining animal signaling: influence versus information in communication. *Biology and Philosophy*, **25**, 755–780.

Rorty, R. (1982). *Consequences of Pragmatism: Essays 1972–1980*. Minneapolis, MN: University of Minnesota Press.

Searcy, W. & Nowicki, S. (2005). *The Evolution of Animal Communication*. Princeton, NJ: Princeton University Press.

Shannon, C. (1948). A mathematical theory of communication. *Bell System Mathematical Journal*, **27**, 379–423.

Skyrms, B. (1996). *Evolution of the Social Contract*. Cambridge, MA: Cambridge University Press.

Skyrms, B. (2010). *Signals: Evolution, Learning & Information*. New York: Oxford University Press.

Stegmann, U. (2009). A consumer-based teleosemantics for animal signals. *Philosophy of Science B*, **76**, 864–875.

Wagner, E. (2011). Deterministic chaos and the evolution of meaning. *British Journal for the Philosophy of Science*. Online ahead of print at doi:10.1093/bjps/axr039.

Commentaries

The conclusion that partial mutual benefits can result in stable communication is perhaps formally equivalent to the conclusion that both sender and receiver must benefit on average, as discussed in my chapter. The examples analysed by Godfrey-Smith all resemble cases of deception, when signals sometimes, but not always, evoke responses disadvantageous for the receiver, or eavesdropping, when signals sometimes, but not always, evoke responses disadvantageous for the sender. On other occasions, these same signals have compensating advantages for the receiver or sender.

Godfrey-Smith's analysis, like many other treatments of the evolution of communication, focuses on the persistence (stability) of communication. Another important question is its origin (dynamics) or how a new signal spreads. The evolutionary dynamics of communication is dominated by frequency-dependence of benefits for signallers and receivers. The necessary quantitative approach follows naturally from a focus on average benefits. As a result, beneficial signals and responses spread at first slowly, then more rapidly, and finally slowly again (Wiley, 2000). A focus on partial mutual benefits, rather than average benefits, should not lose sight of the evolutionary dynamics, as well as the evolutionary stability, of communication.

Wiley, R. H. (2000). Sexual selection and mate choice: trade-offs for males and females. In M. Apollonio, M. Festa-Bianchet & D. Mainardi, eds., *Vertebrate Mating Systems*. Singapore: World Scientific Publishing Co., pp. 8–46.

R. Haven Wiley

Godfrey-Smith uses the notion of information in a way that allows for disjunctive informational content. On his usage we could say, for example, that fever in a child, taken just by itself, carries the information that the child has measles or flu or chicken pox or strep or pneumonia … and so forth. In my usage (this volume), information corresponds to what the (natural, or intentional-and-true) sign carrying it is a sign of. So we would say that the child's fever either carries information that the child has measles or carries information that the child has flu or carries information that the child has strep … (Retrieving information from signs is not as easy as just looking at their shapes. Perhaps a good doctor would be able to tell of which one the fever actually is a sign.) Now Godfrey-Smith's distinction between informational content and adaptive content would seem to run parallel to my distinction between the content of 'natural signs' and the content of 'intentional signs'. I prefer to think of disjunctive content as arising only in the case of intentional signs, where there are alternative explanations of the utility of the sign, given the adaptive response to it. The question seems worth investigating whether one of these usages will help solve problems that the other will not.

Ruth Millikan

Response

Wiley notes a connection between my treatment of partial common interest and the requirement that signalling behaviours benefit, on average, both senders and receivers. If the interaction did not benefit both sides on average, then either sending or attending would degrade, and the other would follow. He suggests that a requirement of partial common interest is “perhaps formally equivalent” to the requirement of benefits on average to both sides. I think, instead, than the analysis I gave of partial common interest is lower-level that the analysis that Wiley refers to. This can be seen by noting that many different combinations of arrangements of sender and receiver interests, together with facts about the probabilities of states of the world and other factors, can yield the same relationships between average payoffs. When one asks whether a trait will increase or decrease in frequency, it is the average payoffs that matter, rather than the lower-level basis for these payoffs. In addition, only some kinds of partial common interest can stabilise signalling. In my chapter I gave an example of a case where sender and receiver agree about the ‘worst-case’ outcome in each state of the world, and this enables them to maintain partially informative signalling to avoid those outcomes. But there are other situations with similar payoffs and agreement on the ‘worse-case’ outcomes that move instead (from the same initial state) into cycles. I think that Haven Wiley’s criterion and my analysis are complementary rather than equivalent.

Millikan opposes a treatment of informational content that allows that content to be disjunctive, so that a sign’s informational content can be given by something like a disjoined list of possible states of the world that might give rise to the sign in normal conditions. (I agree with Millikan that informational content need not be about causes, but I will stick to those cases here.) A disjunction of this kind is a compression of a distribution of conditional probabilities – the probabilities of those states of the world *given* the state of the signal. Millikan has for some time been critical of the casual use of conditional probability by philosophers writing about information and content, and she raises these problems in her chapter in this volume. She has been right to be critical, and the foundational problems are difficult. I help myself in my chapter to a mode of probabilistic description about signals that seems both useful and reasonably continuous with the most unproblematic descriptions of macroscopic physical events in probabilistic terms (such as events in casino games, for example), and this underlies what I say about informational content.

Suppose, for example, that one species of animal has an alarm call that is used in very discriminating ways and is never produced in the absence of a predator, and an otherwise similar species has an alarm call that is on a 'hair trigger' and is often produced in response to harmless birds flying by. Then I think the alarm calls of these species have different informational properties, and the informational content of the second species' calls is disjunctive – something like *predator or harmless bird* – whereas the informational content of the other species' calls is not disjunctive. The two calls may have the same functional content: *predator*. The difference in informational content is a consequence of the different facts about what the signal makes likely, and these are a consequence of many features of the local set-up and the physical laws operating – just as in a casino. Sometimes selection processes lead to a match between functional and informational content, and sometimes they don't. A theory might be developed of when they can be expected to match and when they will diverge, and this theory is naturally developed in a way that recognises that both kinds of content may be disjunctive.

Peter Godfrey-Smith

PART V FROM ANIMAL SIGNALS TO HUMAN LANGUAGE

17

Information, meaning and animal communication

FRED ADAMS AND STEVE M. BEIGHLEY

17.1 Introduction

Wittgenstein (1953, p. 223) once said, "If a lion could speak, we could not understand him." As with many Wittgenstein quotes, no one really knows what he meant (though many think they know). What does 'speak' mean? Does it take a fully articulated language with a compositional syntax and semantics? If so, what use is the 'could' in Wittgenstein's aphorism? As far as we can tell, non-human animals communicate not by speaking, nor by language. Their vocalisations (or other signals) carry information and allow communication, but their signals lack meaning (if meaning is something that can be true or false and is something an animal might communicate stimulus independently). That genuine meaning requires stimulus independence of a type not shared by animal signalling will be a major theme stressed throughout what follows.[1]

Recently there has been much discussion in the animal communication literature about whether information is the right tool for understanding animal communication (Cheney & Seyfarth, 2003, 2007; Owren & Bachowroski, 2003; Rendall, Owren & Ryan, 2009; Stegmann, 2009; Owren, Rendall & Ryan, 2010). We think it is. There are several objections to using information as a basis for understanding animal communication, and there are some interesting alternatives on offer. We think the objections are misguided and that the alternatives actually require a notion of information, as we understand it. So in this chapter,

[1] In this view, we find ourselves aligned with Pinker (1994), and possibly opposed to Allen and Saidel (1998).

Animal Communication Theory: Information and Influence, ed. Ulrich Stegmann. Published by Cambridge University Press.

we give an account of information and meaning, how the first relates to the second and how the two are different. We consider some cases of what are sometimes called 'false signalling' and explain why these do not qualify as cases of linguistic meaning. Then we will turn to some objections to using the notion of information to understand animal communication. We explain why these objections are misguided. Many of them are based upon thinking of animal signals as linguistic (as language). Animal signals clearly are not language and probably do not have meaning of the type that language requires.[2] However, neither of these facts disqualify them from conveying important information (as we understand information).

17.2 Information

In the view we develop below, the sense in which animal signals convey information is in the sense of indication. We elaborate this view in the following sections. Now we will connect information with indication.

Information is not meaning. In fact, when a signal or symbol has meaning (and is capable of being falsely tokened), it loses its pure informational value. Shannon and Weaver (1949) worked out ways to quantify amounts of information generated by a message and carrying capacity for how many 'bits' or 'bytes' can be sent felicitously over a communication channel. These are very important matters and have led to the technological revolution that we enjoy everyday with our computers and cell phones. But what the notion of information helps us understand for the purposes of animal communication is neither the mathematical formulae nor ways to measure reduction of uncertainty or negative entropy. The reason the notion of information is useful is because it helps us grasp the indication relation (that one event may tell us about another because of a *lawful correlation* between the events). This is the import of the notion of information for understanding animal communication. The time-worn examples used in the naturalised semantics literature (Stampe, 1977; Dretske, 1981,1988; Adams & Aizawa, 1994, 2010) still hold true. Rings in a tree stump indicate seasons of growth the tree experienced because of the lawful correlation between growing seasons and rings of growth in the tree. Smoke in the forest indicates fire, and on and on.

Now there are two more things about this notion of information – the indication notion – that are worth reminding ourselves about. The first is that

[2] The usual case to be made for why animal signals are not language is based on lack of compositional syntax. Here we are adding further considerations based upon lack of stimulus-independent meaning. See also Anderson (2004, 2008).

there is no falsity here. Smoke in the forest indicates fire. It never falsely indicates fire. Of course a Hollywood movie set might artificially produce smoke, but that is not the setting in which smoke indicates fire. When people say "smoke means fire", of course, what they 'mean' is 'indicates'. It does not mean 'mean' in the way that a word or a sentence of a language has meaning. It means 'indicate', in the way that a look on your wife's face can mean you are now in big trouble. So only against a certain set of background conditions (so-called 'channel conditions') do natural signs (Grice's 1957 term) indicate things ('naturally mean' things, also Grice's term). A nice and easy way to draw the distinction we are now pointing to is this. There is a crucial difference between an indication (or a natural meaning) relation between two things and a semantic (or meaning) relation. Consider the following.

Information: Smoke means fire (indication, cannot be falsely tokened)

Meaning: "Smoke" means smoke (semantic, can be falsely tokened)

When there is smoke, there is fire (somewhere nearby). But when someone says "smoke" there may or may not be smoke near by. One can lie. One can be mistaken. One's saying "smoke" is not stimulus-dependent upon smoke nor upon fire. One can say "smoke" or "there is smoke", when there is no smoke and no fire. This is one of the upsides of meaning. We can engage in discourse about the world or things in it when those things are not present – or perhaps do not even exist. There is no stimulus dependency.[3] Ah, but with the pluses comes the minuses. Although we can, with meaningful symbols, discuss what is not true or not present, we also lose the tight and reliable connection with the world that comes with pure information (indication).

Smoke cannot arise without fire (in natural settings). So one measure of the true value of information (in the sense of indication) is its nomological connection with the world (with what it indicates). This is one reason information (indication) has been so central to tracking theories of knowledge (Dretske, 1981; Adams, 2004, 2005, Adams & Clarke, 2005) and naturalised theories of meaning (Dretske, 1988, Adams & Aizawa, 1994, 2010). Of course, the downside of things that have only information or indicational value is that they cannot be falsely tokened. That may sound strange because falsity is seldom a benefit. But natural signs cannot be cut free from their environmental origin. So they cannot, as can symbols with meaning, be used to talk about what is not the case, or not yet the case, or what might become the case and so on. Symbols with meaning open the door for error. They also open the possibilities of expression

[3] See also Sterelny (2003) on 'de-coupled' representation and its role in the evolution of cognition.

and thought, and free the mind from stimulus dependence. This stimulus independence, we claim, is essential to understanding the origin of meaningful tokens of symbols for purposes of communication in a population of individuals. Hence, we agree strongly with the following claim of Tomasello and Call (1997, p. 232):

> To the extent that communicative signals are produced automatically whenever an individual is in a certain mood or state or perceives a certain stimulus (without flexibility, strategic choice, or voluntary control), they are not cognitive phenomena for the signaller...[4]

17.3 Informational origins of meaning

An interesting and very important question is how a signal can lose its informational guarantee when it makes the jump to meaning. Suppose an animal shrieked "fire" when and only when there was fire. Then "fire" would at best naturally mean or indicate the presence of fire no differently than does the presence of smoke. In that case, "fire" would not mean fire the way that "smoke" means smoke, but it would be capable of informing one that there is fire (the same as smoke).

How does the jump from the level of information (indication) to genuine meaning take place? There are several competing theories available for how thoughts do this (Adams & Aizawa, 2010). For our purposes here, we will look only at one very plausible scenario for language-like expressions. Suppose an animal that shrieks "fire" at the presence of fire gains voluntary control over its behaviour and shrieks.[5] Suppose further that it comes to realise that it can manipulate the behaviour of others by its shrieks. There may be advantages to doing so (no fire, yet others run away and this animal gets the spoils). So at first fire causes the animal involuntarily to shriek "fire". These shrieks cause this animal and the other animals to scurry away. Over time this animal acquires voluntary control over whether it produce a shriek of "fire" even when there is no fire and still it can cause the other animals to scurry away (but voluntarily learns to override its own tendency to run away when it shrieks "fire"). Whereas originally, fire and only fire (in the correct context) caused shrieks of "fire" in this animal, now what explains its shrieks of "fire" is that it can voluntarily produce (whether fire is present or not) what before was only involuntarily

[4] Note that we are agreeing with the conditional 'to the extent that', and not saying that all animal signals are involuntary. Even if stimulus-dependent, they could be voluntary. And even if voluntary, they still may not be linguistically meaningful.

[5] Of course it would not literally be "fire". Substitute your favourite fire-induced shriek.

produced by the presence of fire. In such a case, "fire" would actually come to mean fire in much the way that "smoke" means smoke. Both can be falsely tokened. Both can say something true (when there is fire) and both can say something false (when there is no fire). And very importantly, the informational origin and value that explains why "fire" means fire and not something else (because originally it was tied to fire) is not compromised. That is, although a token of "fire" no longer guarantees the presence of fire, the explanation of the original connection between fire and "fire" is preserved. Equally important, now an utterance of "fire" might *not inform* others of the presence of fire, even if it can cause them to react in the same way or to think there is fire.[6] With the jump from information to meaning, there is some disconnection with reality brought on by the possibility of false tokening, and hence the possibility of misrepresentation.[7]

Notice that this scenario is possible only if the animal is no longer in the grips of tight stimulus dependence on conditions that involuntarily produce its signalling. For genuine linguistic meaning to be established, the animal must be able to break free from the stimulus triggers of the signalling. What is more, notice that the *meaning* of the signal must be established *prior* to the ability of false tokening, not the other way around. Some seem to have believed that if we can find cases of deception (even one-off cases of emitting signals that fool the hearer) then that shows a kind of linguistic meaning. Not so. If I make tracks in the snow to mislead my pursuers about where I am, this is deceptive. But the tracks in the snow do not have linguistic meaning. They are not false tokens. They do accurately represent where my foot was even if they mislead you about where I am. It gets the order wrong to think that a few misleading or deceptive uses of signals count as establishing meaning. The practice would have to be widespread and free of stimulus triggers, and the content of the signal would have to be fixed prior to the 'false tokening' in order to establish linguistic meaning. We will have more to say about this below.

[6] In a song, Tommy Smothers once explained that he yelled "fire" when he fell into the chocolate because no one would come to help if he yelled "chocolate". Nonetheless, "fire" is connected in meaning with fire (not chocolate) because it traces its informational origins to fire (not chocolate). See Adams and Aizawa (2010) for theories of how this historical connection to what is formerly indicated is preserved after the jump to meaning.

[7] This is loosely modelled on some suggestions by Grice (1957), Dretske (1988) and Pinker (1994, p. 352). Dennett (1983) and Tomasello and Call (1997, pp. 269 ff) give anecdotal examples of a chimp giving an alarm call during a fight and then watching the participants scatter.

17.4 Linguistic reference

Animal signals have genuine linguistic reference only if (1) animals utter sentences or (2) their utterances fit a pattern of mutually understood intentions and patterns of linguistic activity or language games (Perry, 1994). But neither is the case. Frege and Davidson maintained that words have reference only within the context of a sentence that expresses a complete thought. Perry (1994) explains (again borrowing from Wittgenstein) how this might be false, but in place of complete sentences substitutes something like Wittgenstein's slab-language game.[8] In the builder scenario, when the builder says to his assistant "slab", this is actually a one-word sentence with the content "Bring me a slab." "Slab" may mean slab, but only against a background of mutually understood intentions, beliefs and desires. And on either account, there is more to reference than an involuntary, stimulus-dependent evocation of a call or signal. Although animal signals do not have genuine linguistic reference (meaning), because they do not have the background context of mutually understood beliefs, desires and intentions (essentially no theory of mind[9]), they do have *aboutness.*[10] Signs or signals that convey information have aboutness and that is enough to communicate about *indicated* objects in the environment (Cheney & Seyfarth, 2003).[11] Notice that rings in the tree stump

[8] Perry does not reject that there is only reference within the context of a complete thought.

[9] We are inclined to agree with Tomasello and Call (1997, p. 340): "... with regard to understanding the less observable aspects of behavioral functioning, there is no solid evidence that nonhuman primates understand the intentionality or mental states of others." This ability is absolutely essential to establishing linguistic meaning and thereby linguistic reference in a community of signallers. Elsewhere, Tomasello, Call and Hare (2003) distinguish a kind of 'perceptual' theory of mind from an 'epistemic' (false belief type) theories of mind and argue in favour of primates having the former, but we think this is largely gaze-following (Ristau, 1998) and not the more interesting epistemic variety that could support meaning. Allen and Saidel (1998) require a kind of 'joint attention' model necessary to connect signaller with recipient of the signal, but can only speculate about the existence of such cognitive mechanisms in non-human animals. For similar skepticism about non-human primate theory of mind see Güzeldere Nahmias and O'Denner (2002).

[10] There is a common association between the mental property of intentionality and aboutness, due to Brentano. On our view, the aboutness of intentional states is inherited from the aboutness of the informational states upon which they are built. See Dretske (1981).

[11] Cheney and Seyfarth (2003, p. 238) are themselves aware of this worry – that their talk of 'meaning' may be vague. Thus they realise that folks like us may step in and say they are really talking about something else – indication and natural meaning or information. The aboutness of information is also likely sufficient to satisfy the notion of 'reference' that Allen and Saidel (1998) defend, as well. Even though we think we disagree with

indicate and are *about* the seasons of growth. Indication is quite sufficient to serve the purposes that Zuberbühler, Cheney and Seyfarth (1999; Cheney & Seyfarth, 2003) and others need to explain about animal signalling. An "eagle" alarm call has aboutness because it carries information *about an eagle* overhead (again, in the way that smoke indicates fire, not the way that "smoke" means smoke or "eagle call" means eagle).

Lastly, when we say that animal signals do not have linguistic meaning, we do not mean to imply that receivers of animal signals respond only to the perceptual acoustic properties of the signal. The receivers may well understand the informational value of the signal (what it indicates about the world) even if the signal has not elevated to the level of linguistic meaning. So even informational value of signals may reach the level sometimes (Zuberbühler *et al.*, 1999) called "conceptual", without rising to the level of linguistic meaning. That is, in the mind of the hearer there may be a conceptual connection between the sign and what it signifies in the same way that the smeller of smoke knows smoke indicates fire. This is a conceptual connection. The animal has the concept of smoke and the concept of fire and learns to associate the two. Similarly, for example, a vervet may have the concept[12] of an eagle alarm call and the concept of the eagle and cognitively associate the two even if the alarm call does not

Allen and Saidel about whether there is sufficient stimulus independence in animal signalling for genuine reference, we seem to agree with them on what it would take. What we call genuine reference they call 'conceptual reference', and they say about vervet alarm calls: "...only after the vervet can refer to absent objects in false signals could it engage in the kind of reference that we have labeled 'conceptual'". Notice that their first use of 'refer' has to be a weaker sense that they call "proxy", where signals elicit the same kinds of response that the object with which the signal is paired normally elicits. For us, that is not genuine reference in the way "slab" means (refers to) slab.

12 In our view, non-human animals can think. Since they can think they have concepts. Concepts do have what Grice would call non-natural meaning. We agree with Cheney and Seyfarth (2003, p. 236) about that. So when a Diana monkey or a vervet thinks about an eagle, its thoughts mean eagle and its thought *eagle there* refers to an eagle. This can all be true even if the calls that come out of the vervet's mouth only have indication or natural meaning, not linguistic meaning. Indeed, this is our view of the matter. This commits us to there being more required for animal signals to acquire genuine meaning and reference than thoughts themselves, and in this chapter we are attempting to get at what more is required. We notice that Cheney and Seyfarth (2003, p. 251) seem to acknowledge the same thing – the evolution of thought is prior to the evolution of language, suggesting that they too accept that more is involved in the latter. Dretske (personal communication) asked us why, if their thoughts mean eagle, can't they express their thoughts? Can't they express their thoughts in behaviour? It is not that they *cannot* express their thoughts in speech, but that they *do not*. To do so, they would need to intend to convey a message. But what comes out is not intended to convey information *because* it is stimulus-driven.

linguistically mean *eagle*. What is more, there need be nothing physically intrinsic to the signal for it to communicate information about what it signals. So the animal is not picking up only on the acoustic-perceptual properties of the signal.

17.5 False tokening

An important concern for the picture we present is false tokening. Is there false tokening sufficiently stimulus-independent to constitute a basis for genuine linguistic meaning and reference? Are there cases more like "smoke"–smoke and less like smoke–fire, among cases of non-human animal communication? And if there are, aren't these genuine cases of linguistic meaning and reference?

First, flexibility in signalling is not the same thing as stimulus independence and voluntary control. Many animals produce food calls the rate of which varies with the presence or absence of their mates, or alarm calls which vary in rate or intensity with the presence or absence of offspring, a phenomenon known as 'audience effect' (Tomasello & Zuberbühler, 2002; Di Bitetti, 2005; Karakashian, Gyger & Marler, 1998). The fact that calls can change with the presence of mates or offspring does not show stimulus independence or that control of signalling has been handed over to a voluntary cognitive control system. Instead, it shows that the stimulus conditions that control the signalling may be varied and complex.

Second, several types of cases are cited in the literature about voluntary signalling. Cheney and Seyfarth (2003) detail many complexities surrounding animal calls and signalling, and they convince us that there is wide variation among the conditions that produce the signalling. But they do not convince us that animal signalling is so stimulus- and context-free that you find anything like the possibility of 'free tokening' of a signal that retains its meaning: for no reason at all Steve can yell, "Your pants are on fire", and I know exactly what he means. He can randomly talk about lions and snakes and eagles, free of their presence or threat. One just does not find anything like that in the wild – nor in any of the cases Cheney and Seyfarth or others cite about move grunts, alarm calls or anything else.[13]

[13] Cheney and Seyfarth (2003, p. 227) note that in laboratory conditions some vocalisations can be brought under operant control. We do not dispute that. Still, operant control is not equivalent to stimulus-free production. They also suggest that some animals choose to remain silent. But they add that the male Thomas Langur monkeys who did this "only ceased calling . . . after every other individual had acknowledged the predator's presence" (p. 228). This too is not stimulus-free or context-free signalling

Stegmann (2009) cites purported examples of fireflies (*Photinus macdermotti*) and false tokening. Females produce flashes of light to signal preparedness for mating. The male signals back until they find each other and mate. False tokening exists when other female (*Photuris versicolor*) fireflies, who prey upon the *P. macdermotti* fireflies, falsely signal to the males. When males signal back, there is a fatal rendezvous.

Stegmann thinks that these are examples of false tokening that count as instances of misrepresentation. It would be a short step to take these to be what Grice (1957) would call non-natural meaning or what we are calling linguistic meaning. Stegmann buys into consumer-based theories of meaning. So perhaps for Stegmann, the false tokening has the (false) content *for the consumer*, "Conspecific mate over here."

We think this does not count as genuine meaning. Instead, it is a case of evolutionary exploitation of natural meaning or indication. The predator firefly, as a species, has evolved the practice of imitating the mating signal of another type of firefly. This is very similar to the case of the viceroy butterfly whose colouring imitates that of the foul-tasting monarch. In both cases, there is evolutionary selection over a trait where the selection is at the level of the species (not the individual). What we mean by this is that this does not involve individual learning or recruitment in the individual's lifetime and there is no stimulus-independent production under voluntary control of the individual. For example, the predator females only signal in this way to the males of this species, even though they could prey upon the females just as easily. Food is food. If the so-called false tokening were under voluntary control, the predators could easily *learn* to go after the females as well.

(withholding). Its conditions of signalling are just complex. What is more, the fact that signalling is "not impossible to suppress" does not show that they are voluntarily produced, as Cheney and Seyfarth surely seem to imply (p. 233). Even if, as they say, baboon vocalisations often depend upon their own motivation, the particular situation at hand and who else is involved, this still falls short of stimulus- and context-free utterances with fixed meaning and reference. In the end, Cheney and Seyfarth (2003, p. 234) accept this as a possibility. However, we would be remiss not to mention the puzzle that Cheney and Seyfarth present to us – that in virtually all mammals, the striking differences between (highly constrained) signal production and (quite open-ended) signal perception constitutes one of the primary puzzles when comparing language to animal communication. Why should a monkey that can attach almost any kind of meaning to a sound in its environment through learning and experience be so utterly prevented from producing calls in a manner that is equally flexible? After all, every individual is both a producer and a perceiver. As to Dretske's question, our reply is not that they *cannot* but that they *do not*. Cheney and Seyfarth's puzzle relates to the important question of why they don't. We do not have that answer and think that is where attention should turn going forward.

Güzeldere *et al.* (2002) develop useful categories in order to determine the kinds of cognitive abilities necessary for some kinds of deception. Their first category is 'hard-wired' deception. This could include deceptive colouration (viceroy/monarch) or deceptive motor programmes (a mantis shrimp pretending it is ready to fight, when shell-less it is vulnerable to attack). In each case in this category, there is an evolutionary-level explanation of the selection for the deceptive signal or behaviour. The explanation lies not in the lifetime of the individual. Still in cases of deceptive behaviour, the behaviour is stimulus-dependent. Its onset occurs inflexibly and automatically with the presence of a predator or environmental condition. Stegmann's fireflies fall in this classification.

Their second category involves 'behaviouristic learning'. These cases involve learning transfer; that is, a piece of behaviour appropriate to one context randomly occurs in another and then is rewarded and reinforced in the new context.[14] They give an example of a monkey crying for help and then being comforted and suckled by its mother. Then later the monkey gives a "help" cry, but this time to be suckled. Here the explanation is not at the level of selection across generations but of learning within the life of the individual. Güzeldere *et al.* (2002) insist that even in this case the deception is not intentionally planned or conceived. The animals do not understand why this works, only that it does.

Their third category is 'intentional deception'. This is of the kind so familiar to humans, where the deceiver understands only too well why and how it works and engages in it for that reason. Of this category they say:

> In fact, it is unlikely that any non humans, even the great apes, have a well-developed understanding of how intentional deception works ... The reason is quite straightforward. These definitions generally hold that intentional deception requires a theory of mind, the ability to understand that others have beliefs and desires, and there is no persuasive evidence that any non human animals are capable of this.

Interestingly to us, O'Deaner set up an experiment using the Menzel paradigm with lemurs (Güzeldere *et al.*, 2002). In this paradigm a lesser-ranking individual is shown where a cache of food is and then is put back into a group with dominant individuals, the aim being to see if the subordinate will engage in deceptive behaviour to keep the large cache of food for him or herself. In

[14] We are not sure why they did not call this 'operant learning'. We think this would also be a place to add the examples that Cheney and Seyfarth (1985) give of youthful vervets making mistakes of giving eagle alarm calls to various things in the sky (but correcting for this by adulthood).

O'Deaner's case the food was grapes. The subordinate male was shown where the grapes were cached but did not regularly attempt to deceive the dominant females about the location of the grapes. He did employ what appeared to be a deceptive pattern of search on a very few occasions, but over 56 trials he did not employ deceptive strategies with increasing regularity (even though the time he did, they worked). Why? It may be that he could not break the stimulus-driven motivation to go straight to the highly valued food. This is the explanation Güzeldere *et al.* (2002) adopt.

Now some final worries about our explanation, going back to the case of the fireflies. One could object to our explanation in this way. We say that the predator fireflies are only exploiting natural meaning (information, indication) when they falsely token, and that there is no genuine meaning in their signalling (Grice's 'non-natural meaning'). One could easily object that if the predator signals do not indicate (truthfully) that there is a willing mate sending the signal, then the natural meaning connection has been broken. Whatever the physical flashes are, they no longer naturally mean "Willing mate over here." Perhaps one would say they have 'disjunctive' natural meaning ("willing mate here" or "predator here").[15] Yet, if that were so, it still would not show that the firefly signals had risen from the level of natural meaning (information, indication) to the level of linguistic meaning and false tokening. It would just show that, once the predators exploit the code, the code has disjunctive content at the level of natural meaning. A tokening by a predator is not a false tokening with the meaning "willing conspecific here". Instead it truly indicates "predator here or willing conspecific here". In this case, there will not even be false tokening. And if there is no possibility for false tokening, there is no possibility for linguistic meaning.

What is more, this is a familiar type of case in epistemology (Adams, 2010). Suppose some misguided individual makes a fake deer-track maker in order to confuse deer hunters. If he makes false tracks where deer normally move through the woods, does that prove that tracks made by genuine deer no longer carry information that deer are nearby? Not necessarily. What it shows is that normal deer hunters may not be able to tell the genuine tracks from the fakes. If not, they will be misled by the false tracks. However, it still

[15] See also Skyrms (2010). He too claims that animal signals convey information. He too notes that animal signals can break free from their normal contexts (as in cases of deception). He too says of the firefly signals that the informational content they convey is 'mixed'. He too does not attribute the false tokening to linguistic meaning. He gives a slightly different way to measure amounts of information (that we do not have space to go into here), but his overall view is consistent with our overall view about animal signals, information and meaning.

will be true that genuine tracks naturally indicate the presence of deer. The difficulty will be distinguishing the fakes from the genuine tracks. This may well be what is happening in the case of the fireflies.[16] The *Photinus macdermotti* cannot differentiate the copy-cat signals from those made by genuine conspecifics. Yet, if there were not still a genuine informational connection to exploit, the copy-cat signals would be ineffective. The fact that they are not ineffective shows that the natural meaning has not been lost even though the *Photuris versicolor* has come to exploit that connection. There is still some physical difference in the *Photinus macdermotti* signals, but the fireflies are not able to distinguish them.[17] So the tokenings from the conspecifics of *Photinus macdermotti* are *not false*. On either explanation above, there is no false tokening of the kind needed for genuine linguistic meaning. There is nothing on the order of "smoke" meaning smoke.[18]

17.6 Objections to the use of information to understand animal signalling

Owren and others object to using information to understand animal signals. A good many of these objections depend on blurring the distinction between information, meaning and reference carefully distinguished above.

Owren *et al.* (2010, p. 759) object that authors in the animal communication literature use the notion of information but have "uniformly failed to define this construct". The complaint is that people cite Shannon and Weaver (1949) and then move on without explanation. We do not intend to join in on a game of 'pin the tail on the donkey'. People who invoke the notion of information in discussing animal signalling may well be guilty as charged. As we emphasise, the crucial notion needed is that of indication or Grice's natural meaning, and for that, nothing fancy in terms of definitions is needed. We have explained the crucial relationship that signals have to the world when they indicate events or

[16] Of course, if there is absolutely no difference in the physical properties of the signals, and if both sources of signals are widely available in the population, then the first option holds: that is, the signals have disjunctive indicator content.

[17] Counterfeit bills may look like legal tender to the consumer, but they still have physical differences and do not have the same monetary value.

[18] One might ask (indeed Stegmann asked) about occasions upon which animals do signal when there is nothing signified in the environment that would be naturally indicated by the signal. Our view is that these are akin to performance/competence errors (infants learning the natural signs), mistakes or other competence failures. If they become too common an "*x*" may occur in response to *y*s not *x*s, then one finds cases of disjunctive indication (and still not falsity).

have natural meaning or carry information, and that is *lawful correlation*. Fancy mathematical ways of calculating or quantifying amounts of information or carrying capacity of a channel, although extremely important for some purposes, are less important for understanding animal signals as conveying information.

Continuing, Owren *et al.* (2010, p. 759) complain: "Nor is it explained what is meant by saying that information is conveyed from one individual to another." However, they themselves go on to say: "Signals can thus be said to be informative in the sense that they allow perceivers to draw inferences about their environments, other individuals, and the like." If an animal smells smoke in the forest, that indicates fire. If one wants an explanation of how smoke's presence conveys to the animal the presence of fire (danger) that is surely done in terms of the fact that the animal can *exploit the regularities* in the natural environment between fire and danger. The one (smoke) is followed by the other (fire) on a very uniform basis and can be *used to predict* the other. Smell smoke – best to flee! The same holds for the mating call or the warning threat of a rival. Information is conveyed via the regularities in the environment that can be exploited by both the sender and the recipient (perhaps for competing purposes).

Next Owren *et al.* (2010, p. 759) complain that researchers who base their interpretation of animal signalling upon information move from the statistical relations between signal and world to the content of the signal:

> Information no longer refers to correlations among events, but rather becomes an entity unto itself . . . this metaphorical view of information is primarily based on intuition and everyday conceptions. It has no connection to Shannon and Weaver's definition, and is not a scientifically grounded construct.

Now something seems to have gone horribly wrong. Owren *et al.* (2010) seem to be complaining that information has *content* – perhaps even propositional content. But that is hardly news (Dretske, 1981; Floridi, 2005). Suppose two events are statistically correlated such that Shannon and Weaver's account would allow there to be an informational (statistically relevant) connection between them. Objects have lots of properties, but suppose a's being F is correlated with b's being G in a lawful way. Then b's being G tells one (who is suitably equipped to exploit that correlation) *that a is F*. That is, *to say that there is information available* is to allow that there is *content*, a *message*, something to learn about the correlation. So there *is* more than mere correlation. There is correlation *about some fact* and the correlation about that fact *does generate a message*, the "entity unto itself" that is referred to in the quote above. This is perfectly consistent with the mathematical treatment of information by Shannon and Weaver. It even has a name: the 'surprisal' value of a signal.[19]

Next is the objection that on standard communication theory there is discussion of messages being 'coded' (Owren *et al.*, 2010, p. 760). This is certainly true for human communication theory. Think of Morse code or Braille. But think of the rings in the tree stump. What is the code there? Or smoke in the forest? In cases where correlations are set up by human convention (Morse code, Braille), the codes are invented. In cases where correlations follow nature's regularities, there are no conventions. Nature's regularities are exploited as they are found. In the case of animal signalling, especially where the signalling is not under the voluntary control of the agent but is involuntary and stimulus-dependent, the correlations between the signal and the state of the animal and world is a natural regularity. There is no need for a special conventional code there any more than there would be for tree rings and seasons of growth or smoke and fire. As far as we can tell, there are no animal signals that conform to conventional voluntary coding (Cheney & Seyfarth, 2003). Vervet calls are different for predators on the ground or in the trees or overhead. But these are not different *by convention.*[20] Whatever the evolutionary explanation of the calling patterns, they are much more like the relation of smoke to fire than of "smoke" to smoke.

Another worry that Owren *et al.* (2010, p. 761) correctly highlight is the tendency to confuse information with meaning.[21] It is quite right that such confusion in the literature is a distinct worry and that is why we have been very careful not to confuse them (Adams & Aizawa, 1994, 2010). What is more, we hope that we have shown here how keeping them distinct helps with worries being raised about the use of information as a basis for interpreting animal signalling.

[19] By the way, we think there are some important places in the literature where authors go out of their way to differentiate the amount of information a signal carries (reduction of uncertainty measured as the log of a reduction in a number of possibilities and measured in bits or bytes) from the content of the message that carries this information. Any transmission of information requires both message content and, given that, a computation of the amount of information conveyed. To assume that Shannon–Weaver information is all reduction of uncertainty with no message content makes no sense. Some message content is required to reduce uncertainty. But that content is, as we are at pains to point out, only indication or natural meaning. Compare Krebs and Dawkins (1984).

[20] Throughout, by 'convention', we mean something that at least operates via shared intentions.

[21] Randall *et al.* (2009, p. 234) seem to us to be guilty of this themselves. They say, "Studies of primate communication are often couched in the metaphor of language where *meaning* is the central explanatory construct . . ." In our view, this is just the mistake to be avoided. They should have said "information (indication)". This would remove their complaint.

Rendall *et al.* (2009, p. 234) represent the informational view as requiring some kind of representational ideation on the part of the signaller that is translated into a message whose content is then encoded in a signal and transmitted to the receiver, who then decodes it and recovers the relevant representational content. In this view, the communication depends upon a packet of information flowing from signaller to receiver. Non-human primates "routinely show little intention to inform others through their calls" (Rendall *et al.*, 2009). But of course, it is incorrect to be using the human model in comparison. Consistent with Cheney and Seyfarth's idea that non-human animals have no theory of mind or understanding of intentions, it is a mistake to model animal communication on this particular model of the use of information in communication. Animal vocal behaviour is modulated primarily by involuntary processes (Rendall *et al.*, 2009, p. 235).

One last objection (Owren & Bachowroski, 2003, p. 187) is that frustrated youngsters scream again and again, vocalising distress to their mothers. The representational view says the initial vocalisations convey information about distress. So why do the youngsters scream again and again? The objection suggests that if it were for informational value (news) that the youngsters scream, there would be no need for additional signalling. Mother should have got the message the first or second time. The answer given by Owren and Bachowroski is that the multiple screaming activates the mother's affect system, initiating a response (not news). First, we do not see that these are mutually exclusive. Indeed, only if the youngster 'gets through' to its mother will it get what it wants. Second, it is very likely that with repetition comes a ramping up of the screams. Elevated screams indicate increasing distress. There is news in this (not just activation of the mother's affect system). A mother can detect how serious things are by the pitch or amplitude or frequency of the distress signals.[22]

17.7 Alternative views of animal communication

The new view (Owren *et al.*, 2010) is that the primary function of vocalising is to influence the listener's attention, emotion and arousal, rather than inform or transmit information. Now we do not see that these are mutually exclusive and, what is more, we think the new view requires information as indication for it to be correct that signalling is about manipulating the listener. For example, about courtship signals, Owren *et al.* (2010, p. 767) say:

[22] Adams' daughter once fell off the couch on her arm. Adams knew how serious was the pain by the pitch and intensity of his daughter's cries.

> ... critical aspects of communication have little to do with encoding and decoding of representational information. Instead, the broader view is that courtship signals do not evolve to carry information about signaler quality, but rather to influence perceiver mating behavior by any and all available means.

In this quote Owren *et al.* were responding to discussion of 'signal honesty'. Now as Cheney and Seyfarth (2003) correctly point out, to influence a mate it is at the very least necessary to let the potential mate know *where you are*. To influence your behaviour or affect system, at least this much information (indication) is an absolute essential, not to mention that it is also to let the mate know that *you are ready* for mating.[23] Indeed, any signal that so influences is guaranteed to indicate this readiness.

We think objections to these obvious points may be clouded by the prospect of signalling involving conscious voluntary packaging of messages in a pre-set code and then receiving and breaking or unpacking the possibly encrypted message on the other end. Indeed, Rendall and Owren (2002) emphasise the intimate connection of the information-based model of animal signals with the linguistic model of information communicated by human words (stressing the arbitrary connection to signal design and so on). This is, of course, what Claude Shannon was interested in when developing the mathematics for communication channels for voluntary communications. It is not, however, the proper way to conceive of information being conveyed by animal signals that largely are not even under voluntary control, much less language-like. When they suggest that "The significance of such signals lies not in *what* is said, but rather *who* says it and *how*. Hence, linguistic constructs, like meaning, may have limited application to animal vocalizations", we think they are conflating the distinction with which we began that separates information from meaning: smoke indicating fire from "smoke" meaning smoke.

When they insist that animal communication is not necessarily intentional, we could not agree more. This is central to our claim that not much of animal signalling is under voluntary control and to Cheney and Seyfarth's (2003) point that there is no theory of mind at work in animal communication. And similarly while the content, or meaning, of human word use hinges on intentional agents – *meaners* to mean what they say – non-human primate communication evidently does not. By extension, then, they are left to wonder whether there can ever truly be *meaning* in primate vocalisations without there being a

[23] Of course, in cases of so-called 'false tokening' the information conveyed may be disjunctive, as we explain above in the case of the fireflies.

meaner – again, we could not agree more.[24] But this does not make the case against the information-based model for interpreting animal communication. This is because it is natural meaning (indication) not semantic meaning.

Now again, think about the new view itself – that animal signals exploit evolved sensitivity to involuntary brain responses. On this view, vocalisations in non-humans are said to function primarily through their influence on the affective systems that guide behaviour, including subcortical sytems like the brainstem and limbic structures that control attention, arousal and affect (rather than higher ingredients of information or indication that we outlined earlier for systems like conceptual and language representation and comprehension). Yet, for such systems to operate and be successful at manipulating the affect systems of the listeners there must be a stable channel of communication for the signals to travel over. There must be lawful regularities to be exploited by the physical properties of the vocalisation and the neural properties of the listener. These exploited lawful regularities are the very essence of natural signs, indication and information in the relevant sense.[25]

Owren *et al.* (2010) see evolved auditory sensitivities to certain kinds of sound as creating opportunities for senders to use vocalisation to engage others, thereby influencing affective states that are concomitants of behaviour of the listeners. As they say: "Among non-human primates, one entire class of vocalisations that we have labeled 'squeaks, shrieks, and screams' appears to capitalize on this potential." And they go on to list functions such as to "advertise identity". They claim that vocalisations in these species thus often contain conspicuous cues to caller identity, and listeners are demonstrably responsive to such cues. Acoustic analyses reveal clear identity cues in the 'contact' calls used to coordinate activity among dispersed group members in several species (reviewed in Rendall, Owren & Rodman, 1998; Rendall, Cheney & Seyfarth, 2000). Field experiments involving the playback of these calls have confirmed that different group members can be distinguished by voice and that identity cues form the basis for differential responses by

[24] Seyfarth correctly reminds us that even if there were no meaners that would not necessarily count against the informational view that the hearer can get significance from a signal even if the signaller did not intend or mean to send a message with that significance. Still, for us, this is information (indication) and not linguistic meaning.

[25] The regularities exploited are not only those between the world and the animal signal but also those between the animal signal and the affect system of the hearer. There are no doubt lawful relations between the acoustic properties of, say, an infant's vocalisations and a mother's affect system. Even if these are hard-wired they are lawful and if lawful, there is an information channel being exploited. Lawful regularities are the medium along which information travels.

listeners (e.g. Waser, 1977; Snowdon & Cleveland, 1980; Mitani, 1985). Here clearly information (as indication) is being exploited. It is through such lawful correlations that these affective interactions are even possible.

17.8 Conclusion

We still think that information (properly understood) is the right tool to use to analyse animal communication. We join those before us in distinguishing information from meaning, but go further in suggesting that genuine meaning (linguistic meaning) has semantic requirements not met by animal signalling. Meaningful signals must be stimulus-free, must establish meaning and then must permit false tokening.

The notion of information relevant is that of indication or what Grice called 'natural meaning'. This notion of information includes that signals are *about* objects or events in the environment and this *aboutness* is sufficient for the purposes of explaining animal calls and signals. There is no genuine linguistic meaning or linguistic reference in animal calls, but they are *about* things in virtue *of indicating* them.

There probably is no legitimate false tokening in animal signals, if false tokening presupposes linguistic meaning and reference, as we maintain. There surely are cases of deceptive signalling, but these can all be explained in terms of exploitation of natural signs or indication relations.

We consider alternative approaches to understanding animal communication that claim to eschew the use of information. The objections used to motivate the alternative accounts are mistaken, and even the alternatives presuppose something like indication or information, as we understand it.

Acknowledgements

Many thanks to Robin Andreasen, Ken Aizawa, Colin Allen, Fred Dretske, Marc Hauser, Robert Seyfarth, Ulrich Stegmann and one anonymous reader for comments on earlier versions of this chapter.

References

Adams, F. (2004). Knowledge. In L. Floridi, ed., *The Blackwell Guide to the Philosophy of Information and Computing*. Oxford: Basil Blackwell, pp. 228–236.

Adams, F. (2005). Tracking theories of knowledge, *Veritas*, **50**, 11–35.

Adams, F. (2010). Epistemology. In L. McHenry & T. Yagisawa, eds., *Reflections on Philosophy*, 3rd edn. San Diego, CA: Cognella/University Readers, pp. 107–134.

Adams, F. & Aizawa, K. (1994). Fodorian semantics. In S. Stich & T. Warfield, eds., *Mental Representations*. Oxford: Basil Blackwell, pp. 223–242.

Adams, F. & Aizawa, K. (2010). Causal theories of mental content. *Stanford Encyclopedia of Philosophy*.

Adams, F. & Clarke, M. (2005). Resurrecting the tracking theories. *Australasian Journal of Philosophy*, **83**, 207–221.

Allen, C. & Saidel, E. (1998). The evolution of reference. In D. Cummins & C. Allen, eds., *The Evolution of Mind*. New York: Oxford University Press, pp. 183–202.

Anderson, S. R. (2004). *Doctor Dolittle's Delusion: Animals and the Uniqueness of Human Language*. New Haven, CT: Yale University Press.

Anderson, S. R. (2008). The logical structure of linguistic theory. Presidential address to the Linguistic Society of America Annual Meeting, Chicago, Illinois, 5 January. *Language*, **84**, 795–814.

Cheney, D. L. & Seyfarth, R. M. (1985). Vervet monkey alarm calls: manipulation through shared information? *Behaviour*, **94**, 739–751.

Cheney, D. L. & Seyfarth, R. M. (2003). Signalers and receivers in animal communication. *Annual Review of Psychology*, **54**, 145–173.

Cheney, D. L. & Seyfarth, R. M. (2007). *Baboon Metaphysics*. Chicago, IL: University of Chicago Press.

De Bitetti, M. S. (2005). Food-associated calls and audience effects in tufted capuchin monkeys (*Cebus apella nigritus*). *Animal Behaviour*, **69**, 911–919.

Dennett, D. C. (1983). Intentional systems in cognitive ethology: the 'Panglossian paradigm' defended. *Behavioral and Brain Sciences*, **6**, 343–390.

Dretske, F. (1981). *Knowledge and the Flow of Information*. Cambridge, MA: MIT Press.

Dretske, F. (1988). *Explaining Behavior*. Cambridge, MA: MIT Press.

Floridi, L. (2005). Is information meaningful data? *Philosophy and Phenomenological Research*, **70**, 351–370.

Grice, H. P. (1957). Meaning. *Philosophical Review*, **66**, 377–388.

Güzeldere, G., Nahmias, E. & O'Deaner, R. (2002). Darwin's continuum and the building blocks of deception. In C. Allen, M. Beckoff & G. Burghardt, eds., *The Cognitive Animal*. Cambridge, MA: MIT Press.

Karakashian, S. J., Gyger, M. & Marler, P. (1998). Audience effects on alarm calling in chickens (*Gallus gallus*). *Journal of Comparative Psychology*, **102**, 129–135.

Krebs, J. R. & Dawkins, R. (1984). Animal signals: mind-reading and manipulation. In J. R. Krebs & N. B. Davies, eds., *Behavioural Ecology: An Evolutionary Approach*. Oxford: Blackwell Scientific, pp. 380–402.

Mitani, J. C. (1985). Sexual selection and adult male orangutan long calls. *Animal Behaviour*, **33**, 272–283.

Owren, M. J. & Bachowroski, J. (2003). Reconsidering the evolution of nonlinguistic communication: the case of laughter. *Journal of Nonverbal Behavior*, **27**, 183–200.

Owren, M. J., Rendall, D. & Ryan, M. J. (2010). Redefining animal signaling: influence versus information in communication. *Biological Philosophy*, **25**, 755–780.

Perry, J. (1994). Davidson's sentences and Wittgenstein's builders. Presidential address, Pacific APA. *Proceedings and Addresses of the APA*, **68**, 23–37.

Pinker, S. (1994). *The Language Instinct*. New York: Morrow.
Rendall, D. & Owren, M. J. (2002). Animal vocal communication: say what? In M. Bekoff, C. Allen & G. Burghardt, eds., *The Cognitive Animal: Empirical and Theoretical Perspectives on Animal Cognition*. Cambridge, MA: MIT Press, pp. 307–313.
Rendall, D., Cheney, D. L. & Seyfarth, R. M. (2000). Proximate factors mediating 'contact' calls in adult female baboons and their infants. *Journal of Comparative Psychology*, **114**, 36–46.
Rendall, D., Owren, M. J. & Rodman, P. S. (1998). The role of vocal tract filtering in identity cueing in rhesus monkey (*Macaca mulatta*) vocalizations. *Journal of the Acoustical Society of America*, **103**, 602–614.
Rendall, D., Owren, M. J. & Ryan, M. J. (2009). What do animal signals mean? *Animal Behaviour*, **78**, 233–240.
Ristau, C. (1998). Cognitive ethology: the minds of children and animals. In D. Cummins & C. Allen (eds.), *The Evolution of Mind*. New York: Oxford University Press, pp. 127–161.
Shannon, C. E. & Weaver, W. (1949). *The Mathematical Theory of Communication*. Urbana-Champaign, IL: University of Illinois Press.
Skyrms, B. (2010). *Signals. Evolution, Learning, and Information*. Oxford: Oxford University Press.
Snowdon, C. T. & Cleveland, J. (1980). Individual recognition of contact calls by pygmy marmosets. *Animal Behaviour*, **28**, 717–727.
Stampe, D. (1977). Toward a causal theory of linguistic representation. In P. A. French, T. E. Uehling Jr. & H. K. Wettstein, eds., *Midwest Studies in Philosophy*, Vol. 2. Minneapolis, MN: University of Minnesota Press.
Stegmann, U. E. (2009). A consumer-based teleosemantics for animal signals. *Philosophy of Science*, **76**, 864–875.
Sterelny, K. (2003). *Thought in a Hostile World: The Evolution of Cognition*. Oxford: Blackwell Publishing.
Tomasello, M. & Call, J. (1997). *Primate Cognition*. Oxford: Oxford University Press.
Tomasello, M. & Zuberbühler, K. (2002). Primate gestural and vocal communication. In M. Bekoff, C. Allen & G. Burghardt, eds., *The Cognitive Animal: Empirical and Theoretical Perspectives on Animal Cognition*. Cambridge, MA: MIT Press, pp. 293–299.
Tomasello, M., Call, J. & Hare, B. (2003). Chimpanzees understand psychological states – the question is which ones and to what extent? *Trends in Cognitive Science*, **7**, 153–156.
Waser, P. M. (1977). Individual recognition, intragroup cohesion and intergroup spacing: evidence from sound playback to forest monkeys. *Behaviour*, **60**, 28–74.
Wittgenstein, L. (1953). *Philosophical Investigations*. Oxford: Blackwell.
Zuberbühler, K., Cheney, D. L. & Seyfarth, R. M. (1999). Conceptual semantics in a non-human primate. *Journal of Comparative Psychology*, **113**, 33–42.

Commentaries

Terrence Deacon in *The Symbolic Species: The Coevolution of Language and the Brain*, p. 61 and 71, also used 'indicates', in this case to differentiate between words (and sentences), which have meaning, and human laughter, which he argues does not have meaning (he also uses the smoke example, p. 77). Laughter *indicates* something, e.g. about a person and context, but it has no meaning. Human laughter is apparently innate, like most animal signalling. Our curiosity was piqued to know if you view his use of indicate as the same as yours. If so, why do you feel we still need 'information'? Doesn't this concept elevate reference of signals to the symbolic level of reference, far beyond what animal communication is about?

Our perspective on animal signalling is consistent with Adams and Beighley's argument that it does not have linguistic properties. Nevertheless, some signals, like alarm calls, *appear* linguistic in human terms because they engender logically cohesive antipredator behaviour. We view this cohesiveness as characterising prey recognition of Gibsonian affordances – dynamic relations between agents and features of situations yielding specific effects (see Chemero, 2003) – such that vervet monkeys and California ground squirrels both perceive overhead threats as constrained (lowered) by bushes and shrubs that preclude raptors from attacking on the wing. Similarly, alarm calls to leopards engender in baboons and macaques immediate flight to trees and seeking refuge on thin branches that will not support the leopard's weight. How these species understand these constraining affordances of predator hunting ability and safe microhabitats is unclear, but despite innate recognition of some aerial and terrestrial predators, repeated experience in nature probably facilitates a species' understanding of these affordances.

Chemero, A. (2003). An outline of a theory of affordances. *Ecological Psychology*, **15**, 181–195.

Eugene S. Morton and Richard G. Coss

"Yes" to indication versus reference, but what's this 'information' again? Consistent with several other chapters in the volume, Adams and Beighley argue that the *information* concept should remain central in understanding animal communication. They nonetheless avoid any attempt to define or explain this problematic concept. On the one hand, we concur with the authors' argument that the *indication* function of non-human signalling is fundamentally different from the falsifiable *reference* value of human language. On the other hand, Adams and Beighley fail to address the deeper issue that information

is not a scientifically useful construct if understood only as folk-intuition and metaphor.

Michael J. Owren and Drew Rendall

This chapter contends that information is "more than mere correlation" between signals and the states or contexts of signallers and receivers, because "there is correlation about some fact and . . . that fact does generate a message". As I emphasise in my chapter, deciding what such facts might be (perhaps states of mind) requires empathy with the signaller and receiver. Furthermore, Adams and Beighley argue that encoding and decoding require voluntary participation of signaller and receiver, not just "natural regularity". As my chapter emphasises, this attribution of volition (intention), even to other humans, also requires empathy. Indeed how much of human communication even appears to involve "voluntary control of the agent" over decoding or encoding? Most of us no doubt learn a language because it works for us, not because we voluntarily choose a code. As my chapter explains, I maintain a necessary ignorance on matters that require empathy with others.

R. Haven Wiley

Response

To **Morton and Coss**: Yes. Deacon's use of indication is similar to ours, but our use derives from Dretske and Stampe, not Deacon. No, this does not mean the concept of information is not useful. Information theory is about indication and more and the concept of information connects the two (connects indication to the more mathematical treatment of measurements of amounts of information). And no, indication alone does not yield reference in a symbolic sense.

To **Owren and Rendall**: We define by example the portion of the concept of information that we need: indication. There is nothing more to explain about indication as an information relation. You admit that indication is a scientifically useful concept and it is connected to the mathematical treatment of information. What more could one want?

To **Wiley**: When we say "voluntary" we don't say "conscious". When children over-generalise "goed" as the past tense of "go", it is voluntary even if they are not conscious (ignorant) of the rule they over-generalise. As for whether turning signals into symbols requires empathy, this surely is not the case for concepts. One need not empathise to learn what a dog is. To learn a public language, one does need to understand intentions of others, but then we stress that in our chapter. If that is what Wiley means by empathy, then we are on the same page.

Fred Adams and Steven M. Beighley

18

Information, influence and inference in language evolution

THOMAS C. SCOTT-PHILLIPS AND SIMON KIRBY

18.1 Introduction

The various chapters that appear in this volume reflect a range of perspectives on a question of contemporary and interdisciplinary debate: the nature of communication. There are several reasons (surveyed elsewhere in this volume) why this issue has arisen at the present time. One of these is the growing research interest in the origins and evolution of human language, which has highlighted the need for a general framework and vocabulary with which to describe communication, since the development of such a framework would assist cross-disciplinary discussion of the transition(s) from non-human primate communication to language (Rendall *et al.*, 2009). In addition, several protagonists in the current discussion have argued that comparisons to language have, depending on your perspective, either hindered or enabled research on animal communication (e.g. Rendall Owren & Ryan, 2009; Seyfarth *et al.*, 2010). Despite these motivations, the discussion has mostly taken place in the animal communication literature, and the contributors to it have mostly been experts in that same field. Consequently, debate can be advanced by a detailed discussion of how linguistics, and the study of language origins in particular, conceives of communication. This chapter will address these needs.

First, we will briefly chart the development of language evolution research, with a particular focus on how the discipline has tended to conceive of communication (Section 18.2). We then describe a distinction, commonly made in pragmatics (the branch of linguistics that deals with language use in context), between two different approaches to communication (Section 18.3), and discuss

Animal Communication Theory: Information and Influence, ed. Ulrich Stegmann. Published by Cambridge University Press.

the implications of this distinction for language evolution (Section 18.4). We will explain why consideration of language highlights the need for discussion about the nature of communication to develop an account that is sufficiently general to describe a communication system that is heavily context-dependent. We then provide a set of definitions that are able to do this, and that hence provide the foundation for a general account of communication (Section 18.5). Our overall objectives are thus to present a unified, consilient account of communication, and to discuss the implications of that account both for language evolution research, and for the more general issues that have motivated the present volume.

18.2 Communication in language evolution research

Those unfamiliar with recent research into the evolution of language are often struck with an obvious question: how is it even possible to study the origins of a behavioural trait that is apparently unique to one species and leaves no direct fossil remains? In other words, where are the data for those interested in language evolution going to come from, and what are the appropriate methodologies that should be employed? Perhaps because for a long time there were no clear answers to these questions, the field has sometimes been viewed as one that leads to unconstrained speculation, giving rise to an abundance of theories with little other than personal taste to help choose between them.

It was in this context that the use of computer simulations was pioneered in the late 1980s (in particular Hurford, 1989, 1991), as a way to tackle the problems of unconstrained speculation. Although we cannot study real evolving populations of communicating hominids, we can create populations in computer-simulated environments, and use these as a test-bed for evaluating different hypotheses about the mechanisms, selection pressures and so on implicated in the origins of language. This general methodology proved highly influential through the 1990s and 2000s, when computational modelling became an established methodology for language evolution, with a large proportion of papers in the regular international conferences and edited collections using such simulations (e.g. Briscoe, 2002; Cangelosi & Parisi, 2002). This foundational research often conceived of communication in a very idealised way, typically for practical, implementational reasons – but these assumptions shaped much of the subsequent thinking in the wider field of language evolution. Because of this, it is worth going into some of the detail of a typical early model in order to see how such models bear on the topic of this volume (for more thorough reviews of the early modelling literature, see Kirby, 2002; Steels, 2003).

In a typical simulation, there would be a set of independent simulated 'agents' implemented using very simple algorithms. The interesting behaviour of these models arose from the consequences of interactions between these agents. For example, the agents might engage in a communication task, taking turns as a producer of a signal and a receiver of a signal. The agents might tackle this task in a range of different ways, each particular response arising either because the agents learned their behaviour from each other or because it was encoded for each as a set of idealised 'genes' in the specification of the agents. Populations of the agents might be static or change over time, and could be used to examine hypotheses about the cultural and biological evolution of communication systems.

The very first simulation models of language evolution focused principally on the biological evolution of signalling systems (e.g. Werner & Dyer, 1992; MacLennan & Burghardt, 1993; Ackley & Littman, 1994). Models that addressed other concerns, such as the social transmission of language through learning, and the consequent cultural evolution of linguistic systems, came later (e.g. Batali, 1998; Kirby, 2001; K. Smith, 2004; Brighton, Smith & Kirby, 2005). In one of these early models, agents are born with a set of genes that specify directly what their behaviour is, and this behaviour does not change throughout their lives (Oliphant, 1996). Agents engage in a communicative task with each other, and their success at this task determines their fitness. In other words, better communicating agents were more likely to pass on their genes to future generations of agents. The particular concern of this piece of research is the way in which fitness could be calculated in these models, and the details of the communication task are not a central concern. Accordingly, a set of simplifying idealisations about how communication works is made for the purposes of modelling. At each time-step of the simulation, one of the agents is prompted to produce a signal for a particular meaning. To do so, it consults a table determining its transmission behaviour, which is specified directly by the agent's genes. This signal is then transferred to another agent, which consults a corresponding table determining reception behaviour. This results in a response to the signal received. If this response is appropriate then communication is deemed to be successful; see Figure 18.1.

In this work, signals and meanings are, respectively, referred to as *observable behaviours* and *states of the world/appropriate responses* (Oliphant, 1997, pp. 15–16), yet in the model there is none of the richness that this might imply. Signals and meanings are simply members chosen from a finite set. Success relies on signaller and receiver having coordinated mappings from meanings to signals, and signals to meanings. This work was influential in the modelling community (as were others like it) in that it set the scene for much future computational

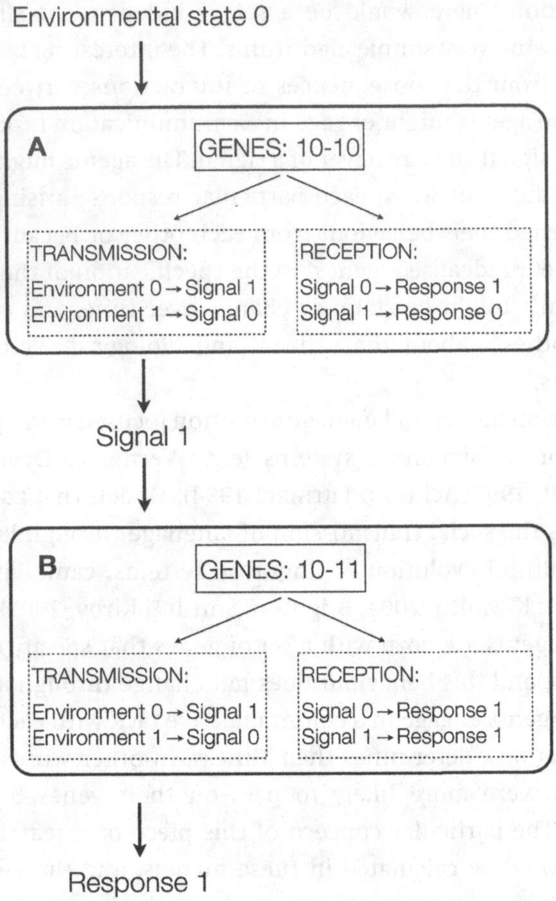

Figure 18.1 A sketch of Oliphant's (1996) model of an innate signalling system. Individuals' communicative behaviour is divided into transmission and reception. Transmission relates distinct states of the environment to signals, whereas reception relates signals to particular responses. (In the literature more broadly, the environmental states and responses are typically both glossed as 'meanings'; we follow this convention in the main text.) These relationships are determined by a string of heritable genes, the first half of which give the transmission behaviour, and the second half of which give the reception behaviour. There are two components to each of these: the first figure describes the output given an input of 0; the second describes the output given an input of 1. In this example, agent A signals to agent B. The environmental state is 0, so agent A signals 1 (the first part of the signalling genes '1 0'). Agent B then receives this input, and so produces response 1 (the second part of the signalling genes '1 1').

work on language evolution. It provided a backdrop which focused on the evolution of mappings between sets of possible signals and possible meanings in which communication was about individuals encoding meanings as transmittable signals and others decoding those signals into meanings.

Later work loosened various parameters of these models. In particular, models were built that added contexts in which to ground symbols, showing how agents can converge upon stable meaning–signal associations using techniques such as cross-situational learning (disambiguation across multiple contexts) and even that communication can be successful when agents do not represent meanings in the same way as one another (e.g. Steels, 1999; Vogt, 2002; Smith, 2005). Although such research can be described as inferential (Smith, 2005) because meanings are not given directly, the basic paradigm remained one in which producers are prompted to transmit signals for particular meanings, which receivers then decode.

More recently, language evolution has seen a rapid growth of experimental approaches, much of it informed by the previous modelling work (Scott-Phillips & Kirby, 2010). In particular, the general framing of communication in terms of a system that encodes and then transmits signals with fixed 'meanings' has persisted in much (but not all) of this experimental work. For example, in one study participants learn to associate strings of syllables (signals) with coloured shapes (meanings). They then go on to produce strings for particular shapes that they are prompted with. The resulting language collated from one participant's output is used to train the next participant in the laboratory. In this way, cultural evolution of language is modelled in a way that is entirely analogous to the computational simulations (Kirby, Cornish & Smith, 2008). The analysis of the results is even conducted in the same fashion, treating the data as a matrix of signal–meaning associations. This way of thinking about communication is sometimes called the *code model*, because it assumes that communication consists of the encoding of a message into a signal, which is then transmitted along some channel, to be decoded (subsection 18.3.1 below).

18.3 Two models of communication

18.3.1 *The code model*

The code model is an idealisation of communication in which signal–meaning mappings are the primary representation: the signaller 'looks up' the correct signal to use for a given meaning and produces it, and the receiver then takes that signal and 'looks up' the associated meaning in order to interpret it. Any approach that models communication in this way is using the code model, even if the representations of meanings may be different in signaller and receiver. As far as we are aware, the term *code model* was coined by Dan Sperber and Deirdre Wilson in *Relevance: Communication and Cognition* (1986), in an effort to distinguish it from the *ostensive-inferential model* that they wished to promote, and which we discuss below. But the code model itself has a much longer, if often unrecognised history, particularly in theoretical linguistics (Blackburn, 2007). Although there is no definitive definition of the code model, perhaps because its use often goes unrecognised, the foundational assumption is that communication consists of the encoding of a message into a signal, which is then transmitted along some channel, to be decoded. The communication system is the set of mappings (i.e. codes) between messages and forms – and these codes exist independently of any given user. When applied to language, this way of thinking about communication leads to the belief that languages are codes that define a correspondence between sound and meaning.

A historical analysis suggests that the code model combines at least two metaphors of how communication works (Blackburn, 2007). The first is the conduit metaphor, in which signals are packaged up and sent along some channel, to be unwrapped at the other end (Reddy, 1979; see Figure 18.2A). This view pervades our everyday language about communication (e.g. "Send me your ideas"; "Get your message across"), and it has been hugely influential in the animal signalling literature, where many textbooks define communication in this way (see Rendall *et al.*, 2009 for a critical review).

The second metaphor is the telecommunications metaphor. It has its roots in Claude Shannon's information theory (Shannon, 1948; see Figure 18.2B). This was designed to address a particular set of electrical engineering and telecommunication problems, in particular how to transmit digital strings along noisy channels. The metaphor is to treat language as if it operates in the same probabilistic, context-independent way. Yet there is no attempt in Shannon's work to relate the structure or semantic aspects of any underlying message to the real world (Blackburn, 2007), and Shannon himself is explicit about this: "these semantic aspects of communication are irrelevant to the engineering problem [that this work is concerned with]" (Shannon, 1948, p. 5).

Despite its influence, the code model is plainly an insufficient characterisation of linguistic communication. Much of what is meant is not encoded in what is said (that is, the utterance *underdetermines* the speaker's meaning). In sarcasm, for example, the 'encoded', literal meaning of an utterance is the opposite of the speaker's intended meaning. More generally, linguistic communication often leaves much implied, and both speakers and hearers lean heavily upon context to ensure that communication is achieved successfully (Grice, 1975; Sperber & Wilson, 1986; Carston, 2002; Atlas, 2005). For example, if Ann asks John, "Where's Bill?", and John replies, "There's a yellow VW outside Sue's

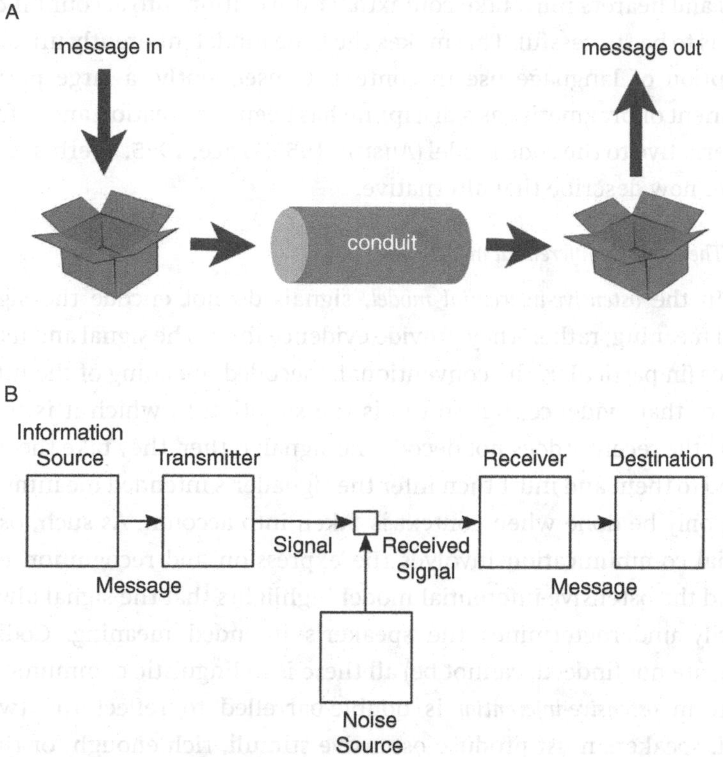

Figure 18.2 Two metaphors for communication. **A**, The **conduit metaphor**, in which information is packaged up and sent along a channel, from signaller to received. **B**, The **telecommunications metaphor**, in which communication is conceived of as the transmission of digital strings along noisy channels (from Shannon, 1948). While both approaches are intuitively appealing, it is important to keep in mind that they are metaphorical, and should not be taken as a complete description of what is involved in communication.

house", then John has not explicitly stated that he thinks (or at least has reason to believe) that Bill is inside Sue's house; this is only implied (example from Levinson, 1983). Furthermore, important contextual information is required if Ann is to comprehend John's utterance appropriately. Specifically, Ann must know that Bill drives a yellow Volkswagen, and perhaps that Bill knows Sue, and hence it is plausible that he is visiting her house. If Sue does not know this or, worse, believes otherwise, then it becomes difficult for her to make sense of Bill's utterance. The study of how such contextual factors affect meaning is called pragmatics.

This underdeterminacy is ubiquitous: there is *always* a distinction to be made between what a speaker says and what they mean (Carston, 2002). As such, both speakers and hearers must take contextual information into account if communication is to be successful. This makes the code model inherently unsuitable as a description of language use in context. Consequently, a large part of the development of pragmatics as a discipline has been the creation and refinement of an alternative to the code model (Austin, 1955; Grice, 1975; Sperber & Wilson, 1986). We now describe that alternative.

18.3.2 *The ostensive-inferential model*

In the *ostensive-inferential model*, signals do not encode the signaller's intended meaning; rather, they provide evidence for it. The signal and its various properties (in particular, the conventional, 'decoded' meaning of the utterance) are part of that evidence, but so too is the situation in which it is produced. Similarly, the receiver does not decode the signal; rather, they take the evidence presented to them and must then infer the signaller's intended meaning – a task that can only be done when context is taken into account. As such, ostensive-inferential communication involves the expression and recognition of intentions, and the ostensive-inferential model highlights that the signal always and necessarily underdetermines the speaker's intended meaning. Coding and decoding are not (indeed, cannot be) all there is to linguistic communication.

The term *ostensive-inferential* is double-barrelled to reflect the two tasks involved: speakers must produce ostensive stimuli, rich enough for their purposes, and listeners must draw context-dependent inferences from those stimuli (Sperber & Wilson, 1986). Note that although the model is typically presented in terms of vocal linguistic communication (with 'signaller' and 'receiver' replaced by 'speaker' and 'listener'), that need not be the case; the model applies to any forms of ostensive communication, vocal, linguistic or otherwise. A classic example of non-vocal, non-linguistic yet ostensive behaviour is pointing (see e.g. Tomasello, 2008).

Because it emphasises the fact that both parties are doing some work in this process, the ostensive-inferential model contrasts with the conduit metaphor, in which listeners are characterised in a more passive way, as recipients of pre-packaged pieces of information. Nevertheless, ostensive-inferential is a wordy term, and so *ostensive communication* or *inferential communication* are sometimes used as shorthand. One question that follows from this discussion is how these different ways of thinking about communication (the code model and the ostensive-inferential model) inform the current debates about the nature of animal communication. In Section 18.5 we will discuss how the ostensive model relates to a view of communication predicated on influence. Before then, we wish to highlight the importance of ostension and other pragmatic factors for the study of language evolution itself.

18.4 The relevance of pragmatics for the study of language origins

Although pragmatics is an active branch of linguistics, and indeed forms part of any typical undergraduate curriculum, there are many other areas of core linguistics, such as syntax, phonology and so on, that can and do operate largely without consideration for the role of ostension, inference and other pragmatic concerns. Moreover, it would not be inaccurate to say that for many linguists pragmatics falls at the periphery of the discipline. However, although it may not be part of the core of linguistics, pragmatic factors are of critical importance for the study of language origins (Hurford, 2007; Tomasello, 2008). Language is the archetypal example of ostensive communication, and hence any comprehensive explanation of the origins of language must, in our view, account for why this form of communication has apparently emerged in only one species. We consider this to be a central question for current language evolution research (Scott-Phillips & Kirby, 2010).

To this end, comparative research has begun to identify the similarities and differences between the social cognition of humans and other primates (Tomasello *et al.*, 2005), and has suggested some of the selection pressures that may explain these patterns (Humphrey, 1976; Byrne & Whiten, 1989; Dunbar, 1998; Dunbar & Schultz, 2007). Thus one of the present challenges is to focus on the social cognition of ostensive-inferential communication in particular, in order to make this account more precise. What are the specific cognitive mechanisms involved, and how did they evolve? Recognition of the importance of this question is reflected in recent trends in the comparative literature, which has seen a move towards studies focused on the psychological and cognitive mechanisms involved in non-human primate communication, rather than their surface form (e.g. Cartmill & Byrne, 2010).

Indeed, one of the main criticisms made of the informational approach is that it borrows constructs from language and attempts to shoehorn them into descriptions of animal communication (Rendall *et al.*, 2009; Owren *et al.*, 2010). For example, the development of the notion of *functional reference* can be seen as a way to bring the idea of reference, developed in the study of human communication, into animal (and particularly non-human primate) communication. In this light, it is worthwhile to point out that when we consider the role of pragmatics, it becomes clear that the conduit metaphor is an insufficient characterisation of even human communication, where, as discussed above, reference and other factors that contribute to literal meaning are only part of the story. Context-dependent factors are also critical. This is why the trend towards investigation of the underlying cognitive mechanisms required for ostensive communication is to be welcomed. The picture that appears to be emerging is that non-human primates possess and use some but not all of these mechanisms (Hurford, 2007). For example, evidence of intentionality (widely defined as behaviour that is directed towards another, with the apparent objective of obtaining a goal, and which is employed flexibly, depending on the audience response) has been observed in the communication of several non-human primate species, particularly in the gestural modality (e.g. Pika, 2008; Tomasello, 2008; Cartmill & Byrne, 2010; Holbaiter & Byrne, 2011).

Such results present a significant theoretical challenge. Specifically, they suggest that ostension and inference are not all-or-nothing phenomena. The characterisation of human communication as ostensive and non-human communication as not ostensive may be too simple. Rather, it seems that there are shades of grey here; there may be forms of communication that are 'somewhat' ostensive and inferential. Therefore an important research problem for language evolution (and indeed for pragmatics) is to develop a theoretical framework with which to characterise such systems, in order to compare them against one another. This is a highly interdisciplinary problem. One way in which it might be approached is in the context of a more general account of what communication is, at its most basic level.

18.5 A general framework for communication?

The code model has been a dominant framework not only for the study of language and linguistics, but also for studies of animal communication (Rendall *et al.*, 2009; Owren *et al.*, 2010). The strengths and weaknesses of this approach have been recently debated (Rendall *et al.*, 2009; Seyfarth *et al.*, 2010), and are a central concern of the present volume. What the preceding discussion highlights is that regardless of its utility for the study of animal communication, the code model is certainly an insufficient description of human ostensive communication, including language, and therefore cannot be sufficient to describe communication in the most general sense. This section presents an alternative approach, one predicated on functionality, that is able to describe both coded and ostensive communication. The implications and applications of this framework are then discussed.

18.5.1 Definitions

We adopt functional definitions of communication and associated terms. We are inspired by definitions developed in evolutionary biology (Maynard Smith & Harper, 2003; Scott-Phillips, 2008), but here we express them in more general terms, so that they can be applied whether we are concerned with ultimate or proximate sources of design. A signal is any behaviour that satisfies the following three conditions: (i) it causes a reaction in another organism; (ii) its function is to cause the reaction; and (iii) the reaction's function is to be caused by the action. If these conditions are all satisfied, then the action is a signal; the reaction is a response; and the overall interaction is communicative. If only conditions (i) and (ii) are satisfied, the action is coercive; and if only conditions (i) and (iii) are satisfied, the action is a cue. (Interestingly, a similar view, expressed in terms of manipulation and exploitation rather than actions and reactions, was developed by some of the pioneers responsible for the early computational models of the evolution of communication and language (e.g. di Paolo, 1997; Oliphant, 1997). However, a detailed discussion of the way in which different definitions of communication have been used in the literature is beyond the scope of this chapter.)

If, for example, an individual deliberately pushes a colleague from her chair, and she then falls to the floor, then this satisfies criteria (i) (the push caused the colleague to fall) and (ii) (the fall was the intended outcome of the push). Criterion (iii) is not satisfied, however, and the interaction is *coercive*. If the pusher's boss, unbeknownst to the pusher, observes the incident, and subsequently acts on it (by punishing the pusher, for example), then that interaction between the pusher and the observer is a *cue*: it satisfies criteria (i) (the push caused the boss to punish the pusher) and (iii) (the function of that punishment was to take account of what had been seen), but not (ii) (since the pusher did not intend the boss to see the incident). Now suppose that there is one further colleague, and that the pusher had actually intended this second observer to see the incident, perhaps as part of a practical joke. Then criterion (ii) is satisfied, and the push is a *signal* to this colleague. Note that these examples also illustrate how the same event can involve several different interactions, each with a different communicative status (see Figure 18.3).

In these examples, the required functionality comes from the intentions of the individuals involved. However, we have in mind a more general notion of functionality (see Millikan, 1984). Specifically, a trait or behaviour's function is the task that it performs that at least in part explains why it is reproduced from one generation to the next (Millikan, 1984). For example, hearts make noise, contribute to body weight and pump blood, amongst other things. Yet it is only the last of these that is their function, since it is their capacity to pump blood, and the contribution this makes to survival, that explains why hearts are reproduced from one generation to the next. This notion of functionality applies to any adaptive system, including (amongst others) human cognition, and natural selection, whose dynamics produce traits and behaviours whose function is to maximise an organism's inclusive fitness (Grafen, 2002, 2006). Hence these definitions work across multiple domains in the sense that they accurately

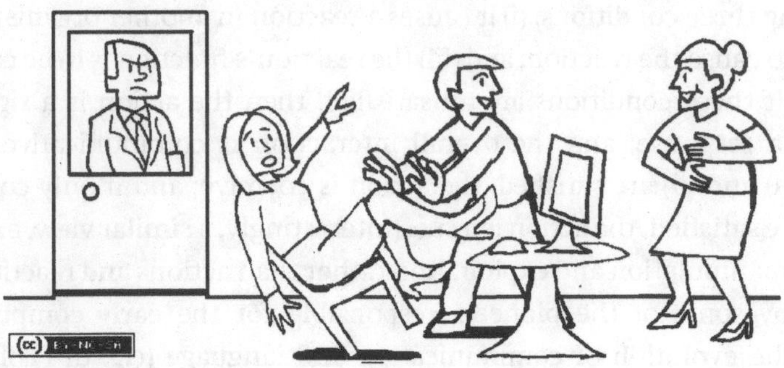

Figure 18.3 Functional definitions of communication.
This illustration shows one man (in the centre of the image) in three different interactions, each of which is of a different type *vis-à-vis* communication. In one, he is pushing a colleague from her chair. This is **coercion**. In another, he is seen pushing his colleague by a second colleague (on the right of the image), and he intended for this to be the case. This is **communication**; the push is a signal, and the laugh of his colleague is a response. In a third interaction, his boss (on the left of the image) has also seen him pushing his colleague, but this was not the man's intention; indeed, he does not know that his boss has seen him. The pushing is a **cue** for the boss; it guides the boss's future action, but this was not the function of the push. See main text for further discussion.

capture various *prima facie* cases of communication and non-communication, whether these cases occur in human communication (as in Figure 18.3, above), animal communication (see Maynard Smith & Harper, 2003; Scott-Phillips, 2008 for discussion and examples of how this definition applies to animal communication) or elsewhere (e.g. computer-to-computer communication, where the source of the functionality is the software engineer that designed the program). The result is a set of definitions that make no commitments regarding the mechanisms involved in any particular instance of communication, and as such allow for discussion of communication in general terms.

18.5.2 *Communication is a matter of effects*

Can the above definitions be used to inform the present debates about how best to conceptualise communication? Our definitions, which are centred on the effects that signals have upon receivers, plainly align with the view that communication should be seen, at the most basic level, as a matter of influence (Dawkins & Krebs, 1978; Rendall, *et al.*, 2009). However, this does not mean that information should be rejected from the study of communication (linguistic or otherwise). On the contrary, it is possible to integrate information into our approach (Carazo & Font, 2010). In fact, we suspect (but do not know) the following: that once the functionally interdependent relationship between signal and response described above (subsection 18.5.1) is established, then a necessary corollary will be a correlation between some properties of the signal and some properties of the world (e.g. there is a negative correlation between a deer's size and the formant dispersion of its roar; Fitch & Reby, 2001). If this is correct, then it will be possible to identify something we may wish to term information (others have termed this *functional information*; Carazo & Font, 2010).

Our point is only that functional effects are what lie at the heart of communication, by which we mean: it may be possible to observe and/or quantify information transfer, but we can only do this in a post-hoc way, after we have specified what the effects of a signal are (Scott-Phillips, 2008). Indeed, this is a general point about communication, be it animal communication or human language. First and foremost, signals *do* things. Only once we know what they do can we identify information, conventional meaning and other associated phenomena – since these things simply do not exist until there is functional symbiosis between signals and responses. Effects are methodologically prior.

We will not labour this point, since it has been discussed at length previously, in a range of different contexts (di Paolo, 1997; Blackburn, 2007; Scott-Phillips, 2008; Rendall, *et al.*, 2009), and is discussed further elsewhere in this volume. What we do wish to emphasise is that our insistence that effects are a general, fundamental property of communication aligns with the point made by the discipline of pragmatics that linguistic communication is about more than conventional meaning. Utterances are behaviours that cause others to do things; conventional meanings are simply part of the story of how these effects are achieved (Origgi & Sperber, 2000; Scott-Phillips, 2010a). Indeed, one of the founding texts of pragmatics is entitled *How To Do Things With Words*, with the emphasis very much on the *do* (Austin, 1955). Moreover, there have been recent calls in the pragmatics literature for *all* types of linguistic utterances to be reconceptualised as acts of social influence (Reich, 2010). One of the arguments presented in favour of this view is that it is particularly compatible with evolutionary theory, and hence that it allows for comparison with non-human communication. This emphasis within pragmatics on the social, interactive aspect of linguistic utterances in turn aligns with the ostensive-inferential model of communication, in which utterances have effects only by virtue of the inferences they cause others to make.

18.5.3 *Applications and implications*

In this subsection we highlight three ways in which the functional approach to communication outlined above has already provided insights into various questions and topics about communication, and speculate about how it may do so in the future.

First, this approach has allowed microbiologists to investigate the communicative nature of bacterial social behaviour (Diggle *et al.*, 2007). Many bacterial cells use a process known as quorum sensing (QS), in which individual cells produce small diffusible molecules, and once the concentration of these molecules reaches a threshold level they bind to their cognate receptors, causing changes in the expression of QS-dependent genes. This allows the population of cells to behave in a coordinated way. The functional approach described above has allowed microbiologists to determine when behaviour associated with QS should be considered communication, and when it should be considered a cue, or coercive. These differences matter, because they make different predictions about how bacterial cells should behave. In addition to this direct application to the study of bacterial social behaviour, the functional approach also allows evolutionary biologists to integrate two disparate literatures: one on the evolution of animal signals, the other on the social behaviour of microbes (Diggle *et al.*, 2007).

Second, a functional account brings the question of how communication systems emerge into focus. Signals and responses depend upon one another to explain their existence, and this interdependence produces a chicken-and-egg problem: how does such mutual dependency emerge in the first place? A recent mathematical model that explicitly adopts the functional approach describes the different ways in which this problem can be overcome, and explains their relative frequency in nature (Scott-Phillips *et al.*, 2012). As such, the functional view has been shown to provide a comprehensive explanation of the ways in which communication systems can emerge.

Third, the functional approach has been used to choose between different theoretical approaches to pragmatics itself. Like any discipline, there are several different theoretical proposals around the central questions – in this case, how listeners are able to interpret utterances in context (and how speakers are able to construct context-appropriate utterances) – and these accounts compete with one another to varying degrees (e.g. Horn, 1984; Sperber & Wilson, 1986; Levinson, 2000; Bara, 2010). One criterion that we can use to choose between them is compatibility with evolutionary theory, and the functional approach has been used to pursue such a project (Scott-Phillips, 2010b).

Finally, we wish to return to one of the major desiderata for future research identified above: the development of a theoretical framework for pragmatics that is richer than a simple ostensive/not-ostensive dichotomy. The reasons why this is desirable were discussed in Section 18.4: although it is still at an early stage, the evidence from the comparative literature on cognition and pragmatics suggests that some non-human primates possess at least some of the cognitive foundations of ostensive communication. Thus if we wish to understand how ostensive communication evolved, we need a theoretical framework and a vocabulary with which to discuss different possible grades of pragmatic competence. We believe that the functional approach described here is well suited to this task, because it is expressed in general terms, and hence makes no particular commitments regarding the mechanisms involved in communication. This means that researchers in this area are able to develop such frameworks unencumbered by terminology that is weighted towards one or another conclusion. In contrast, the conduit metaphor, and other related approaches to communication, can, by virtue of the language they adopt, lead researchers to think about animal communication in terms of representations and other aspects of human communication when the empirical data do not necessarily warrant this (Rendall *et al.*, 2009).

18.6 Concluding remarks

We started this chapter by surveying the history of computational thinking about the evolution of language. Primarily as an approach to simplifying the problem of modelling the complex adaptive systems underpinning language emergence, modellers naturally gravitated to a form of the code model to implement communication among simulated agents. Given the central role that simulations played in the development of evolutionary linguistics, it is not unreasonable to say that the information-centric code model is taken as a default idealisation by many within the field, extending beyond modelling work and into experimental approaches. Whilst we believe that much important progress has been made with this approach, we hope to have demonstrated that it is plainly incomplete, and that there is much to be gained from thinking not merely about *information* but also *influence* and *inference* in the evolution of language. It is likely that future breakthroughs in the field will come when the theoretical work on ostension and inference in language evolution inform modelling and experimental frameworks. This aligns with arguments that at the most basic level, communication is fundamentally a matter of influence, in which signals and responses are functionally symbiotic. This does not mean that we should seek to remove all talk of information – but neither should we confuse information transfer with a complete description of what communication is about.

Acknowledgements

T.S.P. acknowledges financial support from the Leverhulme Trust.

References

Ackley, D. H. & Littman, M. L. (1994). Altruism in the evolution of communication. In R. Brooks & P. Maes, eds., *Artificial Life IV*. Cambridge, MA: MIT Press, pp. 40–48.

Atlas, J. D. (2005). *Logic, Meaning and Conversation: Semantic Underdeterminacy*. Oxford: Oxford University Press.

Austin, J. L. (1955). *How to Do Things With Words*. Oxford: Oxford University Press.

Bara, B. (2010). *Cognitive Pragmatics: The Mental Processes of Communication*. Cambridge, MA: MIT Press.

Batali, J. (1998). Computational simulations of the emergence of grammar. In J. R. Hurford M. Studdert-Kennedy & Knight, C., eds., *Approaches to the Evolution of Language: Social and Cognitive Bases*. Cambridge: Cambridge University Press, pp. 405–426.

Blackburn, P. (2007). *The Code Model of Language: A Powerful Metaphor in Linguistic Metatheory*. SIL International e-books.

Brighton, H., Smith, K. & Kirby, S. (2005). Language as an evolutionary system. *Physics of Life Reviews*, **2**, 177–226.

Briscoe, E. J. (2002). *Linguistic Evolution Through Language Acquisition: Formal and Computational Models*. Cambridge: Cambridge University Press.

Byrne, R. W. & Whiten, A. (1989). *Machiavellian Intelligence: Social Expertise and the Evolution of Intellect in Monkeys, Apes and Humans*. Oxford: Clarendon Press.

Cangelosi, A. & Parisi, D. (2002). *Simulating the Evolution of Language*. London: Springer Verlag.

Carazo, P. & Font, E. (2010). Putting information back into biological communication. *Journal of Evolutionary Biology*, **23**, 661–669.

Carston, R. (2002). *Thoughts and Utterances: The Pragmatics of Explicit Communication*. Oxford: Blackwell.

Cartmill, E. A. & Byrne, R. W. (2010). Semantics of primate gestures: intentional meanings of orangutan gestures. *Animal Cognition*, **13**, 793–804.

Dawkins, R. & Krebs, J. R. (1978). Animal signals: information or manipulation? In J. R. Krebs & N. B. Davies, eds., *Behavioural Ecology*, 1st edn. Oxford: Blackwell, pp. 282–309.

di Paolo, E. A. (1997). An investigation into the evolution of communication. *Adaptive Behavior*, **6**, 285–324.

Diggle, S. P., Gardner, A., West, S. A. & Griffin, A. S. (2007). Evolutionary theory of bacterial quorum sensing: when is a signal not a signal? *Philosophical Transactions of the Royal Society of London Series B*, **362**, 1241–1249.

Dunbar, R. I. M. (1998). The social brain hypothesis. *Evolutionary Anthropology*, **6**, 178–190.

Dunbar, R. I. M. & Schultz, S. (2007). Evolution in the social brain. *Science*, **317**, 1344–1347.

Fitch, W. T. & Reby, D. (2001). The descended larynx is not uniquely human. *Proceedings of the Royal Society of London B*, **268**, 1669–1675.

Grafen, A. (2002). A first formal link between the Price equation and an optimization program. *Journal of Theoretical Biology*, **217**, 75–91.

Grafen, A. (2006). Optimisation of inclusive fitness. *Journal of Evolutionary Biology*, **238**, 541–563.

Grice, H. P. (1975). Logic and conversation. In P. Cole & J. Morgan, eds., *Syntax & Semantics III: Speech Acts*. New York: Academic Press, pp. 41–58.

Holbaiter, C. & Byrne, R. W. (2011). The gestural repertoire of the wild chimpanzee. *Animal Cognition*, **14**, 745–767.

Horn, L. R. (1984). Towards a new taxonomy for pragmatic inference: Q-based and R-based implicature. In D. Schiffrin, ed., *Meaning, Form, and Its Use in Context: Linguistic Applications*. Washington, DC: Georgetown University Press, pp. 11–42.

Humphrey, N. (1976). The social function of the intellect. In P. Bateson & R. Hinde, eds., *Growing Points in Ethology*. Cambridge: Cambridge University Press, pp. 303–317.

Hurford, J. R. (1989). Biological evolution of the Saussurean sign as a component of the language acquisition device. *Lingua*, **77**, 187–222.

Hurford, J. R. (1991). The evolution of the critical period for language acquisition. *Cognition*, **40**, 159–201.

Hurford, J. R. (2007). *Origins of Meaning*. Oxford: Oxford University Press.

Kirby, S. (2001). Spontaneous evolution of linguistic structure: an iterated learning model of the emergence of regularity and irregularity. *IEEE Transactions on Evolutionary Computation*, **5**, 102–110.

Kirby, S. (2002). Natural language from artificial life. *Artificial Life*, **8**, 185–215.

Kirby, S., Cornish, H. & Smith, K. (2008). Cumulative cultural evolution in the laboratory: an experimental approach to the origins of structure in human language. *Proceedings of the National Academy of Sciences USA*, **105**, 10681–10686.

Levinson, S. C. (1983). *Pragmatics*. Cambridge: Cambridge University Press.

Levinson, S. C. (2000). *Presumptive Meanings*. London: Longman.

MacLennan, B. & Burghardt, G. M. (1993). Synthetic ethology and the evolution of cooperative communication. *Adaptive Behavior*, **2**, 161–187.

Maynard Smith, J. & Harper, D. G. C. (2003). *Animal Signals*. Oxford: Oxford University Press.

Millikan, R. G. (1984). *Language, Thought and Other Biological Categories*. Cambridge, MA: MIT Press.

Oliphant, M. (1996). The dilemma of Saussurean communication. *Biosystems*, **37**, 31–38.

Oliphant, M. (1997). Formal approaches to innate and learned communication: laying the foundation for language. Unpublished PhD thesis, Department of Cognitive Science, University of California, San Diego.

Origgi, G. & Sperber, D. (2000). Evolution, communication, and the proper function of language. In P. Carruthers & A. Chamberlain, eds., *Evolution and the Human Mind: Language, Modularity and Social Cognition*. Cambridge: Cambridge University Press, pp. 140–169.

Owren, M. J., Rendall, D. & Ryan, M. J. (2010). Redefining animal signalling: influence versus information in communication. *Biology and Philosophy*, **25**, 755–780.

Pika, S. (2008). Gestures of apes and pre-linguistic human children: similar or different? *First Language*, **28**, 116–140.

Reddy, M. J. (1979). The conduit metaphor: a case of frame conflict in our language about language. In A. Ortony, ed., *Metaphor and Thought*. Cambridge: Cambridge University Press, pp. 284–324.

Reich, W. (2010). The cooperative nature of communicative acts. *Journal of Pragmatics*, **43**, 1349–1365.

Rendall, D., Owren, M. J. & Ryan, M. J. (2009). What do animal signals mean? *Animal Behaviour*, **78**, 233–240.

Scott-Phillips, T. C. (2008). Defining biological communication. *Journal of Evolutionary Biology*, **21**, 387–395.

Scott-Phillips, T. C. (2010a). Animal communication: insights from linguistic pragmatics. *Animal Behaviour*, **79**, e1–e4.

Scott-Phillips, T. C. (2010b). The evolution of relevance. *Cognitive Science*, **34**, 583–601.

Scott-Phillips, T. C. & Kirby, S. (2010). Language evolution in the laboratory. *Trends in Cognitive Sciences*, **14**, 411–417.

Scott-Phillips, T. C., Blythe, R. A., Gardner, A. & West, S. A. (2012). How do communication systems emerge? *Proceedings of the Royal Society of London Series B*, **279**, 1943–1949.

Seyfarth, R. M., Cheney, D. L., Bergman, T. *et al.* (2010). The central importance of information in studies of animal communication. *Animal Behaviour*, **80**, 3–8.

Shannon, C. E. (1948). A mathematical theory of communication. *Bell Systems Technical Journal*, **27**, 379–423.

Smith, A. D. M. (2005). The inferential transmission of language. *Adaptive Behavior*, **13**, 311–324.

Smith, K. (2004). The evolution of vocabulary. *Journal of Theoretical Biology*, **228**, 127–142.

Sperber, D. & Wilson, D. (1986). *Relevance: Communication and Cognition*. Oxford: Blackwell.

Steels, L. (1999). *Words and Meanings. The Talking Heads Experiment*, Vol. 1. Laboratorium: Antwerp.

Steels, L. (2003). Evolving grounded communication for robots. *Trends in Cognitive Science*, **7**, 308–312.

Tomasello, M. (2008). *The Origins of Human Communication*. Cambridge, MA: MIT Press.

Tomasello, M., Carpenter, M., Call, J., Behne, T. & Moll, H. (2005). Understanding and sharing intentions: the origins of cultural cognition. *Behavioral and Brain Sciences*, **28**, 675–691.

Vogt, P. (2002). The physical symbol grounding problem. *Cognitive Systems Research*, **3**, 429–457.

Werner, G. & Dyer, M. (1992). Evolution of communication in artificial organisms. In C. Langton, C. Taylor, D. Farmer & S. Rasmussen, eds., *Artificial Life II*. Redwood City, CA: Addison-Wesley, pp. 659–687.

Commentaries

We agree that what signals *do* is primary, and talk of information can serve this stance in several ways (cf. Horn, 1997). Here are three. First, signals only *do* things on average, so talk of information helps us to articulate the best case (normative/selected-for) scenario. Second, because the effect of the signal itself is only one piece of the puzzle of how it *does* things (the rest being context), talk of information helps us articulate what piece the signal contributes (that's what semantics is). Third, if information is inherent in particular manifestations of the physical world (e.g. sight of prey) that, when they are signals, are evolved behaviours of other animals, then surely the clearest shorthand (*not* metaphor) for speaking of both influences in a unified way is to talk of information.

Horn, A. G. (1997). Speech acts and animal signals. In D. W. Owings, M. D. Beecher & N. Thompson, eds., *Communication. Perspectives in Ethology*, Vol. 12. New York: Plenum Press, pp. 347–358.

Andrew G. Horn and Peter McGregor

Communication without perceiver adaptation. Scott-Phillips and Kirby adopt a pragmatic approach to the information construct, emphasising information as correlations between signals and objects or events in the world. We concur with this view, while noting that such regularity exists whether or not anyone attends to it. As elaborated in our commentary on Scarantino's contribution, a conceptual firewall is therefore needed between information as correlations in the world and observer representations of those correlations. In defining signalling and communication, Scott-Phillips and Kirby require both that signallers be specialised to influence perceiver behaviour and that perceivers be specialised to be so influenced. Thus, the authors argue that an interaction is merely coercive if an actor relies on its own physical power to influence the behaviour of another. In contrast, communication involves a signaller-actor who capitalises on the senses and muscles of a perceiver-other. Only if the latter has evolved to respond to the actor's behaviour can one conclude that true communication has occurred. As Scarantino argues, however, even in cases of clearly coercive behaviour, possible perceiver specialisation cannot be ruled out. In fact, one can argue that such cases are particularly likely to create selection pressures shaping reactor responses over evolutionary time. We must also point out that while it is difficult to rule out possible reactor specialisation in coercion, ruling it in even in archetypal cases of communication can be still more challenging. In predator-specific alarm signalling in vervet monkeys, for example, adaptive specialisation is clearly evident on the production side. Vervet infants produce recognisable, predator-appropriate alarm calls without first needing to experience how others use them or to practise making these sounds. In contrast, there is no evidence of specialisation in responding to the calls. The same infants that competently produce the vocalisations initially show no sign of knowing how to respond when others give them. Responding is acquired over the first year of life through evidently standard, generalised learning mechanisms. In other words, there is no indication of perceiver specialisation even in this quintessential instance of animal signalling.

Michael J. Owren and Drew Rendall

The distinction between the 'code model' and the 'ostensive-inferential model' of communication depends primarily on whether a signal uniquely specifies the signaller's meaning or just provides evidence for it: in other words, whether the correlation between signal and meaning is 1.0 or less than 1.0 (but not equal to 0). In both models the meaning of a signal is something (perhaps a state of mind) other than the correlation. This approach is explicit in those simulations of communication that score a successful interaction when the receiver interprets a signal in the same way the signaller does. The authors' new model of communication makes an important improvement by incorporating 'functional effects' (the consequences of producing or responding to a signal). It is then easy to show that communication must have benefits for both signallers and receivers. It is important to emphasise, however, that signallers and receivers must receive benefits only on average. In this chapter, the 'on average' is missing from the accounts of 'functionality'.

R. Haven Wiley

Response

I thank the commentators for their thoughtful and engaged responses to the chapter I co-authored with Simon Kirby. I have divided my responses into three main areas: (i) the difference between the code and ostensive-inferential models of communication; (ii) the role of information in communication; and (iii) various issues around the functionality of signals and responses.

First, I wish to clarify the difference between the code and ostensive-inferential models of communication. **Wiley** interprets the distinction between the two as whether or not a signal uniquely specifies the correct meaning. This is not quite right. In some computational models agents have different meaning–form mappings, and their responses are determined probabilistically (e.g. Smith, 2005). In these models signals do not uniquely specify meaning, but these are still code models – because the basic paradigm remains one that involves 'looking up' signal–meaning mappings, both in production and reception. The ostensive-inferential model, in contrast, involves the expression and recognition of intentions (Sperber & Wilson, 1986). It is this difference in the way that communication is achieved that distinguishes the two models. One view that we wished to express in our chapter was that a potentially profitable avenue for future research is the development of agent-based or mathematical models of the evolution of language that are ostensive and inferential in this way.

Second, I should respond to the comments of both **Horn and McGregor** (H&M) and **Owren and Rendall** (O&R) on information. H&M appear to suggest, with a parenthetical aside, that we think that use of the term *information* is metaphorical, and so I should clarify that this is not the case. What is metaphorical is the code model of how communication works; this is not the same thing as information. Otherwise, H&M, and also O&R, agree with us that although information transfer is, on its own, an insufficient characterisation of communication, there is information in whatever correlations exist between organismic behaviour and features of the world. For H&M, this is a reason to use information as shorthand for the different ways in which external influences can affect organisms. In contrast, for O&R, it is a reason to be very careful about how we use the term information. Both are correct: if we simply want to study how the inputs received by one organism affect its behaviour, talk of information is good shorthand for both signals and other sources – but at the same time, if we are focused on communication, we should not, as our chapter emphasised, equate communication with the use of information to inform behaviour.

Finally, the commentaries raise a variety of issues around the functionality of signals (and responses). The first is the need for the clause 'on average' in our definition of communication. Following Maynard Smith and Harper (2003), we defined communication in functional terms: as any pair of behaviours (or structures) that have symbiotic functionality. This implies that signals should on average be beneficial for both parties. Both Wiley and H&M point out that we neglected to mention this, and they are correct: 'on average' is a necessary clause in nearly all population-level analysis of social behaviour (Davies, Krebs & West, 2012). Our definition of communication is no exception.

As Wiley comments, our definition makes it explicit that communication must (on average) be beneficial to *both* parties. O&R, however, resist this conclusion, and argue that communication can be (but need not necessarily be) maladaptive for the receiver. As I argued in my commentary on their chapter, I do not see how this can be the case. Communication is a symbiotic interaction between two organisms, and if it were not beneficial for both parties then it would collapse (Scott-Phillips *et al.*, 2012). In the specific case of receivers, this means that if responses were maladaptive (on average) then they would be selected against, and the interaction would no longer be communicative.

O&R argue against this conclusion by pointing to some uncontroversial instances of communication in which there is no receiver specialisation (an argument that is reflected in the title of their commentary). They illustrate this with the example of vervet calls, the response to which appears to be acquired through general learning mechanisms. I do not see the relevance of this. Our definition of communication is based upon functionality, not on the specifics of any mechanism, specialised or otherwise. The mechanisms involved in responses produce adaptive outcomes (hiding from predators), and it is at least in part because of this that they are successfully passed on from one generation to the next. This makes them functional as response mechanisms, and that is both necessary and sufficient for our definition (see Millikan, 1984, for extensive discussion of what it means for a trait to have a function). If instead the consequences of the interaction are neutral for the 'receiver', or at least insufficiently strong to undergo selection, then that would be a case of coercion.

Davies, N. B., Krebs, J. R. & West, S. A. (2012). *An Introduction to Behavioural Ecology*, 4th edn. Oxford: Wiley-Blackwell.

Millikan, R G. (1984). *Language, Thought, and Other Biological Categories*. Harvard, MA: MIT Press.

Scott-Phillips, T. C., Blythe, R. A., Gardner, A. & West, S. A. (2012). How do communication systems emerge? *Proceedings of the Royal Society of London Series B*. 279, 1943–1949.

Smith, A. D. M. (2005). The inferential transmission of language. *Adaptive Behavior*, **13**, 311–324.

Sperber, D. & Wilson, D. (1986). *Relevance: Communication and Cognition*. Oxford: Blackwell.

Thomas C. Scott-Phillips

Index

Common/generic species names are used (rather than scientific names)
Locators in **bold** refer to figures/tables

Printed in the United States
By Bookmasters

Printed in the United States
By Bookmasters

Printed in the United States
By Bookmasters